A Longitudinal Study
of Dyslexia

Bergen's Multivariate Study
of Children's
Learning Disabilities

Hans-Jörgen Gjessing
Bjorn Karlsen

A Longitudinal Study of Dyslexia

Bergen's Multivariate Study of Children's Learning Disabilities

With 23 Figures

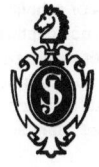

Springer Science+Business Media, LLC

Hans-Jörgen Gjessing, Ph.D.
Professor, Department of Educational Psychology
University of Bergen
5007 Bergen, Norway

Bjorn Karlsen, Ph.D.
Professor Emeritus
Sonoma State University
Rohnert Park, CA 94928
USA

Library of Congress Cataloging-in-Publication Data
Gjessing, Hans-Jørgen.
    A longitudinal study of dyslexia : Bergen's multivariate study of
children's learning disabilities / by Hans-Jørgen Gjessing & Bjørn
Karlsen.
      p.   cm.
    1. Dyslexia—Norway—Longitudinal studies.   2. Dyslexic children—
Norway—Longitudinal studies.   3. Bergenprosjektet. I. Karlsen,
Bjørn.   II. Title.
    [DNLM: 1. Bergenprosjektet.   2. Dyslexia—in infancy & childhood.
3. Longitudinal Studies.   WM 475 G539L]
RJ496.A5G54   1989
618.92′8553′009481—dc19
DNLM/DLC
for Library of Congress   89-4127
                                                                    CIP

Printed on acid-free paper.

Typeset by Publishers Service, Bozeman, Montana.

9 8 7 6 5 4 3 2 1

ISBN 978-1-4612-6452-1   ISBN 978-1-4419-8704-4 (eBook)
DOI 10.1007/978-1-4419-8704-4

Preface

Psychological and educational researchers in the Scandinavian countries have cooperated in a research effort relating to children's learning disabilities for more than a decade. Support has come from the federal governments and other funding agencies in Norway, Sweden, and Denmark through the Secretariat for Scandinavian Cultural Cooperation. A number of independent studies have already been published, dealing with various aspects of learning disabilities in the literacy skills of reading and writing.

The largest and most comprehensive study was the Bergen Project, a longitudinal study of an entire cohort of children, with special emphasis on those who developed specific learning disabilities in reading and writing (dyslexia). These dyslexic children were studied, diagnosed, and treated over a period of nine years, along with various control and comparison groups, which included a large subgroup with general learning disabilities (retarded).

The Bergen Project involved the collection of voluminous data. The children were identified by means of special diagnostic tests and treated using remedial materials and techniques that had been developed to deal with various types of dyslexia. The ophthalmology team not only tested the children, but they also prescribed and provided glasses, and even performed surgery when necessary. The pediatric neurologists did general pediatric and neurological examinations, following up many of the cases with EEGs and CT (computerized tomography, brain x-rays).

Three book length reports on the Bergen Project have been published, along with some articles and, of course, the tests and instructional materials. But these reports have been in Norwegian and thus not available to a broader audience. This book remedies that situation: it is a final report of the entire project in English. Since the project entailed literally hundreds of variables, and since a major thrust of the project was to study how all these variables correlated and interacted, the statistical work-up of the data became quite complex. The data are reported in various tables, but the interpretations in the text are written to reach the large number of people who are vitally interested in this topic. This includes educators, psychologists, counselors, various medical specialists, and other researchers.

Part of the excitement of bringing this report to an international audience is to present the culmination of several decades of work by Professor H.-J. Gjessing at the University of Bergen in Norway. Out of his work has evolved the theory that we are dealing with several types of dyslexia. This research supports the notion that such types can be identified. Of even more importance is the fact that individuals exhibiting the different types must be taught differently; teaching techniques that may be beneficial for some dyslexic children may be *detrimental* to others.

This research project was made possible through the assistance and cooperation of a large number of people over a period of many years: the administration of the Bergen public schools, teachers, special education specialists, school psychologists, and school health services. We must also thank the many who assisted in the data collection: the Departments of Ophthalmology and Pediatrics at Haukeland Hospital (the University Medical School), the Bergen Hearing Institute, and the University Psychology Faculty (especially the Institute for Psychometrics). Our deepest appreciation is also extended to the hundreds of children who participated and to their parents who helped in so many ways.

I personally became involved in this project at an early stage, having done my Ph.D. study in this field and having developed diagnostic reading tests in the United States. Later on, I worked full time on this project for 6 months in Bergen in 1985 and have been solely responsible for all translations and the adaptation of the material for an English-reading audience.

Bjorn Karlsen

Contents

Part I   Introduction

CHAPTER 1

Purposes and Design of the Study; Organization of the Book

H.-J. Gjessing

The Bergen Project was a longitudinal research and developmental study of primary grade children with severe school learning disabilities. It was carried out in the elementary schools of Bergen, Norway, beginning in 1977. Its theoretical goal was the development of a research strategy in which observations and assessments of personal and environmental factors are based more on real life functions and processes than on quantitative scores and products.

The Bergen Project was actually part of a coordinated set of studies of learning disabilities carried out in the Scandinavian countries of Norway, Sweden, and Denmark. It was sponsored, in part, by the Scandinavian council of ministries (Nordisk Ministerråd). This report deals exclusively with the Bergen Project, which was by far the largest and most comprehensive study of learning disabilities carried out in the Scandinavian countries.

Bergen is the second largest city in Norway, having a population of about 250,000. It is located on the west coast and is the main center for higher education in this area. Because of its location, much of its commercial activity relates to the sea — shipping, fishing, and the exploitation of the North Sea oil fields. The population is quite homogeneous and also very stable. This stability is exemplified by the attrition rate of 3% in this longitudinal study.

Objectives

The main objectives of the Bergen Project can be summarized as follows:

1. Describe and analyze the development of an entire regional population of children entering school in a given year with regard to social, emotional, cognitive, and achievement characteristics.
2. Develop procedures for classroom observation and assessment that will identify those learning and behavior characteristics that affect school achievement in the primary grades.
3. Explore a system of individual assessment of children's reading and writing characteristics.

4. Increase knowledge about the many factors, characteristics, and problems involved in school learning problems, in particular underachievement, specific reading and writing disabilities, socioemotional problems, visual dysfunctions, and neurological problems.
5. Develop a set of flexible instructional materials geared to each child's characteristics, problems, and needs.
6. Improve insight and psychological understanding by teachers and other professionals into the nature and effect of children's school learning difficulties.
7. Develop guidance procedures that will result in better self-insight and understanding of learning difficulties by the children themselves, their parents, and their teachers and in more constructive and psychologically sound channeling of parental efforts to help the children.
8. Develop fairly simple professional, administrative, and financial programs that can be incorporated into a school's long-range planning and that fit the school's resources.
9. Collect, coordinate, and evaluate results and experiences from the other Scandinavian countries that participated in this series of research projects.

Research Population

The Bergen Project encompassed every child who entered first grade in the public elementary schools in Bergen in the fall of 1977, including children with mild mental retardation. This population numbered over 3,000 in 69 schools. Children who attended special schools, such as those with severe mental retardation or with extreme disorders of vision or hearing, were not included for practical reasons: we wanted to concentrate on the special and remedial education offerings of the regular elementary school. On the other hand, because of new philosophical and organizational trends (Gjessing, 1969) relating to integration of the mildly handicapped into ordinary schools, research data on such children were sorely needed.

The study covered the first four years of schooling; a final follow-up was done when the children were in the ninth grade. Initial screening tests were administered in the fall of 1977 at the beginning of first grade and repeated in the fall of 1978 at the beginning of second grade. Similar tests were given at the end of grade 3, beginning of grade 4.

Although extensive data were gathered on the entire cohort, the main emphasis of the project was the children who developed learning difficulties. These children were divided into separate target groups: those with specific learning disabilities, referred to in the study as *dyslexics*, and those with general learning problems ("retarded"). The dividing line between the two groups was not always clear. ("Dyslexia" is defined and discussed in Part III; "retarded" is defined and discussed at some length in the Appendix. These two groups make up about 75% of all children who receive some form of special or remedial education in Bergen.)

The main common characteristic of the children with dyslexia was a significant discrepancy between their otherwise normal scholastic aptitude and their school achievement. This discrepancy was particularly pronounced in reading and spelling but sometimes was also present in mathematics.

The problems of the children with general learning disabilities were more diffuse and all-encompassing, and in most cases there was no discrepancy between their level of learning aptitude (as we assessed it) and their achievement level. They had major limitations in both areas; school achievement was usually quite consistent with their assessed intellectual level.

Children in both groups had varying degrees of social and emotional problems. These problems may have contributed to the learning problems, but they may also have developed as a result of the stress and frustration associated with learning difficulties in the school.

Study Phases

Phase 1: Initial Classroom Testing

Initial screening tests were administered to all children (3,200) in the first grade in the fall of 1977. Screening involved systematic pupil observations by school psychologists and teacher evaluation of each child's social interaction, sense of well-being in the school, self-concept, and attitudes toward school subjects; achievement tests in literacy skills and mathematics; and a mental ability test. At the same time, extensive pediatric, neurological, and eye examinations were carried out by the school health services and the departments of pediatrics, neurology, and ophthalmology of the regional hospital (Haukeland Hospital), which also serves as the University hospital. Screening was completed toward the end of spring semester 1978.

Parts of this screening program were repeated at the beginning of fall semester 1978, when the children entered second grade. The duplication was to reduce sources of accidental (random) errors and also systematic errors, for example, regression effects.

The problem of systematic errors is often solved by the use of regression analysis, frequently based on a single assessment. It was decided that such a correction was insufficient, especially when it dealt with individual pupils at the extreme lower end of the frequency distribution. Dual assessment would yield more accurate identification of children with learning disabilities. (This dual screening program had been subjected to a trial run the previous year with a "prescreening group.")

The screening data were analyzed and the results discussed in detail with each teacher, both procedures under the leadership of the school district's school psychology office. This provided much needed teacher input into the identification process, and it facilitated consistency in the treatment of the identified children.

Phase 2: Individual Evaluation of Children With Learning Disabilities

Phase 2 consisted of intensive individual appraisals of pupils who had been identified in phase 1 as being potentially learning disabled. The specific disability target group consisted of 235 children, 7.3% of the cohort. The general disability target group comprise 40 children, 1.2% of the population. (See the Appendix.) This was done while the children were in the second grade.

Individualized instruction plans, similar for both target groups, were carried out under the direction of school psychological services in cooperation with special teachers, psychologists, and social workers. They entailed initial diagnostic workup of the learning difficulty and subsequent evaluations of associated and interacting problems – educational, cognitive, interpersonal, and emotional. Attempts were made to elucidate problems in these areas by means of standardized tests and techniques and by interviews with parents and teachers. On the basis of this process, the school psychology services provided direct services according to their standard procedures. They gave detailed guidance and educational planning for each dyslexic child.

Phase 3: Individual Supplementary Examination

In the third grade, supplementary examinations were carried out for practical as well as experimental purposes. Such examinations sometimes entailed additional tests of vision or hearing, medical examinations, or tests of neurological functioning, plus some highly specialized psychological and neurological tests. This phase required interdisciplinary competencies beyond those available among the psychological researchers and the cooperating school personnel.

Contacts with specialized personnel were initiated during the fall of 1977. Most of the professional competencies needed were available through the school district's health services and school psychology services and their usual referral services. The most systematic and extensive medical research contribution to the Bergen Project involved visual examinations planned and executed at the University-affiliated regional hospital. Pediatric and neurological examinations were also carried out at this hospital.

Phase 4: Follow-Up Evaluation

Follow-up consisted of observations, interviews, and additional testing continuously to the middle of fourth grade. Parents, peers, and teachers helped evaluate the results of the special programs. Teachers were also involved in evaluating the extent to which the individual plans were being carried out and in determining the nature of problems in general as well as those of individual children.

A final, less exhaustive follow-up study was done when the pupils were in the ninth grade.

Organization of This Book

This book is organized into five main sections. The content of each section is described briefly here. Because of the enormity of the Bergen Project, analyses and discussions of related world literature are included in the relevant chapters. The main dyslexia studies are summarized collectively in Chapter 8. Much space has been devoted as well to research methodology, statistical analyses of data from extreme groups, comparisons of clinical and statistical approaches, typology, and medical research. Some new ground has been broken in all these areas.

Part I deals with the objectives of the Bergen Project and its experimental design. It summarizes the content of some early reports involving the entire Bergen cohort and discusses issues relating to intensive research with individuals.

Part II analyzes the school learning characteristics of the total learning disability group. Both the socioemotional and cognitive aspects of learning disabilities and the related research findings are considered. In both of these areas some interesting comparisons are made between the children with specific versus those with general learning disabilities. Comparisons are also made with other groups within the cohort.

Part III delves into both the clinical and more theoretical aspects of specific reading and writing disabilities. It briefly reviews the history of the field of dyslexia and criteria for its definition. The dyslexia types defined and studied in this project are presented and compared with other models and subtypes (Chapter 8). The basic tenets of "function analysis," an approach to diagnosing and analyzing reading and spelling difficulties, and the specific diagnostic tests used, are described. Finally, issues in the research methodology used in the study of learning disabilities and of dyslexia in particular, especially those that relate to the relevance of a clinical versus a statistical information base, are covered.

Part IV presents detailed results of the study of the dyslexia sample in the Bergen cohort—data relating to the many correlates of dyslexia and potential causative factors, the incidences of these correlates among the nondyslexic subgroups of the cohort, and analysis of subgroups selected on clinical and statistical bases. It also details the medical investigations done in conjunction with the project: extensive eye examinations and pediatric neurological tests. The final chapter in this part describes and discusses the results of the developmental data and the efficacy aspects of this study, comparing these with other studies of prognosis and treatment effects for children with learning disabilities (Chapter 14).

Part V summarizes the most important results of the Bergen Project, discusses these results in relation to the proposed dyslexia model and to dyslexia theory, and presents an analysis of the theoretical and practical contributions of the study as seen in its totality.

Finally, the Appendix details the sampling and selection procedure. Much important information has been placed in this appendix to make the book more readable and to prevent excessive details from obscuring the main premises of the project.

CHAPTER 2

Description of Earlier Reports on the Bergen Project

H.-J. Gjessing

There have been two progress reports of the Bergen Project and also some brief summary reports. Most have been in Norwegian. This is the first major publication in English about this project.

The early reports comprise about 450 pages of print. The following is a brief summary.

Report I

Report I (Gjessing, Nygaard, Solheim, & Aasved, 1982) described the theoretical base of the Bergen Project and its experimental design. It gave no research data. It did discuss in detail some of the very complex problems of interaction research and its applications to the study of extreme groups, where parametric statistical procedures based on normal distributions may have limited utility. It also discussed the problems of defining and evaluating such characteristics as self-concept, learning disabilities, and underachievement and a variety of visual problems and other medical factors often considered associated with reading difficulties. The analysis of the variables that had to be considered simultaneously in the project was sufficiently intricate to warrant devoting this report entirely to a discussion of methodology.

Report II

Report II (Solheim, Nygaard, Aasved, et al., 1984) was the sequel to report I. It analyzed the results of the *entire* cohort studied (3,090 children from 145 classrooms and 69 different elementary schools) and also some individual data. (The average classroom contained 21 pupils, quite typical of the primary grades in Norway, where maximum class size cannot exceed 28.) Some analyses covered data from all of the children, whereas other analyses covered slightly fewer children. The longitudinal data gathered in this study appear representative because the attrition rate was quite low (3%) and a statistical analysis showed that the kind of children who dropped out did not introduce any systematic bias.

Predictor variables

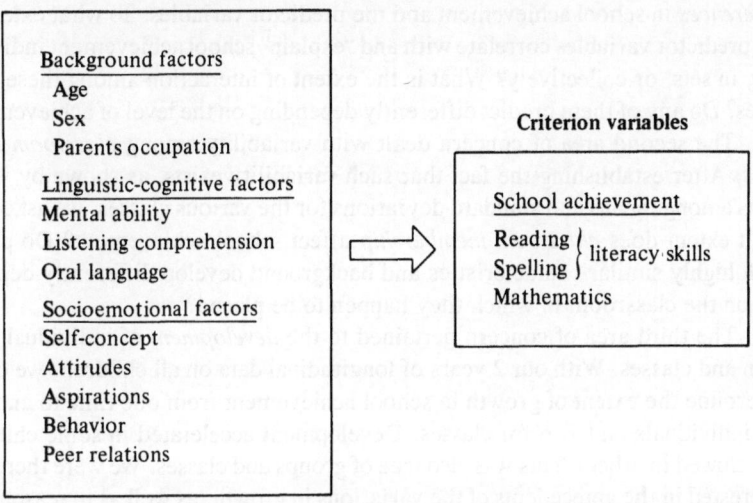

FIGURE 2.1. Predictor and criterion variables.

The assessment tools used to gather the longitudinal, normative data for the cohort included both formal standardized tests and informal inventories. Space limitations prevent the presentation here of a detailed discussion of the many assessment tools and techniques used and the multitude of information collected. A listing of some of the areas subjected to rather intensive study must suffice: school achievement, social interaction, emotional status, self-concept, level of aspiration, school attitudes, sex differences, and socioeconomic variables.

The large number and diversity of variables studied made many analyses possible. However, we limited ourselves to analyses of factors presumed relevant to school learning disabilities, especially in the areas of reading and spelling. The data were therefore analyzed in such a way as to make the achievement variables dependent, or criterion, variables. The others were considered independent, or predictor, variables (see Figure 2.1).

The criterion variables were those characteristics we wanted to explain or predict: growth and variability in school achievement throughout the primary grades. Operationally these were measured by test scores in reading, spelling, and mathematics at two points in time, grade 1-2 ("pretest") and grade 3-4 ("posttest").

The predictor variables pertained to all the data collected in addition to the achievement test scores. By means of the predictor variables we would attempt to predict individual differences in school achievement. As can be seen from Figure 2.1, the predictor variables were classified in three groups: background factors, linguistic-cognitive factors, and socioemotional factors.

Four major areas of concern were explored in report II:

1. We were interested in determining the relationship between *individual differences* in school achievement and the predictor variables. To what extent do the predictor variables correlate with and "explain" school achievement individually, in sets, or collectively? What is the extent of interaction among these variables? Do any of them predict differently depending on the level of achievement?

2. The second area of concern dealt with variability among *classroom averages*. After establishing the fact that such variability exists, as shown by variations among means and standard deviations for the various classes, we asked: To what extent does *classroom membership* affect school achievement? Do pupils with highly similar characteristics and background develop differently depending on the classroom in which they happen to be placed?

3. The third area of concern pertained to the *development* of individual children and classes. With our 2 years of longitudinal data on all children, we could determine the extent of growth in school achievement from one time to another for individuals and also for classes. Development accelerated in some children and slowed in others. This was also true of groups and classes. We were therefore interested in the antecedents of the variations in growth, as well as in reasons for the fact that many individuals and groups remained stable.

4. The fourth set of factors investigated dealt with the relationship between *vision* and reading ability. There is a great deal of controversy regarding possible relationships between reading disabilities and visual characteristics, especially the so-called phorias (exophoria, esphoria). Relatively extensive visual examinations of every child in the cohort, carried out by the Department of Ophthalmology at the University Hospital (Haukeland Sykehus), showed little relationship between the characteristics assessed and scores on reading and spelling tests. These group data are consistent with the results of most other studies of this problem. These statistics do not, of course, preclude the influence of visual problems on certain individuals.

Data from these four major areas were analyzed for the entire cohort. The graphic and statistical techniques used are discussed in detail in report II. Briefly, these techniques included regression analysis, path analysis, interaction analysis, factor analysis, and a variety of techniques for studying change or gain.

A brief summary of the general results and conclusions given in report II follows.

Individual Differences and Characteristics

The school achievement tests in reading, spelling, and mathematics revealed extremely large individual differences among the children, a finding that is quite consistent with other studies of this sort.

We analyzed differences in reading ability by means of a silent reading test for the third grade. The variability was extensive. Reading speed, for example, varied from 4 to 5 words per minute to over 130 words per minute, with all degrees of reading ability in between. We were particularly interested in the borderline between "functional" and "nonfunctional" reading ability. (Such a judgment is of course relative, being dependent on the demands made by the school, the parents, and the students themselves, and also being related to the individual school learning situation. When drawing such a dividing line, however, the error element may not be as large as one might think.) It appeared to us that about 10% of the pupils had a significant reading problem, and that about half of these would have to be considered nonfunctional readers, using rather minimal criteria for "functional" at this grade level.

To determine what factors were associated with these large individual differences in achievement, we first analyzed the *background* factors of age, sex, and parent occupation (see Figure 2.1) in a regression equation. These variables accounted for a very modest 6 to 9% of the individual differences. Thus, knowledge of these three factors alone can explain little about growth in school achievement.

The most important and meaningful set of predictor variables was the second link of the regression equation: the *linguistic-cognitive* factors. These accounted for between 26 and 42% of the variance in achievement, depending on which school subject or combination of subjects was under consideration. The strong relationship between the linguistic-cognitive factors was anticipated, since such a relationship is found universally in studies of this sort. Lundberg (1981b) has published similar findings from the Swedish part of this research effort.

The third part of the regression equation revealed the contributions of the *socioemotional* factors. In comparison with linguistic-cognitive factors, socioemotional factors made a very modest contribution to the prediction of individual variation in achievement: only 1 to 3% of total variance. Because of the very large sample involved in this study, these numbers turned out to be statistically significant, but their contribution would have to be considered quite marginal. Nevertheless, they do add an interesting dimension to our understanding of school achievement. The influence of the socioemotional factors varied with the level of functioning in the linguistic-cognitive areas. This association was particularly perceptible at the lower achievement levels. In the group that made low scores on the linguistic-cognitive tests, we found a significant association between school achievement and scores in the areas of self-concept, level of aspiration, behavior, and peer relations. This finding is a good example of how interaction works, and why we have been particularly interested in this type of analysis in the Bergen Project.

Classroom Differences and Characteristics

Data were collected on classroom averages from the pretest (grade 1-2) and the posttest (grade 3-4). Data were also collected on the extent to which these averages varied from one school subject to another. We tried to determine what factors contributed to the variation among classroom averages found for all characteristics. Of particular interest was to what extent classroom membership per se could be considered a factor in individual differences in achievement:

Does it make any difference which particular classroom or particular type of classroom the child is in?

We analyzed the average achievement for each class in every characteristic studied in the first and the fourth grade in order to study growth, changes, and relationships. We approached these complex problems with a variety of statistical techniques. This particular analysis was considered of great significance, because in the Norwegian school system the children have the same teacher for grades 1 through 3. Thus the effect of the teacher variable would tend to accumulate. In American schools, where children have a different teacher every year, the teacher effect has been shown to be rather minimal. The Bergen data, however, showed that the effects of having the same teacher 3 years in a row were profound.

Correlation of mean scores for each classroom from pretest to posttest resulted in correlation coefficients of just under .80. This result shows a great deal of stability in the *ranks* of the classroom means. However, variability in school achievement increased over time. The classrooms with initial low mean scores showed relatively small gains, while the classes with the higher pretest means showed the largest gains. This conclusion was supported by more complex statistical analyses of actual versus predicted gains.

Despite the general rank stability of the means over time, many classes exhibited either positive or negative changes, some to a large degree. We made a special study of these classes by comparing the 16 classes that showed the largest positive change with the 16 classes that showed the largest negative change. Through complex and admittedly sometimes problematic statistical analyses we concluded that "classroom membership" contributed significantly—6 to 17% —to the variability in all criterion variables. The contribution of this factor to the prediction of school achievement was exceeded only by the linguistic-cognitive factors.

Reasons why classroom membership is a significant variable in school achievement may range from social interaction to teacher variables. Our empirical data can go no further than merely to establish that there is a significant relationship. The problem is a very sensitive one from the standpoint of the participating teachers, and is clearly of considerable interest. This issue fell outside the framework of the Bergen Project and was thus not pursued further.

Development of Children in the Learning Disability Group

The learning disability group, comprising children with specific and general learning disabilities, consisted of 273 pupils, or 8% of the total cohort, at the outset. At the end of the data collection period in the fourth grade, 259 pupils remained, a remarkably low attrition rate of 5%.

Report II gives a detailed accounting of the comparisons we made between the learning disability group and the total cohort, as well as comparisons among the disability subgroups. The purpose of the multivariate analyses carried out

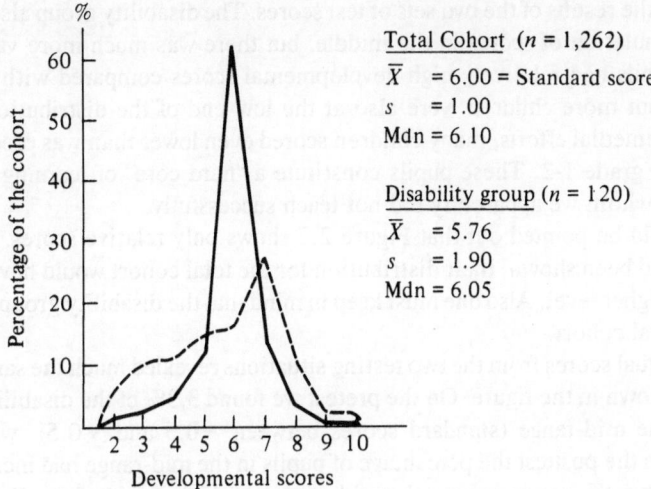

FIGURE 2.2. Distribution of developmental reading scores on the posttest (grade 3-4) for the total cohort (—) and for the disability group (- - -). The superimposed curves show the relative distribution within each of the two groups. See text for explanation of the scoring system.

was to find out what was special or unique about the learning disability group and its subgroups.

Extensive pretest data were collected at the end of grade 1 and the beginning of grade 2 (grade 1-2); the largest amount of posttest data were gathered at the end of grade 3-beginning of grade 4 (grade 3-4). Developmental data were collected on those pupils in the total cohort for whom all pretest and posttest data were available. These data covered the school subjects of reading, spelling, and mathematics and various psychological and medical data. Although 100%-complete records were obtained for only about half the cohort, statistical analyses indicated that the data analyzed were representative of the entire cohort.

Only the developmental data pertaining to reading achievement will be summarized here. The test results were analyzed by the use of standard scores and "developmental scores" (defined as deviations from the anticipated or predicted scores). Figure 2.2 shows the distribution of developmental scores for the posttest, based on the predictions from the pretest. The discrepancy between the scores obtained in grade 3-4 and the scores predicted from the scores in grade 1-2 has been converted to a standard score with a mean of 6 and a standard deviation of 1. A student who obtained a score of 6, therefore, would score as predicted, while scores above or below 6 show the degree of deviation from the predicted score.

The distribution of scores for the total cohort was, as expected, symmetrical around 6 with relatively little variability, indicating considerable stability between the results of the two sets of test scores. The disability group also showed an accumulation of scores in the middle, but there was much more variability. More pupils had relatively high developmental scores compared with the total cohort, but more children were also at the low end of the distribution. Thus, despite remedial efforts, many children scored even lower than was predicted by scores in grade 1-2. These pupils constitute a "hard core" of learning disabled children whom we apparently did not teach successfully.

It should be pointed out that Figure 2.2 shows only relative scores. If actual scores had been shown, their distribution for the total cohort would have been at a much higher level. Also one must keep in mind that the disability group was part of the total cohort.

The actual scores from the two testing situations revealed much the same situation as shown in the figure. On the pretest we found 3.3% of the disability group within the mid-range (standard scores between -0.5 and $+0.5$), with none above. On the posttest the percentage of pupils in the mid-range had increased to 30%, with 5.8% scoring above the mid-range. At the low end of the distribution we initially had 96.7% of the disability group, while this percentage was reduced to 64.2% on the posttest. The disability pupils still seemed to pile up at the lower end of the distribution, particularly at the extreme low end (standard scores below -1.5).

These results may appear discouraging in light of the rather considerable educational effort that was made with this group. Some consolation lies in the fact that careful analyses of similar "efficacy studies" show the results of the Bergen Project to be relatively good (Schonhaut & Satz, 1983). The reasons for the differential growth within the disability group was a central issue in this project.

CHAPTER 3

Methodological Issues in Dyslexia Research

H.-J. Gjessing

Intensive Research With Individuals: Rationale and Problems

The Bergen Project was basically a developmental study of individual children with severe school learning disabilities. It emphasized individual research for two major reasons:

1. On the basis of individual case studies and diagnoses, we designed what in our opinion would be the best possible program of treatment and instruction for each child.
2. We assumed that the children would exhibit varied patterns of educational development, and that collection of individual data would facilitate explaining some of the factors involved in these differing patterns.

The systematic case study material collected in the Bergen Project formed a data bank that we used to describe and evaluate the achievement patterns for (a) the total learning disability group (those with specific and with general learning disabilities), (b) specific subgroups of the total learning disability group, and (c) individual children. (Results of the data pertaining to both the total learning disability group and various subgroups will be given in this volume; the findings from individual children will be given only cursory coverage. The interesting case study material collected will be the subject of a special report later on.)

The use of the term *intensive research* in educational and psychological research is neither unequivocal nor well delineated. The term does imply certain characteristics, primarily those involving intensive analysis of individuals. It also implies the kinds of problems that occur within a practical clinical framework. The extensiveness and large amount of detail usually involved in intensive research tend to result in some restriction in sample size, especially in comparison with surveys and screening testing.

The combination of clinical data and small sample size demands close attention to the research methodology used, especially to research strategies and statistical procedures. Although report I (discussed in Chapter 2) basically dealt with the research methodological problems of screening testing and extreme groups, these problems also apply to intensive research. Statistical interaction, a good example of a type of analysis that can be used with a variety of methods and sample sizes, is particularly useful in intensive research.

Everyday practical and clinical problems also lend themselves to intensive research. When doing a case study, clinicians often find, as they analyze emotional, social, and educational characteristics, that individuals can rarely be understood simply on the basis of normative, quantified data from tests, rating scales, and other evaluation instruments. The individual must be evaluated within the clinician's frame of references.

Problems With Individual Research

The concept of individual research is ambiguous and poorly delineated. Such research does, however, have certain characteristics. One of these is sample size: The depth and breadth of individual research implies a considerable reduction in sample size compared with sample or population research.

Another problem is study design. Highly individual diagnostic testing for the purpose of designing individualized treatment, as done in our project, does not lend itself to the "efficacy study" design, which emphasizes main effects, group differences, and averages. Such a design calls for experimental and control groups and systematic manipulation of treatment variables.

We decided at the very outset that a purely experimental design would be inappropriate for ethical reasons alone. Such a design can only be used when there is reason to believe the results of the study will have limited differential effects. On the basis of past experiences with our approach, we believe that the choice of instructional methodology can have important long-lasting effects, both positive and negative, on the development of learning disabled children in the two vital subjects of reading and spelling. The dyslexia model and its attendant methodology were based on individual planning for each affected child, as defined by the particular type of dyslexia the diagnostic test had identified.

Our stance in this regard is supported by other researchers in the fields of learning disabilities and dyslexia. In a discussion of issues relating to research methodology in the field of learning disabilities, Schonhaut and Satz (1983) stated: "Ideally it would be best to conduct follow-up studies on untreated children. However, to withhold treatment from children at risk could be questioned on ethical grounds" (p. 561).

In addition to the ethical considerations, our research involved methodological issues. We wanted to tackle the problem of learning disabilities in an interpretive and descriptive fashion, rather than in a purely experimental one, and to conduct our research in as naturalistic and nonmanipulative a setting as possible. This approach grew out of our analysis of the results, largely controversial, of many experimental and pseudoexperimental studies of the causes and correlates of reading and spelling difficulties. Studying complex human problems by means of traditional experimental designs – designs based on theoretical assumptions that can rarely be complied with and often requiring rather artificial settings – is certainly questionable.

Obviously, then, our research project could not be an efficacy study in the tradition of experimental psychology. We did not so much want to evaluate and control behavior as to describe, and, to the extent possible, interpret human variability as it presents itself in a naturalistic setting over time. We tried, from this point of view, to get a better understanding of how children function and how they deal with the process of learning the literacy skills. Nevertheless, efficacy data were collected and will be presented in this report.

In addition to comparing developmental trends and background variables for those whose developmental scores were positive, unchanged, or negative compared with predicted achievement, we found additional explanatory material in the various subgroup data. The subgroups were formed along two rather disparate dimensions, generally referred to as *clinical* and *statistical*. We anticipated that these two dimensions would result in both similar and dissimilar results.

Clinical Judgment and Objective Research

Clinical judgment must be viewed as an organic synthesis not only of the elements of a particular case, but also of the general insight required for clinical work. Clinical judgment therefore serves as a supplement, maybe even as a correction, to objective data, which are reductionistic and mechanistic in nature even if subjected to the most ingenious multivariate analyses. On the other hand, one cannot deny that the application of clinical judgment is encumbered by numerous personal characteristics of clinicians such as various biases, wishful thinking, and predetermined professional or ideological viewpoints.

There may even be times when clinical judgment runs counter to findings indicated by the evaluation instrument used. Most clinicians have experienced cases where the diagnosis and suggested treatment would have been erroneous had only quantitative scores been used to determine them.

This brings us to a central issue in research in the social sciences, the contrast between "objective" and "subjective" reality, in our case exemplified by clinical practice and clinical research. It places us in a dilemma. The "objectivity" that clinicians often find to be insufficient and limiting in their practice is often the main data base for clinical research.

The contrast between subjective and objective reality has been analyzed from many different points of view, with varied nomenclature. Without going into great detail one can mention discussions in the literature of such dichotomies as idiographic–nomothetic, heuristic–empirical, epistemological–positivistic, deductive–inductive, qualitative–quantitative, process oriented–product oriented, clinical–statistical. These contrasts have been debated in philosophy, psychology, and science. The debates have not always been productive, perhaps mainly because of a tendency for viewpoints to become polarized.

In his well-known book from the 1950s, *Clinical Versus Statistical Prediction*, Meehl (1954) described this polarization of viewpoints in some detail. Only a few of the issues in this book will be discussed here.

Proponents of the *statistical* approach characterize it as scientific, operational, objective, reliable, replicable, realistic, and reasonable. Skeptics would characterize this method as mechanistic, simplistic, additive, fractionated, artificial, sterile, and academic.

Proponents of the *clinical* approach tend to describe it as holistic, meaningful, dynamic, organic, sensitive, realistic, and natural. Critics of this approach would characterize it as unscientific, metaphysical, subjective, unreliable, nonreplicable, and primitive.

Any further comments on this controversy may be unnecessary; it would appear that people see what they want to see, a situation that has not changed much in the intervening decades.

Clinical Versus Statistical

Meehl described the statistical method as one that classifies an individual through a mechanical combination of pieces of quantified information. One arrives at a probabilistic statement based on empirically determined frequencies of occurrence. Such a description probably still holds, despite the more sophisticated multivariate statistical methods that have been developed since Meehl wrote his book.

The clinical method was described as following a somewhat different pattern, its main emphasis being the hypotheses and conclusions that can be derived casuistically from the total picture. We have viewed this line of discussion with considerably sympathy, since clinical validity is based on systematic casuistic analyses and comparisons.

Meehl viewed his own definition of the clinical method as vague and imprecise. Concrete criteria are hard to establish. This method cannot be characterized as having its base in instrumentation. But statistical and clinical decisions can be made through the application of the same tests and diagnostic tools. And there are no clear lines of demarcation regarding the use of frequency of occurrence as a basis for establishing the likelihood of the presence of a given trait. Such evaluations may not be as explicitly made by a clinician as by a statistician; nevertheless the clinician has certain built-in quantitative concepts, even though the reference base may not be as finely differentiated.

Before leaving this issue it would seem desirable to consider the clinical notion in more depth. Since the concept is so closely tied to the profession of clinical psychology, its relevance to our psychoeducational intensive research study, the Bergen Project, may not be apparent.

Clinical, as Concept and Profession

The term *clinical* is derived, of course, from the word *clinic*, which originally entailed the description of diseases, their symptoms, and treatment from the physician's viewpoint. Within the medical context, the clinical method became synonymous with direct observation, diagnosis, and treatment of patients. And it is the *application* of this method with respect to a person who needs help (patient) where the line is drawn between theoretical and clinical medicine (Dorland's, 1981, p. 278).

Although the clinical concept originated in the field of medicine, it also has a well-established position in psychology. Clinical psychology has typically been the branch of psychology that has applied scientific methods and principles to the study of the personality of a single individual, for the purpose of giving that person aid with respect to problems of personal and social adjustment. This service has been offered in a variety of settings, among them the school, and in situations requiring the help of different specialists, educators among them. The instruments used, tests, and other diagnostic aids have been applied on a very broad base.

Clinical psychology exists on a very large, international scale. According to Bellack and Hesson (1980), clinical psychology is an applied science where psychological principles are used to understand and to contribute to solving or reducing human problems. The work and problems associated with clinical psychology cover a large spectrum, "in addition to psychotherapy and psychological assessment the clinical psychologists design and institute educational and remedial programs for children, for the mentally retarded and for people with serious psychiatric problems" (p. 4).

In principle as well as in practice, we can also use the clinical concept when applying cognitive, psychoeducational, or special educational research findings, theoretical and applied, in dealing with individuals who need help. This gets us to the main point of this entire discussion: The intensive research aspects of the Bergen Project was clinical in nature and as such was favored and encumbered by the same qualitative aspects and problems of research design typically associated with traditional clinical psychology.

Idiographic Versus Nomothetic

In addition to this explicit discussion of the clinical-statistical contrast, we will consider the dichotomy idiographic-nomothetic. From the perspective of time as well as depth, this dichotomy predated the better known clinical-statistical controversy. It was Allport who, in addition to many other ideas, introduced the concepts *idiographic* and *nomothetic* into the behavioral sciences (Allport, 1937).

According to Allport, nomothetic methods are used to find general laws and principles. These methods are the same research procedures as those used in the exact sciences. And there has been a long struggle to make psychology into a nomothetic discipline. The idiographic disciplines, such as history, biography, and literature, emphasize the true nature of events within their total context. A psychology of individuality must, according to Allport, also be idiographic.

Allport defined science in a very broad and inclusive way when he said that "science prescribes no method, it sets no limits, it simply searches for knowledge" (p. 23). To return briefly to the psychology of individuality, it can, of course, also be nomothetic: the person is viewed simply as a member of a group. For example, the reading ability of a 10-year-old could be described as being at the 38th percentile for 10-year-olds.

Among the many issues that have been debated in the wake of Allport's scientific-theoretical writing is the relationship between theory and method. Many misunderstandings might have been avoided had Allport himself differentiated between these two concepts more clearly (Marceil, 1977). A method can be chosen from two points of view, depending on which has the best payoff: (a) the selective examination of a large sample or (b) the intensive examination of a few people. (It can be seen from our experimental design that both approaches have been used in the Bergen Project.)

Similar issues arise with respect to theory. For example, we can refer to Kluck-hohn and Murray's (1949) well-known distinction that every person is like (a) *all* other people, (b) *some* other people, and (c) *no* other people (p. 35). This rather self-evident observation cannot easily be translated into a research strategy. It is perhaps easier to resort to a more convenient dichotomized viewpoint and research method.

Objectivity and Relevance

Applied research in the behavioral sciences often appears to run into almost unsolvable problems in the conflict between the demand for practical relevance on the one hand and the demand for scientific accuracy on the other. Traditionally there has been a tendency to equate scientific accuracy and statistical accuracy. Our concept of objectivity is based on this notion, and our research tradition has shown almost unequivocally that the demand for relevance has been subordinated to the demand for objectivity.

This situation is almost unavoidable in research. Without objectivity it doesn't help much to comply with other basic rules for scientific research, such as the demand for being systematic. A system devoid of objectivity can easily lead us astray, despite its appearance of being scientific. An obvious example would be a review of the literature where one systematically selects only those studies that support one's point of view. Such a review is systematic, but lacks objectivity. Since we must comply with the requirement of objectivity, it becomes imperative that we clarify exactly what is meant by objectivity.

It is generally agreed that physical objects such as rocks, flowers, human bodies, and so on have an objective existence as contrasted with perceptions, opinions, emotions, and motives, or, generally, all traits whose existence and characteristics are determined by the human consciousness. This means that a perceived object is objective only when it has a subject-independent existence. It must exist independent of one's own existence (Tranöy, 1977).

But objectivity can also be viewed from a different vantage point. Objectivity is often ascribed to human knowledge and the demand for such knowledge, in other words, to our assertions and statements regarding that which we seek to understand. In this case we tend to view objectivity mainly as a *method*.

Our demand for methods that result in perfect objectivity is closely related to the demand for relevance. This gets us back to our original problem, the contrast between application of the traditional real and subject-independent concept of objectivity and the demand for relevance, at least when we are talking about research and its application. This contrast and its implied conflict is easily understood. But to approach real and functional solutions to the problems researched in the behavioral sciences, we must accept the fact that individuals can be understood only against the backdrop of the perceived situational reality. Much of what we do would seem irrelevant without such a frame of reference.

Replicability and Reductionism

We now turn to another major issue in research—that research procedures must be replicable and must be reported in sufficient detail to make replication possible. One must accept replication as a major premise of research activity. But again we must ask about the relevance of our traditional view of replication in the context of complex and, to an even greater extent, applied research in the behavioral sciences. Can we really replicate? How many conditions can we actually control?

Any consideration of the problem of replication must also consider the concept of reductionism. This concept is clear: it implies that something is being abbreviated or simplified.

Within the context of research one can speak of reductionism in connection with theory building, operationalizing, evaluation instrument building, data processing, and interpretation (Kragh, 1977; Underwood, 1975). But reductionism does not only represent something incomplete. It also implies a desire for a simplified and concentrated formulation of complex and multifaceted phenomena. In all steps of data reduction, theoretical speculation included, we try to achieve the utmost in economy in our intellectual activity (Underwood, 1975, p. 139). This is all right as far as it goes. But one must not forget that the reality reductionism should represent through its simplification nevertheless is very complex and transitory, especially when it comes to individuals who differ in some way from the "norm."

One will find reductionism in all phases of traditional research procedures of the behavioral sciences—in our theories, operationalizations, evaluation instrument construction, (e.g., norm-referenced and criterion-referenced tests), data analysis, interpretation of the results, and, last but not least, in our modern, abbreviated, and streamlined style of reporting. It is no wonder that attempts at replication often give disappointing results.

Within the context of applied clinical research it appears more and more necessary to focus on descriptions of processes as such instead of attempting, as done in the past, to explain them from a cause and effect model. The latter research model implies that a phenomenon cannot be understood as unique, only as a product of something else.

How, then, does one view replicability within such a qualitative, process-oriented context? The traditional empirical-quantitative replication model should not be discarded, but used as long as it is relevant. We must also accept a replication based on or supplemented by consensus among competent professionals. The question of replication, as with most central issues in research, relates to our own points of view. We have supported an eclectic stance, and agree with Rychlak (1968) that a rapprochement could emerge from an unbiased dialogue among the different points of view.

In general, the need for both points of view appears to be accepted. The problem may be in applying both in a given research project. Projects that do so appear to be relatively rare, perhaps because the design is more demanding, professionally as well as practically, but certainly also because the idiographic, qualitative, clinical approach lacks status in research areas and issues that have traditionally been "nomothetic territory." The issue is generally avoided, or one can try to legitimize a nomothetic or idiographic alternative. But one can also, as was done in the Bergen Project, seek to justify and apply the combined, integrated alternative, despite awareness of its complexities from the very beginning:

We have, of course, been aware all this time that such research is demanding, some may say Utopian. Our attitude has been that we better risk it. All clinical-practical experience tells us that this issue is so complex as to demand it. It would also seem futile to continue research which by its reductionism produces results which are unambiguous and statistically reliable, but in reality are misleading. (Gjessing, 1978, p. 12)

Let us, then, return to our discussion of "the objective and the subjective reality," and to the paradox that the objective reality, in its traditional meaning, continues to be perceived as a relevant verifier of the validity of the clinical reality. To advance requires that we get out of what we are tempted to call a scientific straitjacket. And we must accept a replication where verification and control are based on consensus among competent professionals.

For the professional consensus to be reasonably valid, however, the people carrying out the research project, singly or as a team, need to possess a broad background in research methods as well as substantial clinical competence. The statement of the problem must be precise, and all the usual components of empirical research must be considered to the extent possible. This includes such elements as sampling, construction of evaluation instruments, use of experimental controls, data collection, and data processing. Whenever the clinical observations and analysis supplement or add to the information base, they must be justified and described in detail and collected systematically.

In the Bergen Project we have considered viewpoints and methods that span this entire spectrum. We have tried to detect, describe, and analyze common characteristics in our population as well as in qualitatively defined subgroups. We have applied statistical, multivariate methods in addition to clinical methods in conjunction with our dyslexia study.

Research in Reading and Dyslexia: Discussion and Critique

Because of the viewpoints presented here with respect to ideology and methodology pertaining to research in dyslexia, it should come as no surprise that we have taken a rather critical stance with respect to the procedures traditionally used in this field (e.g., Gjessing, 1966, 1977, 1980a).

One also finds such criticism in the international literature. It has been directed at reading research in general (Weintraub et al., 1974), but more specifically at research pertaining to reading and writing disabilities. Central figures in this debate include such researchers as Wiener and Cromer (1967), Applebee (1971), and Valtin (1978).

Criticism has been directed at the procedures used in defining and selecting appropriate samples for study and at the statistical procedures used in analyzing the data. It has been claimed that the main problem and the basis for learning difficulties and lack of progress in reading is our lack of *understanding* of the nature of the reading process and the problems associated with its acquisition. There seems to be no shortage of definitions and hypothetical models, but we must continue to question their value and relevance.

We have concluded, as have Wiener and Cromer (1967) and many others, that there is no consensus regarding a definition of the reading process. This compounds the problem of defining dyslexia.

Definitions and models of dyslexia vary across a wide spectrum. Such models must take into account central issues such as the presence or absence of more than one form of dyslexia, and the extremely important problem of single or multiple causation. Wiener and Cromer (1967) started out with a model originally proposed by Handlon (1960), a model designed to elucidate the many explanations for schizophrenia. The only modification Wiener and Cromer made in the model was a change in criterion, from schizophrenia to dyslexia. (The application of such a model demonstrates how researchers working with other forms of aberration struggle with the same basic problems.)

Handlon's system considers five different models. They are all expressed in mathematical formulas, and are briefly described here.

Model 1. This model is defined as "a class with one single member, this member having a single radical cause." This model is consistent with the classic model of word blindness. This single-factor theory is not very promising and is rejected by most researchers in the field (Wiener & Cromer, 1967, p. 631).

Model 2. This model is described by Handlon as "a class with a single member, that member having multiple factors constituting the radical cause."

Model 3. This model is the reverse of the situation described as model 2. It is defined as "a class with several members having the same . . . cause." It is very difficult to find this model applied in the professional literature.

Model 4. This model is defined as "a class with several members, each having single or multiple causes that are not necessarily unique to that member." In other words, dyslexia has many antecedents and many manifestations, but the relationship between these antecedents and their consequences (dyslexia) is *unspecified* and *undefinable*. This model has been the most accepted, and the instructional methods suggested by proponents of this view cover the gamut of reading methods (whole word, phonics, linguistic, combination, and various experimental methods), in the hope that one of these will work.

Model 5. Finally, model 5 is described as "a class with several members, each member having a single unique cause." By means of mathematical symbols this model can be expressed this way; if A, then $X1$; if B, then $X2$; if C, then $X3$; . . . where the Xs represent different, specific types of dyslexia, the other letters the antecedent conditions. The model expresses the notion that there are many antecedents and a variety of manifestations within the rubric *dyslexia*, and that the relationships between antecedents and symptoms can be specified. It is this last point that differentiates model 5 from the preceding four models.

Wiener and Cromer preferred model 5: "Model 5 appears to be the only acceptable alternative. . . . It is of utmost importance that researchers try to determine the particular antecedents for special and better defined manifestations." (Wiener & Cromer, 1967, p. 633). Clearly, this point of view coincides with our own.

In his discussion of methodology, Applebee (1971) used as his point of departure the interdisciplinary interest in reading and writing difficulties. The interdisciplinary approach has resulted in illumination of many aspects of the problem, but may have been of limited utility in meeting the clinical and practical needs. Applebee considered the reasons for this situation to be found in the difficulties of defining the problem and in the statistical methods used.

As a consequence of the vagueness of our definitions and our concepts, application of the experimental and control group paradigm becomes irrelevant. Nevertheless, this paradigm has been used with remarkable frequency. It must be of little interest to make experimental comparisons when it is not entirely clear exactly what is being compared. This experimental design also leads to unrealistic hypotheses with respect to homogeneity within the dyslexia population.

From Applebee's discussion of the issues involved in definition of the problem, which involves more ideas than we can review here, we will take a brief look at his views on the statistical models and procedures used in this type of research. He made a very thorough analysis of the various statistical models, since he found this more relevant than presenting a series of experimental data from research which he did not consider particularly fruitful.

The main problem with the statistical analysis is related to the issue of defining "learning disability," particularly with regard to group heterogeneity, something which "everyone admits to obtain but few deal with." (p. 98). The variety of relationships possible between dependent and independent variables would appear to be theoretically unlimited. Applebee considered it reasonable to assume, as did Wiener and Cromer (1967), that the causes of dyslexia are multiple, but that the criterion itself, reading difficulty, can exhibit itself in a variety of different ways. His own approach to the problem appeared strongly influenced by Handlon (1960) and by Wiener and Cromer.

Applebee considered model 2 described above as most typical of past research. He described a situation where "two syndromes have been pooled into an undifferentiated sample of poor readers whose performances on various tests is typical compared with that of a sample of normal readers. In this situation even the best results will confound the underlying true situation" (p. 101).

It was Applebee's contention that qualitative differences can be revealed and considered by subdividing the sample systematically before analyzing the data. But he also emphasized that subgrouping is problematic, and that it is not necessarily a solution. One must first find a relevant rationale for subgrouping. The criteria can be common demographic data such as age, sex, socioeconomic status, and so on, but such a subclassification would not appear to be of primary value. Differences in activity level, learning style, emotionality, and teaching method used have also formed bases for subgrouping of the sample studied. This approach has been used in quite a bit of research, using regression models. "In terms of general explanatory power they have proven most satisfactory in explaining the relative position of individual readers within the middle range of achievement; they have not been very successful in accounting for severe reading retardation" (Applebee, 1971, p. 104).

Applebee felt, as we do, that one must approach this problem through thorough clinical observation. On the basis of such observation, one can attempt systematic subclassification. (This was done in the Bergen Project.) Applebee was fully aware of the complex issues raised by such analyses, but he said that, despite the complexity, "to continue any longer with models which have outlived their usefulness seems as foolish as to abandon any attempts at resolution of the problem whatsoever" (p. 112).

Like the other researchers in this field, Applebee did not have a definitive solution. Since then he has been trying to develop a subclassification system, while also searching for suitable statistical methods.

Use of Typology Models

There is clearly a documented need for a subclassification of the apparently very heterogeneous set of problems encompassed by such designations as *dyslexia* or *specific reading and spelling disability*. The problem seems to be one of finding constructive and dependable procedures for such subgrouping. We have already discussed such attempts. We wind up this discussion with some thoughts and ideas that support a typological approach to the study of human behavior in general.

It has been argued that a behaviorally determined typology is pretty much a statistical artifact. Typological classification according to individual differences is seen as the work of psychologists, not the work of nature. There may be relevant grounds for such a view. But a major concern of psychology throughout its history has been to discover types of people, so as to more generally and simply understand and explain complex human behavior. There is every reason to believe that some psychologists will continue to work along these lines. Some degree of typological thinking is probably involved in behavioral research, even though we may not be aware of it.

It may be helpful at this point to differentiate between *trait* and *type*. A *trait* can be defined as a one-dimensional characteristic that has a range within which every person can be ranked. Trait variability can be expressed quantitatively, and the variability could appear almost infinite. Classification by *type*, however, places each person within a limited number of patterns, where each pattern is defined as a step along a variety of associated qualitative dimensions (Loevinger, 1976, p. 189).

In this connection it would seem reasonable to introduced the concepts *monothetic* and *polythetic*. A typology is monothetic if it assumes that a unique set of traits or characteristics is not only necessary but sufficient to determine membership in a certain cell within a typology. A polythetic typology, on the other hand, groups together those individuals within a given sample who have the largest number of traits or dimensions in common. No single trait is necessary, nor is it sufficient (Sneath & Sokal, 1973).

The monothetic requirement maximizes similarities within each group. But it is unreasonable to expect that by the use of empirical criteria every individual will fall only within one category, since empirical testing is far from perfect and reliable. The polythetic alternative is a compromise based on the empirical reality.

The typology issues are complex, but certainly not of recent origin. They go back at least to the ancient Greek philosophers and their speculation about the unique and the universal, the concrete and its various expressions, and human types in the abstract.

A more current example of typology can be found in our language. It is a well-known observation that we have classwords (e.g., furniture, vegetables) that can represent a large variety of objects. Our conceptual framework with regard to language is basically typological: abstract concepts represent systematically a wide range of concrete concepts. This is experienced and accepted, while we at the same time realize that the subconcepts ("the typology") change meaning, depending on the criteria we choose. For example, a chair can be thought of as a piece of furniture, but can also be considered a part of a home's inventory. Some words can also represent different concepts, depending on the context, without either their spelling or the pronounciation being changed. For example, *pupil* can represent the concept of a *young student* or a part of the eye. The elements of our spoken language as well as its basic nature cannot be understood outside their functional context; this is also true of our written language and its characteristics. In this respect, language probably does not differ from other aspects of human behavior.

The use of typology as scientific method would seem difficult to accept. But to dismiss it totally would be the same as denying the existence of all conceptualization.

It is a very demanding task to develop a theoretical framework for a typology based on phenomenological insight combined with understanding of the relevant application of increasingly complex statistical methods. Every field is a demanding specialty, and the combination is mastered by few, even within the research community (Bailey, 1973). The demand for such dual specialization may be the main reason why one will find extremely few research reports in the dyslexia area based on such combined typological analyses.

Part II School Learning Disabilities

CHAPTER 4

School Achievement

R. Solheim

"Learning disabilities" is a denotation often used to describe a variety of problems that can occur during acquisition of knowledge or skills. The problems can vary considerably in nature and manifestations, degree and extent, and duration and course, and they often have complex causes (to the extent to which these can be detected).

Many decades have been spent in intensive search for explanations of learning disabilities. A variety of theories have been proposed, models have been constructed, and attempts have been made to test the theories empirically. Most of the theories that govern research and practical clinical work today can be categorized under such labels as neurological-psychoneurological, linguistic-cognitive, genetic, or information-theory based. Some definitions are negative, specifying what the given disabilities are *not* associated with (Bateman, 1965; Kass & Myklebust, 1969).

Sensory factors relating to vision and hearing are regularly listed as significant. This appears reasonable. But generally emotional factors are not on the list of intuitively likely explanations. These factors have received relatively little attention. A major goal of the Bergen Project was to collect and present empirical data that would clarify the relationship, if any, between learning disabilities and socioemotional characteristics. What might be the nature of this relationship? What kinds of associations exist? How frequently do socioemotional factors contribute to the development of negative school attitudes among pupils with learning disabilities? How powerful are these variables? Would the prognosis have been better if these problems had been studied and an intervention program been integrated into the treatment program? These are among the issues discussed in the next chapter.

A second major objective of this project was to study the educational development of children after the first grade. How do children with learning disabilities develop compared with children without such difficulties? Does the deviation from the mainstream change during the primary grades? What are realistic goals and expectations? What factors are associated with the educational development of different groups of children? Questions such as these are dealt with in Chapter 6.

Before addressing the issues presented in Chapters 5 and 6 it seems necessary to discuss two underlying frames of reference:

1. Some characteristics of the learning disabled children's learning milieu that make it likely that the children perceived their learning situation as special.
2. A known educational theory, the conceptual framework within which we worked.

Characteristics of the Learning Environment of Children With Learning Disabilities

Hidden Preschool Factors

These are handicaps that manifest themselves in the school learning situation. Not until the child begins formal learning is the learning disability revealed. It then becomes a burden during the developmental period of age 7 to 16 unless an appropriate learning environment is established in a regular classroom.

Difficulty in School Learning Tasks

Teaching of school subjects usually occurs in the regular classroom. It is the school's responsibility to adjust instruction to each pupil's abilities and level of past achievement. Many teachers do this quite successfully. Nevertheless, children with learning disabilities are highly likely to encounter an excessive number of "challenges," which they find very difficult, if not impossible, to master.

Increase in Adult Attention

The high incidence of school learning failures tends to attract the attention not only of the classroom teacher but subsequently of various educational specialists. Children and youth with learning disabilities appear to require, almost without exception, individually adjusted instruction from time to time. A very sizeable part of a school's resources in special education and school psychology is allocated annually to such programs.

Delay in School Readiness

This is probably the most obvious factor in school learning difficulties. Development can be viewed as slowed down in two ways, depending on the particular concept of learning difficulties:

1. In relation to the expectations established by the teacher's knowledge of the pupil's scholastic aptitude.
2. In relation to the norms for certain age or grade levels.

Delayed development, perceived as deviance from the mainstream or norm, results in an idiosyncratic perception of oneself as being handicapped in certain respects. This seems to consist primarily of an accumulation of past learnings and impressions that the pupil must face up to. These impressions have two main sources:

1. Objective information, based on direct experiences with various learning and problem-solving tasks.
2. Social perceptions of attitudes, opinions, comments, body language, and so on transmitted by peers, teachers, parents, and others.

Both sources are complex and are not independent of each other.

Cumulative Effects Over Time

Most learning disabilities are revealed in the primary grades, when the fundamentals of basic literacy skills are taught: to quickly and automatically extract meaning from printed text, and to communicate by means of the printed word. Judging from the amount of time devoted to the teaching of these enabling skills, their acquisition is clearly one of the central goals of the primary grades. As has been documented in this research project, a certain percentage of children do not acquire literacy skills. This lack must become a consideration for the rest of each child's obligatory schooling, as well as in further education and vocational choice.

Our society has reached the point where a diagnosis of learning disability triggers certain rights and considerations with respect to individualized instruction and suitable programs. It is, however, an uncomfortable fact that the plans and good intentions of the special education system do not always succeed. Many secondary school teachers can testify to this, especially those who deal with the aspects of the learning disability they find most taxing: indifference, what's-the-use attitude, carelessness, antipathy toward school learning, lack of effort, low frustration tolerance, and lack of enthusiasm and natural curiosity.

To summarize, in the daily practical world of the school one can often observe a close relationship between school learning difficulties on the one hand and poor motivation and school attitudes on the other, often a stronger relationship than that suggested by some theories. But one is up against the old problem of the chicken or the egg. What roles do socioemotional factors play in the etiology of learning disabilities?

A School Learning Theory

It would seem useful at this point to describe briefly the underlying theory of school learning against which the school achievement of the Bergen children was viewed—S. Bloom's theory (Bloom, 1976). This theory takes a very sensible view of the entire field and covers the same factors studied here. Its "affective" label is similar to the concept of "socioemotional" as it ties in with school learning.

A schematic of the Bloom model is shown as Figure 4.1. It describes three types of outcome of the school learning tasks: level and type of achievement,

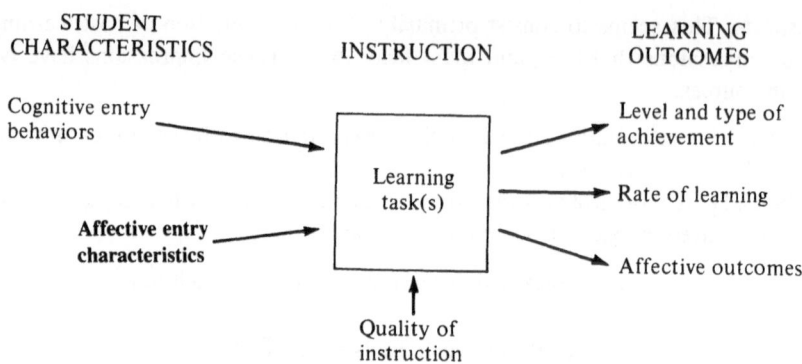

FIGURE 4.1. The Bloom model.

learning speed, and affective outcomes. The first requires little elaboration: it deals with the fund of knowledge and skills that accumulate gradually in the various school subjects in the course of schooling. The variable *learning speed* is a reminder that there is a great deal of individual variation in the speed with which learning is acquired.

Under learning outcomes one finds those easily identifiable changes that take place with regard to students' attitudes toward certain school subjects, particular topics, and school learning in general. Academic self-concept plays a dominant role in this discussion. Self-perceptions and attitudes develop as the result of the student's school experiences, primarily as these relate to competence in various areas and to personal self-worth.

Bloom described the development of this theory as an attempt to identify a small number of variables that can explain the bulk of the variance in school learning. He arrived at three factors. As can be seen in Figure 4.1, each of the three types of learning outcome is determined by an interaction between two initial pupil characteristics, cognitive and affective, and the quality of the teaching process.

A student encounters every new subject to be learned with a particular experiential background. Most school learning tasks are predicated on a set of previously acquired concepts, facts, rules, principles, and so on, which make learning of the new task possible. The *cognitive entry characteristics* (Figure 4.1) are learned behavior, and a central point of Bloom's theory is that knowledge about those previously learned behaviors that are relevant for the learning of a new task makes us better able to explain and predict the outcome of the new learning.

The *affective entry characteristics* relate to the emotional or affective condition with which the learner approaches new learning situations. They include factors such as interest, desire to learn, the perceived usefulness or importance of the new learning task, the degree to which the learner expects to acquire mastery, and the extent to which mastery affects others. Children differ greatly in the extent to which they are emotionally prepared to learn, as indicated by their interest, attitudes, self-concept, and so on. The initial affective characteristics are also determined by past learning and experiences in previous learning situations. Every learning situation begins with a certain set of affective characteristics and ends with another, perhaps quite different, set. Affective characteristics are inextricably integrated into all school learning situations. They are important components; they are also part of the educational fallout or results of direct instruction.

The quality of instruction depends primarily on the degree to which the teaching is based on awareness of each pupil's initial cognitive and affective characteristics. Another factor is the degree to which instruction results in a high degree of mastery.

What has been labeled "socioemotional" in this report corresponds basically with Bloom's "affective" behavior before and after a learning experience. Our study limited itself to an analysis of three specific aspects of affective behavior. These will be described in more detail in the next chapter, which deals with the affective aspects of school learning. Chapter 6 deals with the cognitive domain.

CHAPTER 5

Socioemotional Characteristics

R. Solheim

The study of the affective characteristics of the cohort of children in the Bergen Project covered three different aspects: classroom behavior, peer status, and self-concept. Findings are discussed in detail below, including the methodological problems and the perceptions of these three characteristics by the teachers, peers, and the children themselves.

The Three Problem Areas and Related Research

School Behavior

Are there specific affective problems associated with specific or general learning disabilities? Do children with learning disabilities behave differently in school than other children?

With respect to dyslexic children, questions about classroom behavior relate to the presence of specific, observable behavior problems, the role of the learning disability in classroom adjustment, and so on. Classroom and group learning does depend on the learner's ability to adjust and function in such a context.

In referrals of dyslexics to school psychologists one often finds descriptions like "inattentive," "unable to concentrate," "easily distracted," "disruptive," and "impulsive." Clinical experience leads one to believe that, in general, these children's classroom behavior is problematic. The research literature supports this notion: Children with specific learning disabilities are found to be less task oriented, more distractible, and less independent in school work than others (Bryan & McGrady, 1972; Forman & McKinney, 1975; McKinney, McClure, & Feagans, 1982; McKinney & Feagans, 1983; Myklebust, Boshes, Olson, & Cole, 1969). These problems do not appear to have been dealt with in the Scandinavian research literature.

The situation for children with *general* learning disabilities is somewhat different. These children often are classified as such only after they have been judged not only to have limited intellectual abilities but to be lacking in adaptive behavior (Heber, 1961). Limited intellect is a necessary but not sufficient criterion for this classification; there must also be problems of a more practical, social, and/or affective nature.

The concept "adaptive behavior" is difficult to operationalize and apply in a practical situation. Two areas of behavior have been emphasized as being germane to this concept:

Independence, encompassing a number of practical and functional skills that lead to the ability to manage one's own life.
Adaptation to local standards of behavior (Leland, 1977), including the ability to function in a group and to comprehend and behave in a socially appropriate manner.

This research group was selected solely on a psychometric basis with a somewhat more stringent selection criterion than commonly used—2 standard deviations below the national mean IQ on two tests. The variables involved in adaptive behavior were studied as dependent variables in this research project.

Peer Status

Do the children with specific and general learning disabilities have problems in their peer interaction? Do they tend to be more passive than others in play and study? Do they experience an inordinate amount of rejection from their peers? Are they less accepted socially in the classroom? If they do have these problems, is there a connection between the problems and school achievement? How can we better understand these problems, and how should the insights we gain affect how we deal with these children?

Good peer relations have significance in many aspects of human development. Clinical experience as well as research suggests that difficulties in peer relations are associated with a variety of psychological problems during adulthood (Asher, Renshaw, & Hyme, 1982).

A number of studies of the peer status of dyslexics in the classroom have been carried out with the use of sociometry (e.g., Bruininks, 1978a,1978b; T. Bryan, 1974b,1976; T. Bryan & J. Bryan, 1978; Garrett & Crump, 1980; Scranton & Ryckman, 1979). The results show that dyslexic children have a much higher incidence of being disliked, being unpopular, having low social status, and being socially rejected compared with children without learning disabilities. They also seem less able to gauge their own social status within the peer group.

The peer status of retarded children has also been studied extensively in a variety of settings (e.g., Bruininks, Rynders, & Gross, 1974; Goodman, Gottlieb, & Harrison, 1972; Iano, Ayers, Heller, McGettigen, & Walker, 1974; Lapp, 1957; Rucker, Howe, & Snider, 1969). These children also get lower ratings with respect to a variety of measures of peer status.

The research literature thus suggests rather strongly that social integration and acceptance by peers is a major problem for many of the children in these two groups. It would seem reasonable to anticipate that the Bergen Project would reveal similar findings. On the other hand, because social integration is an educational objective of very high priority in Norwegian schools, will our findings be more positive?

Self-Concept

The research literature regarding self-concept is spotty and ambiguous. An important reason is that this research depends on self-reporting. It is the children's own perceptions, feelings, opinions, and judgments that are recorded.

These data have typically been gathered by some type of group-administered self-reporting instrument. Many such evaluation instruments are available; they differ with respect to conceptualization, format, and psychometric characteristics and quality. The problems of definition and identification of the group studied are other sources of variability that contribute to the difficulties of generalizing from this research literature.

With respect to dyslexics, it would seem reasonable and logical to assume that failure to learn certain school subjects by children who appear intellectually well equipped to learn these subjects will result in loss of self-confidence and negative self-concept. Problems often observed among such children include:

Falling short of personal achievement expectations.
Expressing feelings of inferiority when work is compared with that of peers.
Reacting in a defensive manner to these failure experiences; behaving in anti-social ways.

Some of the better controlled studies reported in the literature support these impressions, documenting significant group differences between dyslexics and normal controls (Black, 1974; Boersma & Chapman, 1981; Chapman & Boersma, 1979; Cullen, Boersma, & Chapman, 1981; Hiebert, Wong, & Hunter, 1982; Larsen, Parker, & Jorjorian, 1973; Rosenthal, 1973). Although we anticipated similar results from our study, we were concerned primarily with certain nuances within this more general domain. This will be detailed later on.

The same hypotheses as stated for dyslexics can be formulated for the retarded group. It appears that similar psychodynamics are operating, and possibly some additional ones. For example, delayed language development may make communication with peers difficult. On the other hand, retardation may "filter out" some of the negative communication. Expressive language disorders may add another stigma. Although we expected results for this target group to be similar to those dyslexics, we were more uncertain about the nature of the self-concept problems in this group.

Methodology

Selection of Target Groups

The research methodology for this aspect of the Bergen Project was of the experimental-versus-control group design. The experimental groups were the dyslexic children and the retarded children. Each group was compared with a separate control group from the cohort. The target groups were selected after the screening testing between first and second grade. The data collected were quite descriptive of the groups selected, that is, the data were to some extent determined by the methodology and criteria used and could conceivably have been quite different if different criteria, methods, and children's ages had been chosen. The identification and group assignments of the children, however, would probably have varied only for marginal cases, the so-called false-positives or -negatives, in the selection process. The most extreme cases would no doubt have been identified at any age.

The control group for the dyslexic group was selected by matching each dyslexic child with a classmate of similar ability and background but with no learning difficulties. No such matching was possible for the retarded group. The four groups are described below.

D Group (Dyslexics)

The selection of these children is explained in detail in the Appendix. This analysis involved 64 girls and 107 boys. All were involved in the intensive study during the second grade and had participated in special individualized instructional programs.

C Group (Control Group for Dyslexics)

Each member of the D group was matched with another pupil on the following bases:

1. Same sex.
2. Member of the same class.
3. Absence of learning difficulties.
4. IQ as similar as possible (test and retest, group IQ test).

The mean ability test score of the C group closely matched that of the D group. The slight differences between the two groups were not statistically significant, so the groups can be considered equal with respect to IQ. They differed markedly, of course, with respect to school achievement variables. (Several other indices of general cognitive development based on (a) teachers' judgment with respect to language development at the end of grades 1 and 3 and (b) an IQ test given at the time of transition from grade 3 to 4 favored the C group, and were all statistically significant.)

R Group (Retarded)

The psychometric criterion we used for the selection of the R group was one now commonly used in many countries—a score of 2 standard deviations below the mean on an ability (IQ) test. This standard was applied by requiring a score of -2 standard deviations or lower on *two* ability tests, given at the end of the first and at the beginning of the second grade. In addition, this classification had to have the concurrence of the teacher and of the parents. (See the Appendix.)

RU Group (Retarded Underachievers)

A few pupils within the retarded group also qualified psychometrically as underachievers; that is, as having specific learning disabilities in addition to being retarded. This group was studied separately.

N Group ("Normal" Comparison Group)

This group consisted of all children in the cohort who were not identified as members of either of the learning disability groups. The R, RU, and N groups were not equivalent with respect to beginning school ability, a fact that makes comparisons like those made between the D and C groups rather nebulous for these groups. The school ability factor simply could not be controlled for the R group. The groups were also very dissimilar in size. The data for the N group are basically norms, showing how average pupils performed on the various tests. The R-N comparison indicates what R-group deviations from cognitive and achievement norms mean with respect to school behavior, peer status, and self-concept.

Dependent Variables: Evaluation Methods Used

The findings in this chapter are based on data gathered at two times: the transition from grade 1 to grade 2 (grade 1-2) and the transition from grade 3 to grade 4 (grade 3-4). The scales used in the three areas studied—classroom behavior, peer status, and self-concept, are described below.

School Behavior: Teacher Evaluation

The idea for teachers' ratings of school behavior came from an American rating scale (Myklebust, 1971), but the scale was extensively modified for use in a Norwegian school. The Myklebust scale has four major parts—listening comprehension, oral language, motor development, and school behavior—but only the last was used in this study. It covers six areas:

1. Acceptance of social norms: evaluates the extent to which the children are willing to cooperate and comply with the usual rules for school behavior.
2. Attentiveness: rates the children's ability to concentrate on school work and to reject external distractions.
3. Degree of maturity: rates the degree to which the child can attend to and complete tasks assigned in school.
4. Social acceptance: determines the extent to which each child is rejected, avoided, tolerated, and accepted by peers, and the child's popularity with classmates.
5. Feeling of security: relates to the extent to which each child feels safe and emotionally secure in school.

6. Self-image: evaluates the degree to which the children reveal self-confidence and belief in themselves, and exhibit feelings that there are some things they can do well in school.

The classroom teachers rated every child in each classroom of the entire cohort. The rating scale had 5 points—a large middle category and two categories on either side. The teachers were asked first to identify the children in the middle category, those who were "typical" or "inconspicuous," and then those at either extreme.

All ratings were basically personal judgments. Although the data were collected during a 3-week period toward the end of the school year, the ratings were undoubtedly affected by the accumulation of impressions and events during the year. There is, of course, the possibility of a "halo effect" when people are rated subjectively, and there are many possibilities for faulty impressions, misjudgments, and biases. It is also quite possible that negative attitudes develop between teachers and "problem pupils," skewing the teachers' evaluations.

However, there appears to be no particular reason to discount the substance of these findings. All of the teachers had been teaching a long time. Teacher judgment is often utilized to advantage in educational and psychological research, including studies of learning difficulties. For example, empirical data from research with Myklebust's rating scales suggest that teacher judgment results in more accurate pupil selection for special learning disability programs than do most other methods (Myklebust, 1971; Myklebust & Boshes, 1969).

When reviewing the data on the dyslexic children one should also keep in mind that for every member of the D group there was a member of the C group selected from the same classroom by the same teacher. This "matched selection" should have reduced the personal idiosyncrasies of the classroom teacher.

These teacher ratings were part of the initial phase of a very comprehensive collection of data for this project. Quite possibly subsequent teacher ratings were affected by teachers' knowledge of pupil classification, since they were aware of which pupils had been selected for special study and special treatment.

Peer Status: Peer Evaluation (Sociometry)

Sociometry is used basically for two reasons:

1. To map peer relationships and preference patterns with regard to social interaction in the classroom.
2. To get a picture of individual pupils' and small groups' peer and social relations. It is this application that we used in the Bergen Project.

Two sociometric tests were developed. Both were administered as group tests in exactly the same way at the end of grades 1 and 3. Each test consisted of a drawing on a single piece of 8½ by 11-inch paper. The drawing for one test showed children playing together (sociometry: play); the drawing for the other showed a group working together on a school project (sociometry: work). The children were asked to write the names of the three classmates they would prefer to play with or work with under the drawings. The number of times each child was chosen was used as an index of peer status. In practice, this index varied from 0 to 16. Some variation was introduced by class size, and this source of error was corrected for statistically.

Sociometry has many advantages. In particular it is time efficient, a quick way of obtaining information regarding patterns of interpersonal relations and social positions in a classroom. It was particularly useful in this study since it was indirect, all children participated, the dyslexic and retarded children were not pulled out for more special assessment, and it was less demanding than most assessment methods.

Self-Concept: Self-Reporting Group Inventory

Grade 1 Inventory

The inventory at this level was patterned after an American inventory by Meyerowitz (1962). It was developed, tried out, and adapted to fit our objectives. In its final form it consisted of 15 items. Each item contained drawings of two children whose words were in "bubbles." One bubble was in the shape of a balloon (the "balloon child") and one was shaped like a flag (the "flag child"). Each item consisted of a statement, one picture illustrating the statement in its positive form, the other the negative. The items were dictated. The teacher would say, for example, "The flag child does not like ice cream. Are you like that?" "The balloon child likes ice cream. Are you like that?"

The children were asked to put an X under the child whom they considered the better description of themselves. Each positive statement marked received a score of 1; each negative one received a score of 0. The theoretical range of scores was 0 to 15.

Grade 3 Inventory

This inventory was developed specifically for the Bergen Project. It consisted of 36 items of the following format:

I enjoy singing   YES   yes   no   NO

The items were an about-equal mix of positive ("I write well") and negative ("I am teased at school") statements. The responses were scored from 4 to 1, YES (strongly agree) being 4 and NO (strongly disagree) being 1. This inventory was analyzed in considerable depth (described later in this chapter).

Results

The results of the various group comparisons are given in the following text and tables. One will find that the number of cases in each comparison group may vary slightly from one comparison to another because of missing data. This is not a

TABLE 5.1. School behavior ratings (percentages) for dyslexic children (D group, n = 164) compared with children in the control group (C group, n = 160)

Characteristics (paired)	Group	Teacher ratings					χ^2	p
		1 (low)	2	3	4	5 (high)		
Learning								
Degree of maturity	D	3	39	49	8	1	38.2	<.01
	C	1	12	63	21	3		
Attentiveness	D	2	34	57	7	0	34.1	<.01
	C	0	14	62	19	5		
Interaction with others								
Acceptance of social norms	D	2	21	68	8	1	15.9	<.01
	C	1	15	59	22	3		
Social acceptance	D	2	34	57	7	0	34.1	<.01
	C	0	14	62	19	5		
Self-perception								
Self-image	D	3	40	52	4	1	31.8	<.01
	C	0	15	74	10	1		
Feelings of security	D	3	26	58	12	1	16.1	<.01
	C	0	17	56	25	2		

problem when dealing with single variables, but in a multivariate study such as this one must have every bit of information from every person. Missing data accumulate as one tries to analyze several variables simultaneously. The attrition reported here was so small that it did not affect the results, but it does explain the slight variations in sample sizes found throughout this book.

School Behavior

The six areas covered in the school behavior ratings were analyzed in pairs by means of a Chi-square test of significance. The pairs were *degree of maturity* and *attentiveness*, relating mainly to the learning tasks; *acceptance of social norms* and *social acceptance*, dealing mainly with how each child interacted with others in a school situation; and *self-image* and *feeling of security*, concerned with how the children perceived themselves and their feelings in the school setting.

D and C Groups

Table 5.1 presents these data for the D and C groups. The chi-square values are given, along with the level of significance (*p* value). [A chi-square value of 13.3 or higher is significant at the 1% (.01) level.]

As can be seen readily from the Table, the trend of the teachers' ratings favored the control group. In the first two characteristics listed, *degree of maturity* and *attentiveness*, three times as many children from the D group were rated as below average (categories 1 and 2) as children from the C group. These two characteristics relate most closely to schoolwork.

The D group was also rated significantly lower with respect to the two social factors. It is noteworthy that about two thirds (68%) of the dyslexics were rated average in *acceptance of social norms*, the difference in their overall ratings being barely significant at the 1% level compared with the controls. The situation was quite different for the ratings in *social acceptance*. The low ratings for dyslexics show that a learning disability had a strong association with social rejection already in the primary grades.

The last two characteristics relate to the children's self-perception. While the control group's *self-image* ratings tended to be about average, the dyslexic children's ratings leaned heavily toward the lower end. The same trend was found with respect to *feeling of security*, but was nowhere near as strong.

It seems reasonable to assume that children who got below-average ratings (1 and 2) on these scales would tend to cause problems in the classroom. These problems would be particularly influential with respect to school learning and, perhaps of equal importance, would tend to result in social rejection and exclusion from social interaction with peers.

In summary, we find that the dyslexics are assigned below-average ratings more than twice as often as the matched controls. The characteristics that showed the largest differences appear to be the ones of particular importance for school learning.

R and RU Groups

Table 5.2 shows data on the same six variables just discussed for the retarded children (R group), the retarded underachievers (RU group), and the rest of the cohort. In this situation, a chi-square value of 20 or higher is significant at the .01 level, although these values may be of somewhat limited utility because of the relatively small number of children in the R group (33) and especially in the RU group (15).

For the first two characteristics rated, *degree of maturity* and *attentiveness*, only one child (3%) from the R group was in the above-average categories, while about one third of the N group were in categories 4 and 5. The difference between the two retarded groups on the one hand and the normals on the other was, of course, quite dramatic. But the difference between the two retarded groups was also of considerable magnitude, the children in the RU group being rated particularly low in maturity.

We find a similar trend with respect to the two social factors, but the differences are not quite as dramatic. The R-group's ratings with respect to *acceptance of social norms* were mainly in the average (3) or slightly below-average (2) categories, while *social acceptance* was lower. The two retarded groups did not differ much with respect to these two social factors. It is also worth noting that only 1% of the N group was given the lowest rating in both characteristics.

Children in both of the retarded groups also rated themselves significantly lower with respect to *self-image* and *feeling of security* than did children in the N group. The difference was particularly large for self-image.

TABLE 5.2. School behavior ratings (percentages) for retarded children (R group, $n = 33$) compared with retarded underachievers (RU group, $n = 15$) and normal children (N group, $n = 2,300$)

Characteristics (paired)	Group	Teacher ratings					χ^2	p
		1 (low)	2	3	4	5 (high)		
Learning								
Degree of maturity	R	9	52	36	0	3		
	RU	53	34	13	0	0	433.2	<.001
	N	1	10	54	29	6		
Attentiveness	R	0	45	52	3	0		
	RU	13	74	13	0	0	117.9	<.001
	N	1	13	55	26	6		
Interaction with others								
Acceptance of social norms	R	3	42	49	3	3		
	RU	13	47	40	0	0	67.3	<.001
	N	1	12	61	23	3		
Social acceptance	R	15	24	61	0	0		
	RU	13	34	53	0	0	160.8	<.001
	N	1	7	79	11	2		
Self-perception								
Self-image	R	12	42	42	0	3		
	RU	20	33	40	7	0	172.3	<.001
	N	1	9	70	17	3		
Feeling of security	R	9	39	49	3	0		
	RU	0	40	60	0	0	63.9	<.001
	N	1	10	62	24	3		

To summarize, the two retarded groups outnumbered the normal group in below-average ratings anywhere from three to five times. By comparison, the dyslexics outnumbered their carefully matched controls about two times. The D group was thus somewhere between the N group and the R and RU groups with respect to the six personal characteristics rated in this project.

Peer Status

The numerical values used to quantify the peer status data are basically proportions: They represent the number of sociometric choices obtained by a pupil out of the total number of choices available. For example, in a class of 25 pupils, Leif was chosen by two pupils. Leif's raw score would thus be 2/72 (each pupil made three choices = 75 altogether, but the children could not choose themselves = 75 − 3 = 72). These proportions were converted to standard scores, using an assumed mean of 0.00 and a standard deviation of 1.00.

The peer status data for the dyslexia and matching control group are given in Table 5.3. The significance of the difference between means was tested with one-way analysis of variance; the F and p values are given in the table.

TABLE 5.3. Peer status values for dyslexic children (D group) and their controls (C group)

Peer status	D group $\bar{X}^a$	s	C group $\bar{X}$	s	F	p
Grade 1: play						
Girls	−.43	0.64	−.02	0.87	8.2	<.005
Boys	−.28	0.76	.10	0.94	7.7	<.006
Total	−.34	0.85	.05	0.94	15.0	<.001
Grade 1: study						
Girls	−.48	0.62	.09	0.87	15.8	<.001
Boys	−.35	0.75	.09	0.94	13.3	<.001
Total	−.40	0.72	.09	0.91	27.5	<.001
Grade 3: play						
Girls	−.51	0.56	−.06	0.87	10.7	<.002
Boys	−.10	1.08	.18	1.04	3.7	<.050
Total	−.25	0.94	.09	0.98	10.2	<.002
Grade 3: work						
Girls	−.60	0.51	−.07	0.88	16.4	<.001
Boys	−.26	1.17	.17	1.08	8.1	<.005
Total	−.39	0.92	.08	0.98	19.0	<.001

[a] Population mean = 0.00, standard deviation = 1.00.

The D group was rated significantly lower than the C group in all instances. The separation of the data by sex brought out some interesting differences, in that the dyslexic girls were consistently rated lower than the dyslexic boys. This difference increased from first to third grade. There was also a slight tendency for girls to be rated lower than boys in the control group; this difference also increased from first to third grade.

A two-way analysis of variance that also took sex into consideration failed to reveal a main effect of sex for the first grade, but the effect was significant at third grade. No interaction was indicated at either grade.

Children with extreme sociometric ratings are usually scrutinized closely in sociometric research. Since the technique used in this study did not involve negative choices (rejections), only the most frequently chosen children and those least frequently chosen were studied in more detail.

In the cohort of 3,090 children, 8 to 11% of the children were not chosen by their peers in any one of the four assessments. On the basis of the sociometric data, the top 10% (most popular) and the lowest 10% were selected for each of the four instances. The low group consisted of children whose scores were zero in practically all instances. They were not chosen for play or work in grades 1 and 3. It was then determined what percentage of the D group ($n = 164$) and of the C group ($n = 160$) were selected the most and the least often. These data are summarized in Table 5.4.

The findings are quite clear: the control group is, as a group, much more popular than the dyslexia group. (The difference is much smaller for the low group in

TABLE 5.4. Percentages of dyslexic children (D groups, $n = 164$) chosen least and most often in sociometric assessment compared with children in control group (C group, $n = 160$)

Peer status	Not chosen		Chosen most often	
	D group	C group	D group	C group
Grade 1: play	17	5	6	11
Grade 1: study	18	7	4	11
Grade 3: play	8	7	5	12
Grade 3: study	15	10	5	12

the third grade.) It is also worth noting that having a learning disability did not prevent around 5% of the dyslexic children from being among the most popular for study as well as for play.

Table 5.5 gives the summary statistics for the retarded children, the retarded underachievers, and the normal children with respect to the four sociometric variables. The two retarded groups clearly were rated below the normal controls, and they also showed much less variability. (The data for the RU group are not entirely consistent with this conclusion, but the irregular statistics are probably the result of the very small size of the RU group.) The fact that the retarded children had low means and small standard deviations means that one should expect very few retarded children with high ratings. This is corroborated in Table 5.6, which shows the percentages of the combined retarded groups that rate in the top and bottom 10% compared with normals. The 2% chosen most often actually represents one child.

The findings regarding peer status can be summarized briefly:

Children with specific and general learning disabilities as groups tend to have lower peer status than children in general, that is, they are less well accepted and they are socially more vulnerable. The problem is more severe for retarded children than for dyslexics.

Girls with dyslexia tend to be rated lower than boys with similar problems.

TABLE 5.5. Peer status values for retarded children (R group, $n = 33$), retarded underachievers (RU group, $n = 15$), and normal children (N group, $n = 2,300$)

Peer status	R group		RU group		N group	
	$\bar{X}^a$	s	$\bar{X}$	s	$\bar{X}$	s
Grade 1: play	−.44	0.50	−.29	0.96	.03	1.00
Grade 1: study	−.55	0.59	.56	0.84	.04	1.00
Grade 3: play	−.48	0.63	−.49	0.80	.03	1.00
Grade 3: study	−.47	0.58	−.19	1.38	.04	1.00

[a] Population mean = 0.00, standard deviation = 1.00.

TABLE 5.6. Percentages of children from the combined retarded (R) and retarded under-achievers (RU) groups chosen least and most often in sociometric assessment compared with normal children (N group)

Peer status	Not chosen		Chosen most often	
	R+RU group	N group	R+RU group	N group
Grade 1: play	9	8	2	11
Grade 1: study	28	10	2	12
Grade 3: play	17	7	2	11
Grade 3: study	19	10	2	11

A few dyslexics rank in the top 10% on sociometric variables, showing that low peer status ratings are not inevitable.

One must assume that the information gathered by sociometry relates to attitudes and feelings. In our situation, children expressed attitudes like "I like you," "You are okay," "I enjoy being with you," "You are one of the three in this class I'd like to play with," and so on. These choices, then, express acceptance and desire for positive associations and contacts with the classmates chosen. It reveals something about the relationship between the chooser and the chosen, as well as information about individual children. The number of times a child is chosen is usually considered a rough index of how that child is perceived within the social system found in every classroom. The zero score becomes a significant piece of information. It is particularly relevant as an indicator of selective discrimination against specific groups. But this information should not be perceived as "diagnostic." It says nothing about causation, and must therefore be perceived as a point of departure for further study.

How reliable is sociometric information? To get a feeling for reliability, data were gathered on two different kinds of social interaction (play and study) at two different grade levels (1 and 3). Various correlations were calculated for the two disability groups (D and R groups) and the two control groups (C and N groups). This information can be summarized rather briefly:

The correlation coefficients between the two social interactions all hovered around .75 for all groups at both grade levels.

The correlations between first and third grade were around .45, except for the dyslexia group, which had a test–retest correlation of .51 for play but .31 for study.

Self-Concept

Both of the techniques used to inventory self-concept—flag child and balloon child in the first grade, rating of statements in the third grade—yielded quantifiable data. Table 5.7 shows means, standard deviations, and the results of tests of significance for the dyslexics and their control group, for the sexes separately and

TABLE 5.7. Summary statistics for self-concept values for dyslexic children (D group) and children in the control group (C group) at grades 1 and 3

Grade	D group		C group		Difference	
	$\bar{X}^a$	s	$\bar{X}$	s	F	p
First						
Girls	−.37	1.02	.09	0.81	7.1	<.009
Boys	−.38	1.07	−.01	0.92	7.2	<.008
Total	−.38	1.05	.03	0.88	13.9	<.001
Third						
Girls	−.67	1.06	−.11	0.92	9.3	<.003
Boys	−.31	1.03	.01	0.99	4.6	<.030
Total	−.44	.96	.05	0.88	12.3	<.001

^{a}Population mean = 0.00, standard deviation = 1.00.

combined. The first-grade C-group means were very close to the cohort means, the girls scoring just a bit above. The D-group values were clearly lower for both sexes, the difference being 0.38 standard deviation. The D group also showed more variability than the control group. All first-grade mean differences were statistically significant.

The control-group means for the third grade were, again, close to the population means, with the girls at this point slightly below. This sex difference was markedly larger with the D group. The difference between these two total groups was clearly significant, with the dyslexic girls contributing the most to the difference. The difference between the boys' means was marginally significant ($p < .03$).

Corresponding data for the retarded students are shown in Table 5.8. Again, the data have been broken down by sex (which has limited utility for the RU

TABLE 5.8. Summary statistics for self-concept values for retarded children (R group), retarded underachievers (RU group), and normal children (N group) at grades 1 and 3

Grade	R group		RU group		N group	
	$\bar{X}$	s	$\bar{X}$	s	$\bar{X}$	s
First						
Girls	−.17	1.2	−1.50^a	1.6^a	.19	0.9
Boys	−.55	0.8	−.84	1.2	−.09	1.0
Total	−.36	1.0	−.95	1.3	.05	1.0
Third						
Girls	−.57	1.2	−.28^a	1.5^a	.14	0.9
Boys	−.57	0.9	−1.08	0.9	−.04	1.0
Total	−.57	1.0	−.93	1.0	.05	1.0

$^a n = 2.$

group, since this group contained only two girls). The data from first grade indicated a somewhat lower self-concept average for boys than for girls within the R group. The RU group average was considerably lower than the R group average, while the latter average was about the same as the D group average at the end of the first grade. By the third grade, mean self-concept scores for boys and girls were equal, 0.57 standard deviation below the population means. The RU group total average was 1 standard deviation below the population mean.

In summary, at two stages in the primary grades, with an interval of 2 years between, dyslexic and retarded children had, on the average, a more negative self-concept than children in general. The retarded children also showed a tendency to develop a more negative self-concept over time than did the dyslexic children. Having a learning disability in addition to being retarded is associated with a lowering of self-concepts.

The Dimensions of Self-Concept

The findings just reported were based on simple total scores. They were generally interpreted as a rough index of "global self-concept," in this particular study "global pupil self-concept." But this concept encompasses a number of unresolved issues of a theoretical as well as methodological nature. These involve, among others, the classic issues within the literature relating to self-concept. Do we have one or several self-concepts? Is self-concept global or of a multiple nature (Gergen, 1971)? In her critical review of the methodology of self-concept research, Wylie (1974) commented on the confusing inconsistency that often characterizes research reports, especially with regard to the relationship between self-concept and school achievement. From a theoretical as well as methodological point of view, the recommendation has usually been to become more specific and delimiting when approaching research in this area. Some developments in this direction have, in fact, occurred in the 1970s and 1980s.

To make a contribution to the question, we carried out a content analysis of the self-reporting scale used in the third grade. The scale, "About Myself," was developed according to standard test methodology. In its final form it contained 36 descriptive items, developed to cover four aspects of self-concept: subject matter mastery, psychomotor skills, social acceptance, and feeling of well being. The idea was to deal with areas in which children have experiences, where they try out various ideas that may or may not have positive results. These four dimensions were perceived as measured variables, and their labels covered only the positive, the educationally desirable aspect of variability within these dimensions.

With this four-factor model as a point of departure, the information gathered was subjected to a factor analysis. We shall limit ourselves here to a brief presentation of the main results. The statistical workup consisted for the most part in testing several different models, including the original one, the purpose being to arrive at a theoretically sound model that would best explain the variability within the collected data. Psychometrically speaking, the model that resulted in the smallest unexplained residual was considered the "best."

We tentatively arrived at an eight-factor self-concept theory: the original four factors plus an additional four. This theory is simply a point of departure for further developments. The eight factors are described briefly as follows (they include some psychometric data):

1. Subject matter mastery (SK-M). The test items for this factor relate to the children's perception, evaluation, and attitudes toward their own abilities to master the school subjects and the school's expectations of them as pupils. The items also relate to experiences of adequacy/inadequacy in relation to school learning situations, such as feeling able to "write," "learn things in school," "get correct answers," "read," and so on.
2. Psychomotor skills (F-M). This part of the scale assesses the children's views and self-evaluation of their own psychomotor skills; for example, "write neatly," "make things with your hands," "play ball."
3. Social acceptance (SO-F). Items in this area attempt to tease out attitudes relating to the degree to which children feel part of the social structure of the classroom and the school as a whole. The children are asked to react to statements such as "feel afraid and anxious," "do foolish things," "blamed for disturbances," "teased," and so on.
4. Social support from peers (SS-B). This factor deals with the combination of, on the one hand, the extent to which children perceive themselves as socially adequate or competent in everyday life and, on the other hand, their perceived peer reactions and attitudes in social situations, such as in statements like, other children "like to play with me" ("like to work with me," "think I'm okay").
5. Social support from adults (SS-V). This factor is similar to factor 4 but has to do with teachers and parents.
6. Self-expression (EKSP). A central dimension in self-concept is a willingness to reveal various characteristics of oneself toward others without defensiveness. This requires feeling secure in social situations, but it will vary somewhat with external factors such as time and place. The items in this area all relate to the classroom situation, for example, "sharing," "do things on the board," "read aloud," "answer questions."
7. Self-actualization (S-AK). This factor deals with the relationship between the perceived self and the ideal self, as in "to be someone else," and "look differently."
8. Feeling of well being in school (TRI). This deals with how children thrive in school, their affective reactions to enjoying or going to school, as in "dread going to school," "wish I could quit school," and "enjoy school."

In summary, we have identified, tested, and described eight different, overlapping aspects of self-concept as it relates to the school setting. This model evolved from a hierarchical factor analysis using the LISREL program, version 5 (Jöreskog & Sörebom, 1974). Some of the main results are shown in Figure 5.1. The correlation coefficients on the lines drawn from the factors to self-concept show to what extent each factor contributes to self-concept. The coefficients vary from .42 to .90. The strongest correlation, .90, is with the factor SS-V, "social

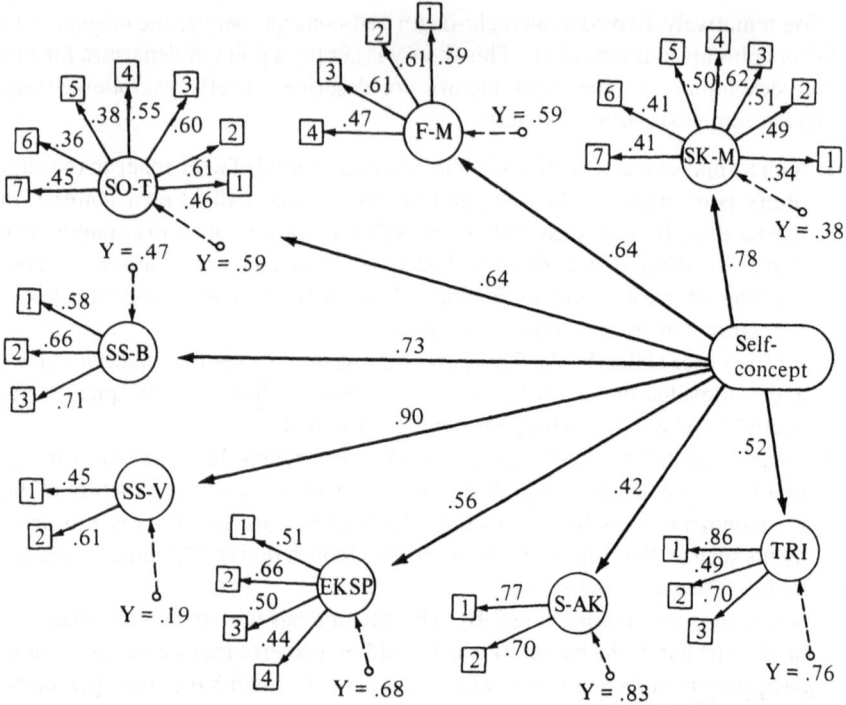

FIGURE 5.1. Self-concept factor structure based on hierarchical factor analysis. Results from children in the third grade ($n = 2,894$). Numbers on lines are correlation coefficients; numbers in boxes are items contributing to factor; Y is residual variance. See text for explanation of abbreviations.

support from adults"; it suggests that the SS-V variance accounts for 81% of the self-concept variance. Several other factors are also highly correlated with the overall characteristic, the correlations being about what one might have expected.

The correlations between each factor and the items contributing to it are also shown in Figure 5.1. There is also an unexplained residual for each factor, indicated as Y at the end of a dashed line.

This factor analysis had a goodness of fit index of .907 and a root mean square residual of 0.054.

Group Comparisons by Self-Concept Factors

After the eight factors were identified through hierarchical factor analysis, group comparisons were made between the dyslexics (D group) and their controls (C group). A two-way analysis of variance was carried out with group membership and sex as independent variables and the eight self-concept factors as dependent variables. The biggest group difference was for variable SK-M (subject matter mastery) for both sexes, in the expected direction. Somewhat smaller but nevertheless statistically significant differences were found for variables SS-V, and TRI; again, the D group scored consistently below the C group. The other four factors showed no significant differences between the two groups.

There were several significant sex differences independent of group membership with respect to the following variables: F-M, SS-B, S-AK, and TRI. All of these differences except TRI favored boys. With regard to group membership, dyslexic girls scored significantly lower than controls in self-actualization (S-AK), whereas dyslexic boys scored nonsignificantly higher than controls.

Problems in Measuring Self-Concept

Every research methodology is based on an explicit or implicit theory regarding the subject under study. It would seem appropriate at this point to clarify our viewpoint and its relationship to the research design.

A major task facing today's schools is transmitting knowledge and organizing learning experiences that develop the desired skills and insights in pupils. Children not only have to learn about the world around them but also must acquire knowledge about themselves. They acquire concepts and attitudes with attendant value systems. The school is to a large degree responsible for this entire learning process.

The outcome is what we may label self-image or self-concept, a very intricate and complex pattern of concepts and perceptions. This pattern continuously changes as a result of environmental changes and of learning experiences. This is particularly true of how primary grade children perceive themselves as pupils, since their new social situation necessitates the establishment of entirely new patterns of person interaction.

The school plays a central role in developing early affective characteristics of self-concept, that is, the school establishes goals and expectations, effort and standards with respect to school work (Bloom, 1976). Self-concept is closely tied to experiences of task mastery and failure. It contributes to the sequence and outcome of events while at the same time being part of the outcome. It affects personal events, and at the same time is affected by them. It can act as "cause" and "effect" within a set of events.

Obviously, the task of developing a methodology that can reveal the pattern of concepts and perceptions in the mind of a human being is extremely difficult. The following are some of the methodological problems involved in our study of children's self-concept.

Test Content

Our self-reporting assessments were group-administered tests of self-image. The items were pairs of statements, and the children were asked to indicate which statement best described them. The first-grade test contained 15 pairs of statements read by the teacher, to which the children responded by marking one of two stick figures. The third-grade test contained 36 statements, also dictated, and the children marked YES, yes, no or NO. The two tests were designed for the developmental stages of the children involved.

The two tests contained items relating to the four factors initially hypothesized: subject matter mastery, psychomotor skills, social acceptance, and feeling of well being. The second test contained more than twice as many items as the first, which resulted in a somewhat uneven distribution of the four factors. This undoubtedly had some effect on reliability and validity.

Reliability

No test-retest data were collected, but internal consistency in the form of coefficient alpha was determined to be .78 and .80, respectively, for the first- and third-grade scales. The subscales arrived at through factor analysis had, of course, lower reliability, ranging from .42 to .74, the median being .68.

Validity

Several pieces of information gave evidence of validity for these tests. First, the tests did differentiate groups that our theory had predicted would be different. Second the self-concept scores had concurrent validity with some other tests used to assess school attitudes, the correlations being .40 and .41. And finally, the two scales correlated significantly with each other as well as with IQ and achievement scores. In the first grade the correlations ranged from .14 to .18, while the third-grade correlations were between .22 and .29.

Sources of Error

Self-concept has been described as a pattern of value-determined concepts about oneself. It is part of our psychological makeup and exhibits itself through a variety of behaviors: verbal, or nonverbal, play, body language, artistic expressions, and so on. Answers on a self-reporting inventory are but one kind of a universe of behaviors that could be sampled. Such an inventory is subject to many sources of error, which should be considered when interpreting our data:

1. Most children in the primary grades are open and free in self-expression. Nevertheless, replies on a self-reporting inventory may reflect defensiveness or wishful thinking or perhaps even guesses at the "correct" answers.
2. Self-reporting involves verbal communication. Even though vocabulary and sentence structure are carefully controlled and items and instructions carefully thought through and studied empirically beforehand, there are still many possibilities for misunderstanding, ambiguity, and idiosyncratic interpretations of wordings and expressions.
3. It seems reasonable to assume that the items in the scale used refer to concepts and ideas that are quite central within the configuration we think of as self-concept, and yield information about the importance of these ideas for individual children. We assumed that the various aspects of the school experience were of major importance to the children studied; undoubtedly there is in reality much intraindividual variability. The total score on such a

scale tells us nothing about this variability. (This is perhaps more of a built-in methodological weakness than a source of error.)

Brief Summary of Results

Analysis of our data reveals that certain aspects of the socioemotional reactions of primary grade children with learning disabilities to their school situations differ when compared with reactions of their peers who do not have such disabilities.

1. According to *teacher evaluations*, children with learning disabilities have a much higher incidence of:
   Behavior assumed to have a negative effect on school learning processes.
   Behavior that indicates negative self-concept and limited self-confidence.
   Behavior that results in rejection by peers.
   Self-expression that is inadequate and unacceptable.
2. According to *peer evaluations*, these children are characterized as:
   Having significantly lower peer status, as a group.
   Being grossly overrepresented at the negative extremes on sociometric variables.
3. According to *self evaluations*, these children express:
   More negative attitudes regarding their own school abilities and skills.
   Less feeling of well being, less desire for expressing themselves in class, less sense of support from the adults around them, and—at least as far as the girls are concerned—a lesser degree of self-acceptance.

Discussion

Two sets of group comparisons have been reported in this chapter. The first type was purely descriptive. A group of retarded children was compared with the non-retarded population and the differences noted were identified and tabulated without much interpretation. They showed that retardation is associated with a variety of socioemotional characteristics.

The second group comparison attempted to explain certain socioemotional characteristics of a group of dyslexic children by comparing them with peers who were matched for such characteristics as sex, mental ability, age, and classroom membership. The purpose of the comparison was to maximize the probability that observed differences could be attributed to or at least associated with the learning difficulties. The discussion here will focus on this comparison.

How valid are the conclusions drawn with respect to the psychological aspects of dyslexia? What alternative explanations are there? What other factors, not controlled for in this research project, could help to explain the observed group differences?

There is no doubt that the research methodology we employed has weaknesses. The matched-group design can handle a great many factors—socioeconomic status, teacher competence, classroom dynamics, achievement level of the class, and so on – that conceivably contribute to group differences. However, the inclusion of classroom membership as a matching variable limits the number and type of matching variable employed, since the matching process has then to be done within the same classroom.

In the earlier phases of this large research project we documented that in the primary grades the most powerful correlates of school achievement are intellectual ability (IQ), sex, and classroom membership (Solheim et al., 1984). (American research has found a high correlation between school achievement and socioeconomic status, but this was not true for the Bergen cohort. This raises some interesting issues, but they are beyond the scope of this book.) The choice of matching variables, then, was based on empirical data. Use of more than the three variables chosen would probably also have been difficult within the same classroom. Although factors not controlled for could and probably did affect the outcome, it is most likely that the connections found between dyslexia and the socioemotional factors studies are of real significance.

Comparative studies are commonly done to gain useful insights into certain problems. The focus is generally group differences, with the tremendous within-group variability being overlooked. From a practical, clinical point of view such a perspective may be somewhat problematic. For example, there was a large, significant difference between the dyslexics and the control group with respect to the self-concept factor of subject matter mastery. The logical conclusion is that dyslexic children have acknowledged their deviant status by the end of the primary grades. That such a conclusion is only partly true is shown by the great variability within each group and the large amount of overlap between the two score distributions. What we have established is that more dyslexic children than control children viewed themselves as less competent in school subjects, which of course, is true. However, some children in the control group reported dissatisfaction with their own competence in school, while some of the dyslexics viewed their school competence positively.

This phenomenon raises a number of questions with psychological and educational aspects. Why do some dyslexic children report positive self-concept with respect to school learning? Why do dyslexic children react so differently to the experiences of school failure? How do school experiences affect self-concepts? What is desirable? What should be our educational objectives in this area? Should we strive for "positive" or "realistic" self-concepts?

We suggest, briefly, some possible interpretations, keeping in mind the problems mentioned earlier with respect to sources of error.

1. *The role of remedial and special education.* The aspect of self-concept relating to success in school – subject matter mastery – apparently emanates from two primary sources: pupils' own perception of the outcome of their efforts and the reactions of others to these outcomes. The former is simply the immediate interpretation of school achievement seen in comparison to the anticipated outcome, experienced as degree of success or failure. The latter is a more complex

and ambiguous conglomerate of formal and informal evaluations, comments, reactions, favorable and unfavorable comparisons with others' results and standards, and so on, from teachers, parents, peers, and others. These two sources are to some extent controllable in the schools. A major educational task, therefore, is to help pupils set goals for themselves and arrange the learning environment in such a way that they have success at their own level of achievement. The school also must arrange for school experiences that result in positive comments, praise, and encouragement, at least to the extent that this happens to children in general.

The need to provide children with positive school experiences has been a major focus of special education for a long time. Whether the school is a humanistic environment that promotes the development of dyslexic children depends to a large extent on whether this major objective has been attained. The efforts and guidance provided for pupils in the Bergen Project by their parents and the school emanated from the offices of the school psychologists, who worked in cooperation with additional special educators. We believe that the provision of this professional help to a cohort of pupils within a specified time frame contributed to the achievement of this special educational goal, and that it explains why not more children had negative self-concepts.

2. *Compensation*. It is quite possible that by the end of third grade some children have developed skills and abilities in other school subjects or outside the school environment in which they invest their time and energy and in which the psychic rewards are much greater than in reading and writing. This could reduce the ripple effect from school failure and help explain why the negative effect on self-concepts is not as severe as one might expect.

3. *Change in frame of reference*. This approach relates to Festinger's theory about social comparisons. A reference group is a group with which we identify, to which we wish to belong, and which shapes our perceptions and standards of judgment. It is quite possible that some children with learning disabilities choose a reference group, spontaneously or at the suggestion of others, that results in personal achievement expectations and personal achievement standards more consistent with the child's level of achievement.

4. *Social relationships*. Our data showed that the children with dyslexia had, as a group, much lower peer status than their classroom peers. The teacher evaluations substantiated this finding. But this perception was inconsistent with the self-reporting data, at least as it related to social acceptance and social support from peers. Dyslexic children did not report feeling stigmatized or rejected by their peers. And they did not ascribe antipathetic feelings to their peers to the extent that the peers refused to play with them, study with them, and so on. This inconsistency in perception can be interpreted in many ways and probably has a variety of meanings. The attitudes expressed by their peers in the sociometric scales were undoubtedly expressed in a variety of ways in everyday social interactions, from passive indifference to relatively explicit, aggressive actions. The sociometric data suggest that such negative signals occurred more often and against more of these children. How many of these signals were received, and how they affected these children, is of course difficult to determine. It is entirely

possible that the signals were perceived as such but were rejected or ignored because of their threatening nature. Another possible and reasonable interpretation is that the signals were not perceived, were only partly perceived, or were misinterpreted. This last hypothesis is supported by a series of research results that suggest that lack of social competence is an important aspect of learning disabilities (Bryan, 1974a, 1974b, 1976,1977,1978; Bryan et al., 1972). What is involved here is the ability to perceive and understand other children's messages and their ways of expressing them, that is, what is being said and how it is expressed verbally.

We tend to support this last alternative. It helps explain the unexpectedly high frequency of problem behavior among learning disabled children. It also contributes toward a nonmoralizing rationale for how we can deal with these children. If their lack of social competence is viewed as a component of a larger syndrome, it ought to be treated as such.

Should we strive for a realistic or a positive self-concept for all children? This may be a "pseudoproblem"; it should not be necessary to consider this as an either-or proposition. Educationally speaking, a certain degree of realism is necessary for the aspiration/achievement balance to function in a psychologically sound way, making it possible for children to have successful experiences at different levels of accomplishment. Although these are very central mechanisms for the development of children's self-concept, they are not easily realized. Our data show quite clearly that by the end of the primary grades, dyslexic as well as retarded children have developed a sense of "realism" with respect to school achievement. We have also found some negative ripple effects relating to self-expression, social support from adults, and thriving in school. Since this occurs quite early in a child's school career, attention should be paid to it, even though it is relatively circumscribed with respect to size and extent. If we had to choose between "realism" and "positive self-concept" for these children, our choice is quite obvious. A school system that fosters negative self-concept and low self-respect among certain subgroups of children does violence to central educational objectives. In addition, it makes the pupils less amenable to special educational offerings and various other treatments.

CHAPTER 6

Cognitive and Achievement Characteristics

H.-J. Gjessing and H.D. Nygaard

This chapter analyzes test data stability and changes over time for various pupil groups. These analyses were based on the data collected for the entire cohort of 3,090 children. Analyses of the individual diagnostic test data, done only for the learning disability group (259 pupils after grade 3-4 testing), are described in Part IV of this book. That part also gives a detailed report by subgroup of the learning disability sample, including the different dyslexia types.

Further Study of Cognitive Factors

Changes in Achievement in Light of the Initial Hypotheses

Changes in achievement in the Bergen Project were assessed by means of "developmental scores," scores developed for this particular project. These scores related achievement test scores obtained in grade 3-4 to the predictions made from the results of the same kind of test obtained in grade 1-2 (Nygaard, 1984a). With achievement test scores in grade 3-4 as the dependent variable and corresponding achievement test scores from grade 1-2 as the independent or predictor variable, a regression line was drawn based on the correlation between the two sets of test scores. Such a regression line could then be used to predict the grade 3-4 scores for each pupil on the basis of the grade 1-2 test results.

For most pupils, grade 3-4 test scores differed from the predicted scores to some extent. Many factors, of course, may influence these changes over time, such as reliability problems relating to the tests and the testing situation, variability in instruction for different classes, and variability in general mental ability. Nevertheless, the results from grade 3-4 have to be perceived as reflecting normative growth for this particular cohort. The correlation between the two points in time reflects relative ranks rather than absolute changes in achievement.

It was impossible to measure absolute growth between grades, since the same achievement test could not be used for both assessments because of the large amount of growth that normatively occurs over the early years. [It should be pointed out here that our (Norwegian) achievement tests provided only relative-position peer norms, such as percentiles, stanines, and normalized scores.

Longitudinal developmental scores such as grade equivalents or scaled scores are not available.] The only comparative data collected related each pupil's score to the scores of the entire cohort, with the expectation that there would be relatively small changes in rank. The extent to which a pupil's scores deviated from the predicted scores in reading, spelling, and math at grade 3-4 was used as a measure of the degree to which that pupil followed the developmental trend. The developmental scores were then basically measures of the extent to which scores in grade 3-4 deviated from the predicted.

One major reason for the analysis of these developmental scores was to search for reasons why some students did not achieve at the predicted level. Results for the three school subjects tested showed that 60% of the entire cohort obtained scores within the predicted band. The deviations of the remaining 40% would have to be ascribed to factors other than those assessed in the pretest. Variables that yielded the most potent predictors were general mental ability (IQ) and listening comprehension. Scores on these two variables correlated positively with the grade 3-4 test results. Other variables that correlated with the outcome data were sex, socioemotional variables, classroom membership (discussed elsewhere), and membership or nonmembership in the learning disability group.

With regard to sex differences, girls did somewhat better than boys in grade 1-2; the difference increased by grade 3-4.

Tests in the socioemotional areas generally correlated positively with achievement test data. It appears that good socioemotional development makes an independent positive contribution to school achievement.

The children classified at grade 1-2 as having learning disabilities showed average developmental scores at grade 3-4 significantly below those predicted from the pretest. A more detailed analysis did reveal, however, that relative status of quite a few pupils from this group had improved.

The conclusion was that, as a group, the children with learning disabilities had not developed on the average as rapidly in achievement as the total cohort, even though they had the benefit of individualized systematic special education programs. This finding is consistent with conclusions drawn from a great many 1960s and 1970s efficacy studies in special education (Goldstein et al., 1965; Østerling, 1967; Stangvik, 1970). These conclusions and the present data led one of us (Gjessing) to propose the following interaction hypotheses in 1974:

1. There are within the learning disability groups, general as well as specific learning disabilities, pupils who profit from special education programs, and whose educational development is dependent on such programs.
2. There are also within these two groups children who are not affected one way or the other by special education programs.
3. There are also within these two groups children for whom the special education programs appear to be detrimental. (Gjessing, 1974a; 1982b)

The Bergen data confirmed the presence of this kind of interaction between learning disabilities and the outcome of special education programs. But it is difficult to determine the reasons why some children react positively, and others negatively, to special intervention. This issue is discussed further in this chapter, and also in Chapter 14.

Incidence of Learning Disabilities and Distribution by Sex

The statistical treatment of the total cohort, procedures, and criteria for identifying children with learning disabilities as well as various control groups are described in detail in the Appendix. The discussion here is limited to brief descriptions of the 195 children with specific learning disabilities (dyslexia)—6.6% of the cohort population—and the 48 pupils with general learning disabilities (retarded)—1.6% of the cohort. The latter group was divided into two subgroups, "low ability low achievers," with 35 pupils, and "low ability underachievers," with 13 pupils. The first of these subgroups had achievement levels consistent with ability levels, while the second group was considered as having specific learning disabilities as well as retardation, since achievement was significantly lower than (low) ability.

The sampling and selection procedure was comparable to that in two other major international studies, the British "Isle of Wight" study (Rutter & Yule, 1970) and the American "Minimal Brain Damage Project" (Myklebust & Boshes, 1969). This made comparisons of incidence data by types and sex possible.

The Minimal Brain Damage Project started with a total population of 2,767 third and fourth graders, from which a group of pupils with learning disabilities was selected for additional study. The main selection criterion was a learning quotient, the ratio between achievement test scores and mental ability test scores expressed in age norms. This quotient resulted in a 15% incidence figure for underachievers. Additional selection criteria were then employed, such as a lower IQ limit—90—and parental consent. The final outcome was that 7.5% of the total population was identified as having a learning disability. Of the total number of boys, 11.9% were selected; the corresponding number for girls was 4.8%. The boy/girl ratio was about 2.5:1 (Myklebust & Boshes, 1969).

The Isle of Wight study entailed a population of 2,334 children aged 9 to 11. The investigators identified 165 children as "backward readers" and "specific retarded readers," or 7.1% of the population. The boy/girl ratio was about 1.7:1, after correction for sex differences in the population.

How do these data compare with the Bergen data? In the Bergen cohort of 2,962 pupils (after attrition), 6.6% were identified as having specific reading and spelling difficulties, not very different from the 7.5% and 7.1% incidence figures just mentioned.

The Bergen Project identified 8.0% of the boys and 5.0% of the girls as having specific reading and spelling difficulties. This yielded a boy/girl ratio of 1.6:1. Table 6.1 compares these ratios for the three studies. Data from both our study and the Isle of Wight study showed much smaller incidence figures by sex at the lower ability levels than did the Minimal Brain Damage Project. The higher incidence in that study for boys may have resulted from the stricter IQ cutting score of 90.

TABLE 6.1. Incidence and distribution by sex of learning disabilities in three studies

Study	Reference	Total population	Percentage with learning disability	Boy/girl ratio
Bergen Project	Gjessing & Karlsen, 1989	2,962	6.6	1.6:1
Isle of Wight	Rutter & Yule, 1970	2,334	7.1	1.7:1
Minimal Brain Damage Project	Mykelbust & Boshes, 1969	2,767	7.5	2.5:1

It should be pointed out that comparisons of incidence figures are problematic with regard to extreme groups, because of differences in sampling and selection criteria. With regard to sampling, very few studies have been based on entire cohorts or populations; the three studies compared here are rather exceptional in this respect. Most studies have been based on "referral samples," that is, the sample is determined by the particular referral policy used. It comes as no great surprise, therefore, that Tarnopol and Tarnopol (1976), in their review of learning disabilities in 20 different countries, reported incidence figures ranging from 1 to 33%. The Bergen data reported here show that when the incidence of learning disabilities is determined for the same population at two different points in time with a 2- to 3-year interval, the incidence remains about the same.

Stability in Achievement Group Membership From Grade 1-2 to Grade 3-4

Results of the tests for scholastic aptitude and for achievement in reading, spelling, and math, administered at the end of third and the beginning of fourth grade, were analyzed the same way as the results from grade 1-2, as described in the Appendix. The purpose was to determine the stability (reliability) of the learning disability classification over a 2-year span.

If the first and second tests had both yielded normal distributions, or if the tests measuring the same attributes had resulted in identical distributions, the same selection criteria could have been used in standard deviation units, resulting in comparable group data. The reading and spelling tests did result in normal distributions in grade 1-2, but grade 3-4 distributions were grossly negatively skewed.

For our analyses it seemed most appropriate to compare groups of the same size, rather than to use certain parametric statistics. To determine if the children who were in the lowest 10% in grade 1-2 were in a corresponding group at grade 3-4, we simply identified those in grade 3-4 who fell below the 10th percentile. An interesting side light of this approach was that if any children in the original learning disability group were no longer in this group at grade 3-4, new cases of "learning disability" would be identified. This side light was beyond the scope of this project.

TABLE 6.2. Overlap in group membership from grade 1-2 to grade 3-4

Group	Grade 1-2	Grade 3-4	Difference
Dyslexia	195 (100%)	119 (61%)	76 (39%)
Retarded	48 (100%)	26 (54%)	22 (46%)

The selection criteria at grade 1-2 were independent of distribution by sex, as were the criteria at grade 3-4. Both selections resulted in about the same number of children, with the same boy/girl ratio and the same degree of underachievement and low achievement in reading and spelling. This outcome formed a very strong basis for the study of stability in group membership.

Table 6.2 shows the degree to which grade 3-4 group membership conformed to grade 1-2 group membership. Of the 195 pupils who in grade 1-2 were identified and treated as having dyslexia, 119 (61%) were still considered in this category in grade 3-4. The number of pupils identified as being retarded showed a much larger shift in group membership: Of the initial group, 46% were no longer considered members, because on the second ability test they scored higher than 2 standard deviations below the mean. We will not explore the data for this general learning disability group any further, but rather take a more detailed look at the 76 children who were no longer identified as having specific learning disabilities in grade 3-4.

Two different factors may account for the "attrition" in this group. It could result from sufficient progress in school achievement to the point where the children scored above the limit for low achievement. Second, the children could still have had a learning disability but could have scored lower on the school ability test in grade 3-4 than in grade 1-2. In other words, the discrepancy between their scores for school ability and for achievement in the literacy skills in grade 3-4 may not have been large enough to qualify for underachievement in reading and/or spelling. Additional analyses revealed that both of these factors were operative. Of the 76 pupils who were no longer identified as having a specific learning disability in grade 3-4, 36 (47%) had achievement test scores above the cutting scores for low achievement. The remaining 40 (53%) still qualified as low achievers, but their scholastic ability was now lower, to the point where they were not considered underachievers. The 36 who no longer qualified as learning disabled at grade 3-4 represented 28% of those chosen because of reading difficulties, 15% of those chosen because of spelling problems, and 11% of those identified as having problems in both areas. If progress had been gauged by the fact that these children were no longer classified as learning disabled, the reading area would have shown the most progress.

The setting of cutting scores and selection criteria for the purpose of classifying or grouping children is always problematic. Since achievement tests are generally constructed to produce normative score distributions, the frequency distribution curve for an extreme group will be triangular, with a piling up of pupils near the cutting score. This increases the likelihood of misclassification for those near the cutting score, as well as of shifts in classification between the two tests. Some children may have changed significantly, but such change would not be detected in a dichotomized classification scheme. Significant change could also take place without change in a pupil's classification. Our approach was also subject to regression effects. The fact that tests were administered twice at grade 1-2 and once at grade 3-4 and that regression analysis was used in the selection process does not preclude the presence of a regression effect. Extreme groups are, of course, particularly susceptible to such effects.

Our analysis of stability of group membership did show changes from grade 1-2 to grade 3-4. Although this is useful information, the problems just described regarding cutting scores and extreme groups make data regarding changes in group membership somewhat nebulous. We thus carried out a more detailed analysis, as described below.

Development of Learning Disability Groups
Based on Predicted Scores

The developmental score previously described expressed the degree to which grade 3-4 scores corresponded to grade 1-2 scores in the same subject. Predicted scores were based on a curvilinear regression analysis of scores of the entire cohort. They were not only corrected for regression effects, they were determined independent of the results of the corresponding scores in grade 1-2.

Data for the total cohort revealed a substantial correlation between school ability and achievement. The correlation coefficients of around .60 were consistent with similar correlations obtained from national samples of American children of the same age.

There was also a significant correlation between school achievement and other variables, specifically language development, age, sex, socioeconomic status (SES), and socioemotional factors. These other variables combined explained about 35% of the variance in reading and also in spelling in grade 1-2. The corresponding percentage for grade 3-4 was 32% in reading and 41% in spelling. On the other hand, about 60% of the variance in reading and spelling in grade 3-4 could be explained by the results of the achievement tests in grade 1-2.

(As an aside, it should be pointed out that the data for the Bergent cohort showed correlations of around .20 between SES and achievement, whereas in the United States these correlations tend to be in the .40 to .50 range. This finding, although interesting, was pursued no further in this project.)

Table 6.3 shows the summary data for the developmental scores of the pupil groups formed in grade 1-2. There was considerable variability among the various groups selected as having learning disabilities, the standard deviations being considerably larger than the cohort's 1.0. The highest and lowest scores also showed rather wide ranges.

It is of considerable interest to compare the data for the various subgroups with those of the entire cohort. The dyslexia group showed some regression, relatively

TABLE 6.3. Developmental scores in reading and spelling in grade 4 for pupil groups chosen by test results in grade 1-2

		Reading				Spelling			
Group	n	$\bar{X}$	s	Mini-mum	Maxi-mum	$\bar{X}$	s	Mini-mum	Maxi-mum
Dyslexia	195	−0.31	2.04	−6.64	4.35	−0.22	1.34	−3.34	3.07
Retarded									
Low achievers	35	−0.12	1.81	−4.75	3.75	0.10	1.26	−2.69	2.67
Underachievers	13	−1.30	2.67	−4.42	2.77	−0.20	1.84	−2.08	4.64
PPT group[a]	16	0.03	1.81	−2.48	2.33	−0.68	0.80	−1.95	0.65

[a] See the Appendix for description of this group.

speaking, in reading from grade 1-2 to grade 3-4. Only the low ability under-achiever group did worse during that time span. The standard deviation for the latter group was also quite large, although not as large as for the former group. The dyslexia group showed the largest amount of variability. Within that group were pupils who developed the most and some who grew the least within the time span. Some of the reasons for this large amount of variability among pupils with relatively high scholastic aptitude but with learning difficulties will be explored in Chapter 14. The low ability low achievers retained pretty much their relative position in this developmental analysis.

The developmental picture in spelling did not differ much from that in reading. All three groups showed about average growth. The two groups of underachievers continued to exhibit the poorest results and the greatest amount of variability. For the low ability low achievers, growth in spelling tended to be slightly better than their general growth pattern. The low ability underachievers showed less decline in spelling than in reading.

Conclusions

This chapter has described characteristics of different learning disability groups with respect to certain cognitive and achievement variables. Data for the learning disability group as a whole have been analyzed, as well as data for three learning disability subgroups: dyslexia (children who are underachievers in comparison with their relatively good scholastic aptitude), low ability low achievers (children of low intellectual ability whose achievement is consistent with their ability level), and low ability underachievers (children of low scholastic aptitude whose achievement is so much lower than their aptitude level as to qualify them as underachievers by our criteria).

The total learning disability sample exhibited somewhat poorer development in the literacy skills than did the total cohort. But they showed a great deal of variability. Quite a few children in the learning disability group showed growth that deviated quite remarkably from that of the total cohort, at the high end as well as the low.

A comparative study of growth in the literacy skills among the three subgroups showed that less progress was achieved by dyslexic children than by retarded children. Although the difference in average developmental scores was not significant, the trend was certainly interesting: the learning disabled children with relatively high scholastic aptitude (IQ) gained less in achievement than those with low scholastic aptitude.

It is generally believed that the prognosis for positive school learning would be better for a group of children with relatively good mental ability than for retarded pupils, if the groups are equal at the beginning. In our study the trend was in the opposite direction. This finding is consistent with earlier data by Karlsen (1954), who found that neither Wechsler Intelligence Scale for Children (WISC) nor Stanford Binet IQs correlated with educational progress of a group of learning disabled children.

In our experimental design, these two main subgroups, dyslexics and retarded, received individually adapted special education based on the same basic model. The group tendency was for the retarded to make slightly better progress in school than the dyslexics, especially in spelling. But the variability was very large for both groups, some pupils in each group making very large gains and some very limited gains in achievement between grade 1-2 and grade 3-4. The variability was especially large for dyslexic pupils (see Table 6.3).

These results confirm our hypothesis that even though learning disabled pupils all receive individualized special instruction, they respond to it in extremely varied ways. Some pupils make very remarkable progress, others maintain their relative rank in school achievement, and others exhibit extremely slow growth in achievement.

What are causative factors in these developmental patterns? Do those who make remarkable progress share some common characteristics, compared with those at the other extreme? Is their progress tied to socioeconomic status, sex, socioemotional status, initial degree of underachievement, or other factor? What is the unique contribution of the special education program offered each student?

Interaction analyses of these characteristics are quite complex, but definitely useful. As can be seen from the data presented here, a simple study of group averages yields very limited answer. This problem is dealt with further in Chapter 14.

Part III   Theoretical and Clinical Foundation of This Study of Dyslexia

CHAPTER 7

Overview of Research on Reading and Dyslexia

H.-J. Gjessing and B. Karlsen

General Trends in Reading Research

Reading instruction has always been a central issue in our schools. Reading is also a central issue in the field of educational research. This century has seen the publication of voluminous textbooks and thousands of research reports. Prior to the 1950s there were already over 3,000 published scientific studies relating to reading, and the rate of publication has accelerated significantly in more recent years (Gray, 1926; Harris & Sipay, 1985; Weintraub et al., 1970).

Despite this enormous effort, few if any would claim to understand fully the very complex process of reading. The definition of reading by Harris and Sipay (1985) is representative of the many attempts to define and explain: "Reading is the meaningful interpretation of printed or written verbal symbols" (p. 12). Such an abstract and all-inclusive definition should be tempered by the fact that reading ability represents somewhat different sets of skills and abilities from one age level to another. Regardless of instructional method, the beginning reader is very much occupied with problems relating to printed symbols and the messages communicated by them. The verbal reasoning process, combined with word recognition and decoding flexibility, makes the written word increasingly meaningful. This, combined with past experiences, results in communication in print.

Reading as a process and as a psycholinguistic function changes character as the reader matures and develops skills. Reading becomes not *one* skill but a set of interrelated characteristics and skills that become more and more sophisticated with age. This fact would seem rather self-evident. But in view of the theories, the research, and the debate surrounding reading and its phenomenology, it apparently is not self-evident; in fact, the opposite may be the case.

The reading process has long been a subject of research. Early experimental psychology toward the end of the 19th century dealt with it. Laboratory research was directed at the psychological and physiological bases of reading, especially through studies of eye movements during reading. Although these studies emphasized some rather peripheral aspects of the reading process, they provided a valuable foundation for later explorations and for better understanding of the central processes, the perceptual and cognitive attributes required for reading.

Between the two world wars much interest and effort were directed toward the practical and applied problems of teaching reading. Objective tests were developed to study reading in a more naturalistic school setting, and the first standardized reading tests became generally available. These early tests revealed a rather remarkable amount of variatioñ among students at any given grade level. This finding was undoubtedly an important impetus toward further study of reading and writing difficulties, becoming a major aspect of reading research in the late 1930s. But the standardized tests also laid the foundation for controlled classroom experimentation relating to a broad spectrum of issues, such as reading readiness, relationships between reading and mental ability, and the outcomes of various instructional methodologies and school organization.

After World War II the emphasis continued to be heavily pragmatic, with development of instructional methods. There was a great deal of faith in the decisive role of methods for facilitating children's growth in reading (Betts, 1946; Gates, 1947; Gray, 1950–1954). Researchers from the fields of curriculum and educational psychology with a strong practical bent dominated this period.

But interest was also growing in the theoretical issues surrounding reading, its complex nature, and its demand for a wide range of individual attributes as well as certain types of educational settings. The reading process began to be studied by people from such diverse fields as cognitive psychology, developmental psychology, linguistics, psycholinguistics, sociology, neuropsychology, and a variety of medical specialties.

From a relatively atheoretical start, reading research became concerned with the development of theories relating to basic reading processes (Holmes, 1953; Kavanagh & Mattingly, 1972; Singer & Ruddell, 1970, 1985; Vellutino, 1979). Accompanying these theories were numerous models (hypothetical constructs), which had many common features and also some unique aspects. Reviews of many of these models can be found in Geyer (1972), Samuels (1977), Singer & Ruddell (1985), and Williams (1973).

But all this theorizing and categorizing has so far had limited influence on the teaching of reading (Doehring, 1983; Lundberg, 1981b). The theories and the models have not lent themselves to practical applications or empirical experimentation except for some peripheral aspects of information processing. Nevertheless, the work with theories and models has led to increased understanding of the complex nature of the reading process and to an appreciation of how reading and other literacy skills interreact with practically our entire perceptual, cognitive, psychomotor, and socioemotional makeup. We still have limited understanding of how this complex interaction takes place. The various theories appear to have become crystallized into two major constellations, the so-called bottom–up and top–down models.

The *bottom–up* models assume that reading is learned as a sequence of hierarchical steps. The reader begins by learning units such as letters. As these are mastered, the units are combined and the learner discovers that the various combinations form known words. As a word is identified it is recoded to a spoken message, which enables the reader to get its meaning in the same way he or she has received spoken messages in the past. Reading comprehension is the result of automatizing an accurate word recognition process and combining it with one's language competence and past experiences. Most proponents of bottom-up models appear to assume, independent of their more general theoretical views, that written language is so intimately tied to spoken language that reading comprehension at the early stages is limited by the degree of language competence the learner brings to the task of reading (Bloomfield & Barnhart, 1961; Fries, 1963; Gagné, 1970; Gough, 1972; Reed, 1965). Processing is assumed to go from the peripheral to the more central aspects of cognition. The sense organs are stimulated by printed symbols, which, though increasingly complex levels in the nervous system, become translated into raised consciousness, interpretation, and comprehension.

The *top-down* model is based on the opposite principle. Here, the higher cognitive processes select and govern the lower-level information acquisition processes.

Most top-down models appear to be based on psycholinguistic theory, on the higher order interaction between language and thought in its broadest sense (Edfelt, 1982; Goodman, 1967; Smith, 1971). Goodman has viewed reading as a "psycholinguistic guessing game." As messages are gradually received through reading, the meaning ascribed to them is confirmed, rejected, or reevaluated as the reading process continues. Top-down models place little emphasis on the decoding process, which is central in the bottom-up models. Top-down theorists prefer to go as quickly as possible from text to meaning, without the indirect involvement of the spoken language. They assume this process to be typical of mature readers.

The theory that good readers can use a direct route from print to meaning has been the strongest argument for the top-down models. But the theory has been strongly contradicted in recent years by significant research findings. The research appears to indicate that even mature readers deliberately us context as an aid to decoding to some limited extent (Mitchell & Green, 1978). Recent eye movement research further suggests that even adult mature readers fixate on the text in considerably more detail than has traditionally been believed (Just & Carpenter, 1980).

These issues will not be discussed any further at this point. Numerous publications provide extensive references on this topic, for example, Singer and Ruddell (1985). In the Scandinavian literature Lundberg (1981b) has described and discussed theories and models in a brief but instructive publication. It is clear, however, that bottom-up models and top-down models produce very different ideas as to how reading should be taught.

There are indications that these either-or positions as they relate to reading instruction are softening. More and more researchers are accepting a third viewpoint—the interactive model. This model considers the reading process as bottom-up as well as top-down. Print interpretation is based on a variety of simultaneous stimuli, such as visual cues, orthographic structure, lexical knowledge, syntax, and semantics (Lundberg, 1981b). Rumelhart (1977) maintained that mature readers apply top–down and bottom–up processing simultaneously and interactively. When comprehension is lacking, the experienced reader will change strategies by, for example, going from a heavy emphasis on context to word decoding.

Our consideration of some rather extreme viewpoints has again led us to what has long been suggested by practical experience alone: The reading process depends to a large extent on the reader's age, ability, purposes, and personal requirements. Such consideration also confirms that reading research is very complex—that reading means different things to different people. Theories are numerous, but relevant empirical data are often lacking.

Trends in Reading Disability Research

From a consideration of the trends in reading research in general we turn now to the large and often dominant area of research on reading disabilities. By *reading disability* is meant inordinate difficulty in learning to read, often combined with writing difficulties, despite adequate instruction. The learner has no apparent problems in the sensory, cognitive, emotional, or social areas.

This problem was first studied by investigators in the medical profession (Pelosi, 1977). Around the turn of this century several British physicians described persons of normal intellect who, despite adequate educational opportunities, failed to learn to read (Hinshelwood, 1896; Kerr, 1897; Morgan, 1896).

That physicians were the first to describe these cases is not particularly surprising—it seems reasonable to expect that when otherwise normal individuals fail to learn to read they must have some sort of visual impairment. But the doctors were unable to find any visual defects or other medical abnormalities that could explain the phenomenon. They proceeded to suggest that this was a disturbance in symbol perception, a congenital defect in the brain's "reading center." Numerous reports emerged in the medical literature, not only from England but also from the Continent and from Scandinavia (Hallgren, 1950; Hermann, 1955; Skydsgaard, 1942; Tamm, 1925) and the United States. A few educators and psychologists had, however, show a serious interest in this area (Fernald & Keller, 1921; Gates, 1927; Gray, 1922; Uhl, 1916).

Both medical and educational-psychological professionals have continued to work on the reading disability problem with varying degrees of interest and intensity. Throughout the years there have been great differences of opinion among these researchers, not only with regard to terminology and symptomatology, but also with respect to theories of causation. Most medical researchers have hypothesized a circumscribed neurological basis for reading disabilities, while most psychological researchers have hypothesized a much broader, multidimensional phenomenon within the normal variability of human characteristics.

Generally the medical research has been dominated by qualitative descriptions of individual cases, with perhaps references to a few other cases, and using a single-cause hypothesis as a base. The educational-psychological research has, on the other hand, typically involved quantitative descriptions of large and representative samples, using a multicausation etiology as a base.

Besides these two main trends one also finds, especially around the time of World War II and thereafter, considerable interest in reading disabilities from psychoanalytic and clinical-psychological viewpoints (Ericson, 1981). Such disabilities were assumed to have an emotional base, the treatment being, of course, psychotherapy. There is little indication that this viewpoint and therapeutic approach have much merit, and there has been little interest in the application of this clinical approach in recent years (Harris & Sipay, 1985).

Recent developments in scientific study in the areas of reading and writing disabilities can be described in a variety of ways. The total body of literature in this area — albeit the studies have been carried out under a variety of labels, a problem that will be discussed later — has become so voluminous that it is doubtful any one person has been able to digest it all (Doehring, 1983). There are, however, several valuable reviews, comparative analyses, and critiques, for example, Doehring (1983), Vellutino (1979), and Torgeson and Dice (1980), as well as Klasen (1972), who gives a good discussion of the German literature.

Despite a certain rapprochement between the medical and the educational-psychological research trends, these two are still quite distinguishable. The premise on which the two trends differ will therefore be considered here in some detail.

Medical Viewpoint

A good place to start taking a closer look at the *medical* viewpoint may be the writing of Rabinovich. In a nosology proposed by Rabinovich (1968), "reading retardation" classified was as primary or secondary, being defined as a significant discrepancy between the assessed reading level and the reading level that could be expected on the basis of mental age as assessed by nonverbal tests. Dyslexia, or what Rabinovich called "developmental dyslexia," was considered one of many causes of reading retardation. He emphasized strongly, however, his premise that dyslexia is a separate entity that is discretely definable from many other causes of reading disabilities.

Rabinovich's nosology included the following classification of reading retardation:

1. Primary reading retardation: Developmental dyslexia.
2. Secondary reading retardation:
   a. Other encephalopathy (specific language impairment, motor-concentration impairments).
   b. Emotional disturbances.
   c. Motivational or opportunity factors.
   d. Deprivation or distortion of language experience.

In his descriptions and comments about primary reading retardation (developmental dyslexia) he emphasized that there is no evidence of definite brain damage either in the case history or in the neurological examination. The disability is mainly the result of how the neurological patterns have developed.

So-called secondary reading retardation was considered secondary to other pathologies. To be classified under "other encephalopathy," it is assumed that (a) there is some evidence of brain damage and that a symptomatic language disorder such as difficulties with symbolic language is part of the total pathology, or that (b) the control mechanisms related to concentration and impulse control are insufficient, impairing the development of reading skills.

With regard to the next type of secondary reading retardation, "emotional disturbances," Rabinovich differentiated between the achievement of skills on the one hand, as measured by educational tests, and the application of these skills in the classroom on the other. On the basis of extensive experience with reading retardation, he was of the opinion that emotional problems affect the *application* of skills more than their *acquisition*.

Many neurotic children, regardless of the severity of the neurosis, function relatively adequately on achievement tests, but they still may obtain failing grades because they can not apply themselves to the tasks at hand. Anxiety, depression, displaced counteraggression, and similar emotional problems tend to affect learning in this way. (Rabinovich, 1968, p. 3)

The "emotional disturbances" and "motivational and opportunity factors" are all attributed to exogenous factors. Children in these categories are considered to have normal potential for learning to read, this potential having been disturbed by negativism, anxiety, depression, emotional blocks, psychoses, insufficient educational opportunities, and other external circumstances.

Among the children in the last category, "deprivation or distortion of language experiences," he reported extremely poor reading ability. But there is no reason to assume that this reflects lack of intellectual abilities to begin with, nor that one can attribute poor reading ability to a neurological dysfunction:

Many of these children have a limited exposure to language, especially abstract language. The question arises as to the process by which this experiential limitation has affected the reading process. (p. 5)

Rabinovich estimated the incidence of reading retardation in the United States to be around 10% among school-age children. But there are great variations from one area to another, with disproportionately large numbers in areas of low socioeconomic status. Within the total incidence figure of 10% he estimated about one-third to one-fourth as cases of primary reading retardation; or developmental dyslexia.

In brief, one can say that Rabinovich considered reading retardation to be primary if there is endogenous causation combined with "normal intelligence and without brain damage." He therefore considered primary reading retardation to be of constitutional origin. Critchley and Critchley (1978) assumed that Rabinovich's primary group corresponded to what they labeled "specific developmental dyslexia." They also seemed to agree that secondary reading retardation is not of genetic or constitutional origin.

Some medical professionals are still interested in the notion that a distinct type of primary reading retardation is the result of a "developmental lag" in neurological development. The problems of lack of a clear-cut etiology and overlap with other phenomena are particularly bothersome in diagnosis as well as in research. (See Rutter & Yule, 1975.)

After a relatively inactive period, medical and neuropsychological research is again making interesting contributions and developing promising research tools for the measurement and evaluation of neurophysiological and biochemical processes. Certain aspects of brain activity can now be observed during cognitive activities such as reading (Galaburda, 1983; Hynd & Cohen, 1983; Knights & Bakker, 1980). These techniques and assessment tools represent enormous progress compared with earlier postmortem studies and the traditional but relatively nonspecific electroencephalographic examination.

Educational-Psychological Viewpoint

Educational-psychological research in the area of reading disabilities was initiated considerably later than the medical research. Some of the early pioneers up to the 1930s have already been mentioned. Among the fundamental researchers of the 1930s and 1940s one must list people like Marion Monroe (1932) and Helen Robinson (1946). Around the 1950s and 1960s we had contributions from Scandinavian researchers with educational-psychological backgrounds (Gjessing, 1958a; Malmquist, 1958; Tordrup, 1967).

In contrast to the more pathological orientation of the medical researchers, the educational-psychological researchers were primarily interested in the large number of children who had great difficulties learning to read. While the medical people worked from a neurological and neuropathological orientation, the educational-psychological researchers had a research orientation that could deal with the interaction of the multiplicity of human factors that must be taken into consideration in the study of cognition and verbal learning. This latter research had, of course, an entirely different character than did the medical research. The classic research model, which is still being used, was a cross-sectional study of a relatively large number of children, consisting of an experimental group with reading disabilities and a control group of normal readers. These two groups were typically compared with respect to a number of factors that could play a role in reading and spelling achievement. However, while most American research was confined to the study of reading difficulties, European research placed almost as much emphasis on problems connected with learning to spell.

Most of the research was confined to the study of reading-disabled children with at least average general mental ability (IQ) and without serious sensory defects. Among the factors studied were vision and visual perception, hearing and auditory perception, language development and speech characteristics, laterality, dominance and spatial perception, personality variables, age, sex, diseases and problems relating to prenatal and postnatal factors, and health and certain specific diseases, as well as such external characteristics as family structure, socioeconomic status, and school attendance, including change of school and absenteeism.

The main purpose of much of this research was to discover correlates that could contribute to an understanding of the etiology of learning disabilities. But the results were contradictory, ambiguous, and disappointing.

Problems of research methodology relating to sampling, experimental control, and statistical treatment have been discussed by many researchers (Malmquist, 1969; Torgesen & Dice, 1980; Valtin, 1978; Vellutino, 1979; Weintraub et al., 1974). (These issues will be discussed further in chap. 11.) Although these are important considerations, it is doubtful that the research methodology per se has been the most important barrier toward increased understanding of learning disabilities. Rather, the greatest barrier may be lack of willingness to accept the consequences of our knowledge about the heterogeneous nature of this problem, relating to the pattern of interaction within the interindividual situation (person-environment interaction) as well as the intraindividual factors (neurocognitive infrastructure).

This problem area has recently become a central topic within the more general research methodology relating to cognition (Cronbach & Snow, 1977; Fisher, 1980), and it has also gained supporters within the field of research in reading disabilities (Doehring, 1983; Torgeson & Dice, 1980). We realize to an increasing degree that quantitative main effects, which undoubtedly have been the dominant concern of educational-psychological research, cannot yield clear-cut answers as long as certain interactions and qualitative nuances are being neglected. This problem is not new, however. It was explicitly pointed out in the 1930s (Monroe, 1932).

Interaction research—the study of the simultaneous effects and interactions of many variables—is difficult and time consuming. This is probably the main reason why educational and psychological research in this area has continued along the traditional lines (Gjessing, 1982b). There is however, an increase in interest in multivariate techniques and interaction analyses, combined with clinical qualitative observations. Along with the development of new techniques for the medically oriented research on dyslexia, this should provide a basis for substantial gains in this complex area of research.

Typological Models

In recent years a promising trend in both medical and psychological research in the study of typological models and subgroups within the reading-disabled population (Lovett, 1984). The basis for such subgrouping has varied. Subgrouping has been based on behavioral observations during the reading and writing process with systematic tabulations of errors (miscues), such errors being considered direct variables in literacy skills. Subgroups have also been formed on the basis of nonliteracy variables of a cognitive or neurological nature (indirect, or nonreading, variables). The subgrouping can also, of course, be done on the basis of a combination of these direct and indirect variables. Systematic grouping can also be the result of clinical analyses based on a priori hypotheses or on purely multivariate statistical techniques that are free of prior hypotheses regarding typology.

Gjessing apparently was among the first to work in this problem area. On the basis of extensive clinical experience with dyslexia, he published detailed descriptions of children with different types of reading and spelling difficulties already in the 1950s (Gjessing, 1953; Gjessing, 1958b). With the Bergen Project he was probably the first to apply clinical analyses of dyslexia types as well as advanced statistical subgrouping techniques to the same representative sample of children. The results of these efforts constitute the central theme of this book.

Terminology, Definitions, and Delimitations

Anyone who tries to study the literature relating to reading disability immediately runs into the problem of the many different labels used to describe or classify people with this problem. The plethora of terms used in this field has caused and is continuing to cause a great deal of confusion. A detailed and systematic discussion of the terminology issue can be found in Harris and Sipay (1985) in the section headed "Terminology" (pp. 134–143).

So far in this book we have used the terms *reading disability, learning disability, reading retardation, reading* and *spelling difficulties*, and *dyslexia*. But we could use many other labels, such as *word blindness, reading disorder,* and *learning handicapped.* "Specific" is often used as a modifier to give the label more precision. Confusion in the American literature has been so extensive that entire articles have been written listing and describing the many labels for what appears to be the same syndrome.

The professional German literature most often uses the term *Legasthenie*, although one also encounters *Lesestörung und Schreibstörung* as well as *Leseschwäche.* (See, e.g., Klasen, 1972).

The term *word blindness* is now obsolete. This is also true of such less known and infrequently used terms as *word amblyopia, thypholexia, amnesia visualis verbalis, analphabetia partialis, bradylexia, script blindness, psychic blindness,* and *symbolia confusion* (Critchley, 1970). Even the term coined by Orton, *strephosymbolia,* never caught on, despite the popularity of his theory (Orton, 1928).

"Reading Disability" Versus "Dyslexia"

Even though a great many terms are still in use, two terms have emerged as the most commonly accepted, *reading disability* and *dyslexia.* As currently used, the two terms are simply descriptive of certain symptoms – they make no assumptions about etiology. But they reflect to some extent the differences in opinion regarding etiology between educators on the one hand and medical and psychological professionals on the other. Physicians typically apply the term dyslexia to mean an etiologically identifiable, distinct type of reading problem, although this use is not universal. Many physicians now use dyslexia to describe all reading difficulties regardless of etiology. The variety presumably caused by constitutional (endogenous) factors is often identified by the modifiers "developmental" or "specific," or even both – "specific developmental dyslexia." But many medical specialists and neuropsychologists now use alternate terms such as reading disability or reading disorder.

Most educational psychologists prefer the term *reading disability*, avoiding the term dyslexia because it implies a certain etiology that can rarely be demonstrated. Harris and Sipay (1985) preferred the former term ". . .because of its relative clarity of meaning." *A Dictionary of Reading* (Harris & Hodges, 1981) published by International Reading Association contains the following note at the end of its dyslexia entry.

Dyslexia in this sense is a term which describes a symptom, not a disease. Due to all the differing assumptions about the process and nature of possible reading problems, dyslexia has come to have so many incompatible connotations that it has lost any real value for educators, except as a fancy word for a reading problem. Consequently, its use may create damaging cause and effect assumptions for student, family, and teacher. Thus, in referring to a specific student, it is probably better that the teacher describe the actual reading difficulties, and make suggestions for teaching related to the specific difficulties, not apply a label which may create misleading assumptions by all involved. (p. 95)

We also have reservations about the premises on which the traditional medical literature used the term dyslexia. But if we use dyslexia as a collective term for reading difficulties with a variety of manifestations and known and unknown etiologies, it represents, in the opinion of the Bergen Project staff, the best label, one that will facilitate communication across the many disciplines working with people having this problem.

To us, the term dyslexia seems to cover the spectrum of processes involved better than any other. The word itself is of Greek origin. The root word, *lexis*, does not mean reading but "word," or perhaps the proper way of using words (e.g., Critchley & Critchley, 1978; Lidell & Scott, 1940). The label can therefore represent difficulties with reading and spelling as well as speech and language disorders in general. This is important, since the broader concept of a *language disorder* has gradually gained ground in research on reading and dyslexia (Kavanagh & Mattingly, 1972; Lundberg, 1983). Even people in the field of reading instruction are now quite often referring to "literacy skills" rather than the much narrower "reading" label. Reading disability has *erroneously* been considered a somewhat isolated phenomenon within the broader field of language competence.

It is peculiar, to say the least, how long it has taken professionals in the English-speaking world to become interested in the connection between reading and writing difficulties (Johnson & Myklebust, 1967). The relationship between these processes has been a central issue in the Scandinavian as well as the German professional literature for a very long time (Gjessing, 1953; Klasen, 1972; Malmquist, 1969; Müller, 1958; Schenk-Danziger, 1959).

A second consideration in preferring the term dyslexia is our practical clinical experience. A "diagnosis" of dyslexia has often resulted in unequivocally positive psychological effects, effects we had not experienced with the more descriptive labels such as reading disability, reading difficulty, or reading retardation. At least with the way we have used the term dyslexia, with its subcategories based on behavioral characteristics, there is a basis for a more concrete understanding and identification of the basic problem. This may sound paradoxical, but from the standpoint of the persons involved it seems more beneficial for their self-concept and self-respect to be a member of a group that has a problem-specific identity, rather than of the more ambiguous learning disability group or simply at the low end of the achievement distribution. The knowledge that there are other seemingly normal youngsters who have the same problem often gives these students some degree of self-confidence and hope.

A further argument favoring the term dyslexia is its almost invariant form across many languages. This is a particularly great advantage for international communication among professionals. Other terms, such as the labels in English — reading difficulties, learning disabilities, learning handicapped — are often difficult to understand and to translate, and they are sometimes used as euphemisms for other problems. Usage varies also, not only from one country to another, but within countries as well. In their valuable review of reading problems in 18 different countries, Tarnopol and Tarnopol (1976) concluded with respect to terminology:

Disparity in terminology exists both among and within states. The lack of universally accepted designations for various types of reading and learning problems tends to handicap anyone attempting to study these problems. (p. 5)

Further Definitions and Criteria for Dyslexia

Our discussion of the research on dyslexia and terminology started and ended with the problem of definition. In the preceding paragraphs we gave our rationale for the use of the term dyslexia. Here we consider this issue in more depth.

Hinshelwood (1917) used the term *congenital word blindness*, defining this condition as a defect resulting in such severe difficulties in learning to read as to be considered abnormal and pathological. He described cases where attempts to learn to read by ordinary methods met with complete failure. His definition contained elements that are still basic when defining dyslexia, even though we may use different words. Over the years his basic definition has been supplemented by others. Skydsgaard (1942) used the term *constitutional dyslexia*, which encompasses congenital and constitutional factors; he pointed out the presence of spelling problems along with the reading difficulties. He also noted that the condition appears to be familial, and that it occurs most frequently among males. He presumed normal intellect, normal speech, and no sensory disorder with respect to vision and hearing. People with this problem make errors in their reading and spelling that are typical, judged qualitatively. Their achievement is particularly low in comparison with their skills and abilities in other areas.

Hermann (1967) maintained, with regard to what he labeled "specific dyslexia," that in addition to reading and spelling difficulties, other problems with printed symbols such as numbers and printed music are also present. These difficulties occur without accompanying environmental problems.

There have also been more recent medical definitions of dyslexia, for example, that of the World Federation of Neurology, Naidoo (1972), and Critchley and Critchley (1978), where dyslexia is ascribed to delayed neurological maturation, or "developmental lag." Critchley and Critchley also used the term *developmental dyslexia* but did not otherwise shed any new light on the problem.

It looks as if the medically oriented research of the late 1980s will concentrate on the importance and relative contributions of the two cerebral hemispheres in the reading process. This research has the potential of illuminating the problems of dyslexia and may affect remedial instructional methods as well.

Definitions of dyslexia from an educational-psychological point of view make no assumptions about causation, in contrast to the medical definitions. But they do agree on the requirement that there must be a significant discrepancy between achievement and potential, although the educational psychologists are preoccupied with the magnitude of this discrepancy. This is probably best illustrated by the classification system of Harris and Sipay (1985). They described five different types.

Disabled reader or **reading disability**: designates individuals whose general level of reading ability is significantly below expectancy for their age and intelligence and is disparate with their cultural, linguistic, and educational experience. The latter part of the definition suggests that factors other than chronological age and intelligence must be considered.

Severely disabled reader or **severe reading disability**: refers to disabled readers whose general level of reading ability is extremely below expectancy. Some writers apply labels such as **dyslexia** or **learning disability** to these cases.

Slow learner in reading: indicates children who, although reading below age level, are generally functioning in reading close to their somewhat limited learning potential.

Underachiever in reading: applies to children who, although reading at or above age or grade level, are reading significantly below their potential or expectancy level, which is often well above average.

Reading skill deficiency or **difficulty**: indicates that, regardless of a child's general level of reading ability, he or she is weak in one or more reading skills. In some cases, the deficiency may be specific and may not lower the general level of reading ability. Naturally, if there are a number of skill deficiencies, if they are in basic skills or if the skills are severely deficient, the child's general level of reading ability will be adversely influenced. (p. 142)

The Harris and Sipay categories have been listed not because this clarifies the problem, but to illustrate the futility of applying quantitative gradations of degree of reading difficulties as a basis for categorization and description.

As can be seen from the preceding, Harris and Sipay seemed to equate "severe reading disability" with '"dyslexia" and "learning disability." Their very broad definition of this category conflicts with other, commonly accepted definitions. For example, the U.S. Office of Education in 1970 used *learning disabilities* to describe

those children who have a disorder in one or more of the basic psychological processes involved in understanding or in using language, spoken or written, which disorder may manifest itself in imperfect ability to listen, think, speak, read, write, spell, or do mathematical calculations. Such disorders include such conditions as perceptual handicap, brain injury, minimal brain dysfunction, dyslexia, and developmental aphasia. Such term does not include children who have learning problems which are primarily the result of visual, hearing, or motor handicaps, of mental retardation, of emotional disturbance, or of environmental disadvantage. (Tarnopol & Tarnopol, 1976)

Harris and Sipay used dyslexia as an alternative to learning disability, while the U.S. Office of Education used dyslexia as one of many types of learning disability. Most American textbooks on reading difficulties and remedial reading reserve the term dyslexia to describe particularly severe and stubborn cases of reading difficulties, while the National Advisory Committee on Dyslexia and Related Reading Disorders (USA) concluded in a paper dated 1969 that the term dyslexia served no useful purpose. We must simply conclude that there is a great deal of ambiguity and confusion surrounding this term.

With this much of a background it would seem appropriate at this time to describe the viewpoints and premises underlying our definition.

Lack of Achievement in Literary Skills

First, there must be present a *severe lack of achievement in the literacy skill*, that is, reading and writing (spelling). Lack of achievement usually encompasses both reading and writing, and the level of achievement tends to be similar for the two areas at the time of the initial diagnosis. During instruction the relative achievement level of the two sets of skills may vary in either direction; some children find learning to read easier than learning to spell, while the opposite may be the case with other children. This difference could be the result of the nature and development of the specific problems, or it may be the result of the kind of remediation used.

What is meant here by a "severe lack of achievement" is to some extent a matter of judgment. It must be viewed in relation to each person's intellect, aptitudes, needs, interest pattern, and past experiences. What may objectively be considered a relatively minor reading and spelling problem may be perceived as a very serious handicap by those to whom it is a major obstacle to the fulfillment of personal goals and aspirations.

It is very difficult to circumvent this subjective judgment in the real world. But for the purposes of research one must set objective criteria so as to make the findings comparable and replicable. This has been done in many different ways, but common to all the studies is the use of various standardized tests. One can choose to view a "severe lack of achievement" in relation to the achievement of children in general at a certain grade level. The criterion for such an achievement problem could be, for example, any reading or spelling score lower than 1 standard deviation below the normative mean (≤ 1 SD). This will result in the identification of about 16% of the total population.

Instead of using relative status one could use the criterion of a certain amount of retardation on a developmental scale such as a grade equivalency scale. (It should be pointed out here that grade equivalency scores are used very extensively in American schools, but are rarely, if ever, used in European schools. There are now some serious attempts to eliminate the use of these scores in the United States because of the difficulties involved in interpreting them, but they are strongly favored by a great many teachers.) It has been quite customary for American educators to consider achievement retardation of 1 year or more as indicative of the presence of a "severe lack of achievement" and a need for remediation. But it is well known that reading development is most rapid in the primary grades, tapering off from then on. One year of retardation in the primary grades would, therefore, have quite a different meaning than would a 1-year discrepancy at a more advanced grade level (Karlsen, 1980). Some writers do differentiate, requiring the differences to become greater as the pupil's grade level increases. There are also differences in the levels at which specific reading and spelling skills are being taught, depending on the school's objectives and the instructional materials used.

To determine the grade equivalents of being below -1 standard deviation, a comparison table was worked out that shows the grade equivalent of being at the 16th percentile. These figures are taken from the 1982 edition of *Stanford Achievement Test* (Gardner et al., 1983) but it is assumed that the figures would be very similar no matter which American achievement test were used.

Since the test was standardized toward the end of the school year, during the eighth month, this was used as the reference point for each grade, from 1st through 10th. (The table goes no further, since beyond this point the higher incidence of dropouts at the lower end tends to distort the data.) As one can see from this table, using 1 year as a cutting score would be consistent with the -1 SD criterion only in the second grade. The grade equivalent criterion is clearly ambiguous. This table also shows that the pupil who remains at the 16th percentile gains only an average of 0.5 year per year in school in terms of grade equivalents.

Any quantitative measure must, however, be coupled with the professional judgment of the teachers, especially, but also of other professionals working with a given child. At the time of standardizing the Norwegian achievement tests, the teachers were asked to evaluate their students with regard to reading and spelling, before they knew the results of the tests. A comparison of the teachers' judgments and the test results showed that the vast majority of pupils whom the teachers thought had severe reading and spelling problems were among the lowest 10 to 15% on the achievement tests. The evaluative judgments and the statistical cutoff scores coincided to a very high degree. But there were some differences. This was particularly true of pupils who scored above the quantitative criterion score. These pupils, because of very high intelligence test scores, would be considered dyslexic because of the wide discrepancy between their intellectual capacity and their school achievement in reading and/or spelling. We also maintain that there are unique *qualitative* signs to be found in their reading and spelling performance. Along this line, a great deal of time and effort have been devoted to the identification and classification of reading and spelling errors. Some of the studies in this

TABLE 7.1. Grade equivalents (GE) of the 16th percentile (PR) for each grade in school

Grade in school	GE of PR 16	Retardation in years
1.8	1.2	0.6
2.8	1.9	0.9
3.8	2.4	1.4
4.8	2.8	2.0
5.8	3.4	2.4
6.8	4.1	2.7
7.8	4.6	3.2
8.8	5.0	3.8
9.8	5.2	4.6
10.8	5.7	5.1
Average gain	1.0	0.5	—

connection have been limited to the tabulation of various specific errors, in order to determine the extent to which pupils with dyslexia make unique kinds of errors. However, there do not appear to be specific reading and spelling errors (e.g., reversals) that can be considered uniquely dyslexic. But if one goes beyond this and analyzes all qualitative data in their *totality*, one will often find patterns and combinations of errors that are characteristic, if not unique and systematically consistent, in people with dyslexia.

Discrepancy Between General Ability and Literacy Achievement

In addition to the criterion of a severe lack of achievement in the literacy skills, we also subscribe to a second and commonly accepted criterion for a classification of dyslexia: There must be a *significant discrepancy* between a pupil's general ability and reading and/or writing ability. General intellectual ability is average and at times above average, while achievement is low or extremely low.

Objective assessment of intellectual ability is, of course, fraught with problems (Harris & Sipay, 1985; Nygaard, 1982; Thorndike, 1963). In research, the discrepancy between intellectual ability and school achievement has typically been determined by the use of standardized tests of intelligence and achievement. In the practical school situation, where this information is used for guidance and educational planning, "clinical judgment," which draws on a variety of information, observations, and impressions, is generally also called upon. The Bergen Project employed a combination of quantitatively measured discrepancies and teacher judgments. This process is described in Chapter 5 as well as in Appendix A.

The discrepancy between ability and achievement is the deciding factor in dyslexia. One would, therefore, expect to find dyslexia at many levels of achievement and ability. this is indeed the case. Despite this fact, it is common research practice to consider only children of average or higher IQ as dyslexic, the criterion score being typically an IQ above 90. There appears to be no professional or scientific justification for such a cutoff point; it has been used simply as a matter of convenience and practicality. We are *in principle* against such an arbitrary decision, the result of which could easily be that reading and writing difficulties of below average-IQ children will not be taken sufficiently seriously. (Normatively, 25% of the population will score below IQ 90.) These problems deserve as much attention as the others, even though they occur among children of lower intelligence or in association with mental retardation. If, at the same time, one maintains the principle that the achievement deficit cannot be explained by low ability alone, the problem becomes more complex, and will probably result in the identification of some doubtful cases. Be that as it may, our desire for scientific neatness and clarification should not prevent us from seeing things as they really are, not even while doing research. We are not alone in expressing such a reality-oriented point of view (Critchley & Critchley, 1978; Doehring, 1983; Vellutino, 1979).

Lack of Other Primary Problems

A third common criterion for a diagnosis of dyslexia involves the so-called *exclusionary principle.* This involves the requirement that the person must possess, in addition to average or higher intelligence, normal vision, hearing, motor development, emotional adjustment, and so on. The practical-clinical application of the exclusionary principle will, in reality as well as in research, depend on what is considered "normal." If the limits are relatively liberal, so that normal is defined to mean that a characteristic has not played a *primary* role in causing the achievement deficits, this principle would be acceptable with respect to vision, hearing, and motor development. But it is less applicable to emotional problems. Quite a few children who would be diagnosed as dyslexic also exhibit rather clear symptoms of social and/or emotional maladjustment. In most cases symptoms are fairly mild, but there are more complex cases of personal and emotional maladjustment. To what extent these problems are cause or effect with respect to dyslexia is often difficult to determine.

Our Definition of Dyslexia

It would seem appropriate to wind up this discussion of criteria for and definitions of dyslexia with a relatively brief formulation of a definition of dyslexia:

By dyslexia is meant an inordinate amount of difficulty with the learning of literacy skills (reading and/or writing), which cannot be assumed to be caused *primarily* by intellectual, sensory, or motor deficits. In most cases, emotional problems do not play a primary, causative role.

The literacy achievement levels must be significantly below expectancy based on the person's intellectual level and educational opportunities.

A qualitative function analysis that considers all factors in a totality will often reveal unique patterns of reading and writing characteristics (Gjessing, 1977).

In summary, our definition of dyslexia does deviate from many others. We do not require average or higher intellectual ability. We do not exclude cases with other problems in addition to an achievement deficit. We do maintain, however, the requirement of a significant achievement-ability discrepancy, especially for research purposes. We have made no assumptions or restrictions with respect to etiology. On this last point we are at variance with the medical writers, but we prefer to limit ourselves to what we can *observe* and what we *know*.

CHAPTER 8

Dyslexia Models and Theories

H.-J. Gjessing and B. Karlsen

Categories and Models

The previous chapter's section on trends in reading disability research differentiated between the two main trends in past dyslexia research, the medical and the educational-psychological. There are some rather clear-cut differences in these trends, especially with regard to etiology. The relatively brief discussion of the main trends in dyslexia research finished with a short discussion of the possibilities connected with the typological studies that have taken place in recent years. Gjessing's early and long-lasting contributions and continued interest were briefly described.

Before continuing the discussion of the Gjessing model and its foundation, it would seem propitious at this point to explore a few more specific directions within the dyslexia research. An alternative to the dichotomy in research emphasis mentioned above, medical versus educational-psychological, is the not-too-uncommon dichotomy of single-factor versus multifactor theories.

Vellutino (1979) differentiated between developmental theories and other single-factor theories. In the developmental rubric, Vellutino mentioned the frequently cited medical pioneers and their interest in cerebral localization theories and aphasia (Kussmaul, 1877), as well as researchers who employ a rather general, psychological model of explanation. They tend to subscribe to the "developmental lag" theory, in which some children are simply slow in their development of perception or cognition or are slow in a more global or organismic sort of way (Bender, 1957; Olson, 1949; Schilder, 1944).

Under the heading "other single-factor theories," Vellutino mentioned Hermann's (1969) belief in the Gerstman syndrome as a causation theory and Hallgren's (1950) heredity model. Other researchers in this category have posited causation theories relating to specific dysfunctions in the area of temporal sequencing and processing (Bakker, 1970; Bannatyne, 1971; Senf, 1969), while yet other researchers have focused directly on phonological processing (Downing, 1973).

Despite their differences, Vellutino found some common characteristics among the single-factor theorists: they have for the most part a medical-organic orientation. They often mention dysfunctions in visuospatial processing. While one faction places the main emphasis on developmental lag or genetic factors, others find the explanation in more specific and circumscribed language disorders. It is not easy to see the commonality among the "other single-factor theories," since they appear to have only one thing in common, the hypothesis that the etiology of dyslexia can be explained by a single factor or hypothesis.

With respect to the multifactor theories, Vellutino differentiated again between two major groups. The first group emphasizes primarily environmental factors and their interaction with the more general cognitive individual characteristics (Malmquist, 1958; Robinson, 1946). Members of the second group are primarily concerned with more specific individual deficits, deficits qualitatively different from the environmental factors. This latter group of researchers also tends to work from a more explicit theoretical base for their working models. The researchers categorized as being in the latter group have been referred to previously in this book as representing the typology trend. With regard to the theoretical base for typological research, one must certainly stress the pioneering work of Herbert Birch as early as the 1960s (Birch, 1962), as does Vellutino. We now turn to a discussion of Birch as well as of many other researchers in the area of dyslexia typology.

Comparative Studies of Dyslexia

Although the Gjessing dyslexia model was published in 1953 (Gjessing, 1953), it was not until the late 1960s that studies of dyslexia by types were published in the Anglo-American literature. Since then, such dyslexia research has steadily increased in volume, to the point where this has become a major trend. Few if any serious researchers have pursued a single-factor model of dyslexia (Miles & Ellis, 1981; Rutter, 1978; Vellutino, 1970).

Whereas up to the early 1970s there were relatively few studies of dyslexia types reported, there are now so many as to defy a detailed analysis of each one here. Several such analyses have been published and are recommended for further study (Doehring et al., 1981; Malatesha & Dougan, 1982; Satz & Morris, 1981).

There are different ways one could try to classify the research that has been done in order to make a systematic summary. One could differentiate along the dichotomy medical-psychoeducational, or within these professions by subcategory such as neurology, ophthalmology, pediatrics, and so on. But one often finds that both the medical and the psychological professions are represented on the research team, as is true of the Bergen Project. Thus, analysis by professional affiliation does not appear to be a helpful differentiation among the many projects reported.

Satz and Morris (1981) did a very systematic analysis of the dyslexia typology studies using two major categories, clinical-inferential approaches versus statistical-classification approaches. Each of these was then subdivided. The clinical-inferential approaches were classified by etiology, nonreading performance variables, and achievement variables. The statistical approaches were differentiated according to the multivariate statistical technique used, such as cluster analysis, factor analysis, Q techniques, and so on. But the problem is so complex, the issues so diverse, that any systematic summary for the purpose of drawing generalizations across studies becomes quite difficult. The fact that different labels have been used for the same types of dyslexia and that the same label may have been used for different types makes this kind of metaanalysis even more complex.

Tabulation of Major Studies

The main body of studies of dyslexia by type are tabulated in Tables 8.1 and 8.2. When we reviewed these studies we found that in about half, the subgroup terminology was similar to ours, that is, audiophonological (A) or visuospatial (V) were the main categories. These studies are summarized in Table 8.1. Studies that did not explicitly use these two main categories are summarized in Table 8.2. These tables should give a brief but fairly comprehensive overview of the literature. Information regarding the type of database (direct or indirect) and professional background (psychology or medicine) is problematic in some cases, since both types of data are often used and professional affiliation may be misleading. That someone works in a medical setting does not necessarily mean a professional background in medicine, since psychologists, neuropsychologists, and educational psychologists often work in such settings. The fact that many reports are carried out by teams makes categorization even more complicated.

The labels for dyslexia given in the tables are the various authors' own. As previously mentioned, the same type of syndrome may have different labels applied to it, and a given label may be used to describe somewhat different syndromes. Also, some researchers have evolved or even changed their theories over time and have tried to some extent to accommodate this by multiple references (e.g., second and third entries in Table 8.2). The intent here is to review research related to the Bergen Project, and we thus consider it important to delineate whether the methodology was clinical or statistical, the database direct or indirect and the professional orientation medical or psychological.

It also seems necessary at this point to consider some of the information from the related studies that is *not* summarized in the tables, particularly the problem of sample selection. The samples used in these various reports are extremely diverse. Most of them are clinic samples, cases that have been referred to clinics for further study. In this situation the investigators have had no control over selection or the sampling process. This introduces an enormous experimental bias, since referrals tend to be based on the "image" of a certain clinic or on its professional orientation. The ages of the clients in the various studies is another confound, since there is much variability within as well as between groups. Mattis, French, and Rapin (1975) reported an age range of 8 to 18 years, while Ingram, Mason, and Blackburn (1970) had a range from 7 to 16 years. Others'

TABLE 8.1. Dyslexia classifications with primary emphasis on audiophonological (A), visuospatial (V), or combinations of A and V, plus miscellaneous types (M)

Entry number	Source	Subgroup terminology	Category	Method[a]	Database[b]	Background[c]
1	Gjessing, 1953	Auditory dyslexia	A	C	D	P
		Visual dyslexia	V			
		Auditory-visual dyslexia	AV			
		Emotional dyslexia	M			
		Educational dyslexia	M			
		Other	M			
2	Johnson & Myklebust, 1967	Auditory dyslexia	A	C	D	P
		Visual dyslexia	V			
3	Schenck-Danziger, 1968	Acoustic difficulties	A	C	D	P
		Optical difficulties	V			
4	Bateman, 1968	Auditory memory deficit	A	C	ID	P
		Visual memory deficit	V			
		Mixed deficit	AV			
5	Boder, 1968, 1973	Dysphonetic dyslexia	A	C	D	M
		Dyseidetic dyslexia	V			
		Mixed dyslexia	AV			
6	Ingram, Mason, & Blackburn, 1970	Audiophonic difficulties	A	C	D	P
		Visuospatial difficulties	V			
		Audiovisual difficulties	AV			
7	M. Smith, 1970	Deficiency in sequencing ability	A	C	ID	P
		Deficiency in simultaneous ability	V			
		Mixed	AV			
8	Naidoo, 1972	Linguistic disorder (nonfamilial)	A	S	ID	P
		Linguistic disorder (genetic)	A			
		Visuospatial disorder (nonfamilial)	V			
		Visuospatial disorder (genetic)	V			

TABLE 8.1. (Continued)

Entry number	Source	Subgroup terminology	Category	Method[a]	Database[b]	Background[c]
9	Denckla, 1972	Visuospatial disorder	V	C	D	M
		Articulatory-graphomotor disorder	M			
		Language disorder	A			
		Deficient verbal memorization	M			
		Right hemisyndrome with mixed language disorder	M			
10	Mattis, French, & Rapin, 1975	Language disorder	A	C	ID	P/M
		Articulatory-graphomotor disorder	A			
		Visual-perceptual disorder	V			
11	Jordan, 1977	Auditory deficit	A	C	D	P
		Visual deficit	V			
		Motor deficit	M			
12	Mann & Suiter, 1978	Auditory deficit	A	C	ID	P
		Visual deficit	V			
		Motor deficit	M			
13	D. Bakker, 1979	Insufficient spatioperceptual processing	V	S	ID	P
		Insufficient synthetic-semantic processing	A			
14	Pirozzolo, 1979	Auditory-linguistic disorder	A	C	ID	P/M
		Visual-spatial disorder	V			
15	Satz & Morris, 1981	Global language impairment	A	S	ID	P
		Specific language (naming) deficit	A			
		Language and perceptual deficit	AV			
		Visual-perceptual motor deficit	V			
		Unexpected learning disability	M			
16	Aaron & Baker, 1982	Anterior dyslexia (language defect)	A	C	D	P
		Central dyslexia (listening defect)	V			
		Posterior dyslexia (visuoperceptual defect)	M			

[a] C, clinical; S, statistical.
[b] D, direct; ID, indirect.
[c] P, psychology; M, medicine.

TABLE 8.2. Dyslexia classifications with primary emphasis on factors other than audiophonological (A) and visuospatial (V) (M = miscellaneous)

Entry number	Source	Subgroup terminology	Category	Method[a]	Database[b]	Background[c]
1	Birch, 1962	Deficiency in intersensory equivalences	AV	C?	ID	M/P
		Inadequate hierarchical sensory organization	V			
		Deficiency in visual analysis, synthesis	V			
2	Zangwill, 1962	Dyslexia with normal hemispheric specialization	M	C	ID	M
		Dyslexia with abnormal hemispheric specialization	M			
3	Kinsbourne & Warrington, 1963	Language retarded	A	C	ID	P
		Gerstman syndrome	M			
4	Bannatyne, 1971	Primary emotional communication dyslexia	M	C	ID	P
		Minimal neurological dysfunction	M			
		Social, cultural, or educational dyslexia	M			
		Genetic dyslexia	M			
5	Doehring & Hoshko, 1977	Linguistic deficit	A	S	D	P
		Phonological deficit	A			
		Intersensory integration deficit	M			
6	Petrauskas & Rourke, 1979	Language disorder (verbal fluency)	V	S	D	P
		Sequencing disorder (visuospatial memory)	V			
		Concept formation (mixed)	M			
7	Satz & Morris, 1981	Global language impairment	M	S	D	P
	Fletcher & Satz, 1980	Global language, perceptual impairment	M			
		Visuoperceptual-motor impairment	V			
8	Aaron, 1982	Simultaneous processing deficit	M	S	D	P
		Sequential processing deficit	M			
		Comprehension dyslexia	M?			
9	DeFries & Decker, 1982	Spatial reasoning deficit	V	S	ID	P
		Symbol processing deficit	M			
		Mixed deficit	M			
		Reading deficit only	M			

[a] C, clinical; S, statistical.
[b] D, direct; ID, indirect.
[c] P, psychology; M, medicine.

samples may have much less variability in age, but may lack comparability because of differences in mean age, which could range from the primary grades to college age.

Sample size can also be a major confound. The nature of the problem and the characteristics of the selection criteria are such as to make large sample studies impractical. Some studies report subtype groups of 4 to 5 people, others as many as 60 to 70. The total samples studied also range in size. For example, the samples of Gjessing (1953) and of Boder (1968) contained 100 dyslexics, whereas Kinsbourne and Warrington (1963) studied 13 cases.

It is quite apparent that detailed comparisons of results and conclusions from such a heterogeneous set of studies is fraught with problems and possible errors.

Discussion of Table 8.1

As early as 1896 Charcot (Freud, 1953) suggested that there are two types of learners, visual (*visile*) and auditory (*audile*), depending on the channel favored for learning. Disabilities in either of these channels became central issues in dyslexia research, not only with regard to direct symptoms in reading and writing but also with respect to behavioral variables of a more general nature in cognition and neurology. The issue of *balance* between the two modalities has been discussed in other contexts as well, such as communication and social behavior (e.g., Bander & Grinder, 1975, 1976).

Table 8.1 shows that the number of subtypes described vary from two to six. Investigators who have used two categories have typically labeled these audiophonological (A) or visuospatial (V), although the specific wording may vary (see entries 3, 12, and 13). It would appear that these are selected cases of fairly "pure" types, using monothetic selection principles. (Note the discussion of monothetic and polythetic methods elsewhere in this book).

Bakker's two types (entry 12) should be described briefly. Instead of concentrating on deficiencies, he referred to his first type as being excessively dependent on syntactic-semantic processing, with insufficient spatioperceptual processing strategies. His second type has the opposite characteristic. The two types are excessively dependent on utilization of the left or right hemisphere, respectively. Supposedly the ideal situation is one in which the first grader is heavily right-hemisphere oriented in order to learn the decoding skills, but left-hemisphere oriented for more extensive use of syntactic and semantic clues and efficient reading. Bakker (1979) has some group data in support of this theory.

Most of the reports with a three-way split typically used A, V, and the combination group (AV) (see entries 2, 5, 6, and 7). These cases have probably also been selected to some extent, the fewer cases that did not fit the model being rejected.

Some researchers have divided the basic subgroups (A and V) further. Mattis, French, and Rapin (1975) divided the audiophonetic group into a "language disorder" group and an "articulatory-graphomotor disorder" group, while Mattis (1978) at a later date added a "sequencing disorder" to the original list of three.

Others have also added another group to the original two, which appears to differ from A and V (e.g., entries 11 and 14). It is quite possible that a group such as "manual deficit" could be a subtype of group A, a conclusion consistent with our data. All cases of dyslexia in our sample with pronounced motoric writing problems have been classified in group A because of similarity in diagnosis and treatment.

Other studies that have arrived at more than three subgroups include Naidoo (entry 8), in which each of the A and V groups is divided into nonfamilial and genetic. Denckla (entry 9) has added several broader, language-oriented categories to the two more common groupings A and V.

We have used a six-way classification (entry 1). The first three coincide with the more typical three-way division A, V, and AV, based on a polythetic selection model. The remaining three groups fall outside the dyslexia classification of the medical tradition. The attempt here was to differentiate between the primary reading and writing problems—dyslexia—and secondary reading and writing problems of a nondyslexic nature (Rabinovich, 1968). We assumed that criteria for such a differentiation would be founded in the study of etiology. But such differential diagnosis does not appear possible with the current state of knowledge. As will be noted in Table 8.2, several other writers in this field have hypothesized subtypes of dyslexia with no organic neurological concomitants.

Discussion of Table 8.2

The studies listed in Table 8.2 do not use the audiophonological (A) and visuospatial (V) breakdown, although some of the types listed coincide more or less with the A and V types. For example, Birch (entry 1) used a breakdown that is so close to those listed in Table 11.1 that he could have been included there. He described three types of dyslexia, all having some sort of sensory integration or organization deficiency. Birch was one of the pioneer scholars in this field in the Anglo-American sphere. He developed a very respectable foundation for this theory. His thinking was based on developmental psychology (Birch & Lefford, 1963), learning (Pavlov, 1927), and neurophysiology (Lashley, 1929). His view on what he labeled "intersensory equivalences" is very much in tune with the hypotheses and theories of the 1980s relating to imbalances of modalities and hemispheres (Aaron, 1982). He was also open to the possibility that dyslexia can be the result of a developmental lag in neurosensory development, where visual perception does not rise to the dominant position that normally comes with age.

Birch's views and hypotheses are still current. His work is discussed in detail by Vellutino (1979) and in his own publications (Birch, 1962; Birch & Belmont, 1964, 1965). He was very interested in the importance of auditory and visual functions and their relevance for the acquisition of reading skills, but he considered the visual aspects of primary importance.

Other reports listed in Table 8.2 assigned primacy to language and auditory factors, placing no emphasis at all on visual factors (entries 3 and 4). The number of types listed by the various writers in this table range from two to four, and the empirical, statistical studies dominate here, whereas studies reported in Table 8.1 were heavily clinically oriented. There is also a big difference in the database of the two tables. Whereas the studies listed in Table 8.1 were based on direct reading-related testing, the studies in Table 8.2 relied heavily on nonreading related (ID) assessment, generally of a neurological nature. There is greater interest in neurological data in recent years because of the advent of new technology such as computerized brain scan (e.g., Hier, Lemay, Rosenberger, & Perlo, 1978). This very promising new technology has great potential for contributing to our understanding of the brain and its neurophysiology (Duffy, Denckla, Bartels, & Sandini, 1980; Lassen, Ingvan, & Skinhøj, 1978; Preston, Guthrie, Kirsch, Gertman, & Childs, 1977).

Conclusions from the Tables

From the data summarized in these two tables we have concluded the following:

A large number of dyslexia typologies coincide with the Gjessing model (Table 8.1, entry 1) with respect to the first three variables. This is particularly true of those who depend primarily on direct (D) observation of children's reading and writing behavior. But researchers who have based their typologies on nonreading (ID) cognitive or linguistic test data have often also arrived at similar categories. The basic auditory-visual differentiation is used by people in the medical as well as the psychological professions, and by people who employ both clinical (C) and statistical (S) approaches.

The audiophonological syndrome (A) has been given a variety of labels. The most common are "auditory deficit" and "auditory dyslexia," but we also find such adjectives as audiophonic, auditory-linguistic, linguistic, and dysphonetic, along with sequencing deficiency and posterior dyslexia. These all represent to varying degrees the same syndrome; different elements and different symptoms simply receive varying degrees of emphasis depending on the types of tests and observations employed and the kinds of samples and situations involved in the various projects.

As can be seen from the two tables, the situation is similar with respect to the visuospatial (V) syndrome. This has also been given a wide variety of labels, but these are the problems of an emerging field where much is still to be learned, a situation that lends itself to a great deal of individual speculation and theorizing. Attempts have been made to consolidate the major findings relating to dyslexia under one unifying theory (e.g., the hemispheric imbalance theory, Aaron, 1982; Bakker, 1979),but such a theory will probably have to await more basic research.

A Basic Reading Model

Without going any further with these classification schemes of dyslexia theories, it would seem appropriate to give an example of a rather "basic model," which can

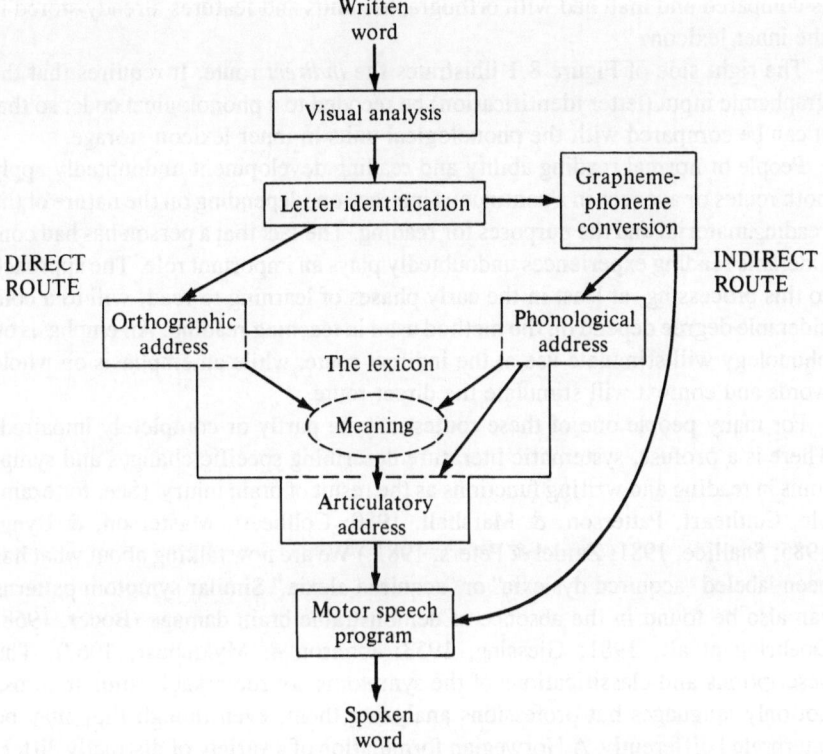

FIGURE 8.1. A two-way model of the reading process.

be derived from neurology, cognitive psychology, and clinical educational-psychological observation and experience. A relatively well-accepted theory states that written language is basically processed two different ways: on the one hand, the more direct visuosemantic way, and on the other, a more indirect phonological way, between print and meaning (Johnson & Myklebust, 1967; Kavanagh & Mattingly, 1972; Marshall & Newcombe, 1973; McCusker et al., 1981). This basic hypothesis is contained in a variety of theories. Rather than provide yet another theory along this line we will simply review the "two-way model" by Marshall and Newcombe (1973), presented in Figure 8.1.

This model proposes, as do most later models, that two relatively distinct mechanisms are involved in getting the message from the printed word. On the left side the model illustrates the *direct* route to the "inner lexicon," where the previously learned elements of the printed word, such as the orthographic, phonological, syntactic, and semantic features are stored, to be mobilized for future use in new encounters with the printed word. This inner lexicon is well elucidated by Lundberg (1981b). The direct route can be characterized by the fact that the printed word is identified by its orthographic features, and it is compared and matched with orthographic units and features already stored in the inner lexicon.

The right side of Figure 8.1 illustrates the *indirect* route. It requires that the graphemic input (letter identification) be recoded to a phonological code, so that it can be compared with the phonological units in inner lexicon storage.

People of normal reading ability and reading development undoubtedly apply both routes or avenues in a continuous interaction, depending on the nature of the reading material and the purposes for reading. The fact that a person has had considerable reading experiences undoubtedly plays an important role. The approach to this processing, at least in the early phases of learning to read, will to a considerable degree depend on the method used in teaching reading. An emphasis on phonology will stimulate use of the indirect route, while an emphasis on whole words and context will stimulate the direct route.

For many people one of these routes may be partly or completely impaired. There is a profuse, systematic literature describing specific changes and symptoms in reading and writing functions as the result of brain injury. (See, for example, Coltheart, Patterson, & Marshall, 1980; Coltheart, Masterson, & Byng, 1985; Shallice, 1981; Zaidel & Peters, 1981.) We are now talking about what has been labeled "acquired dyslexia" or "acquired alexia." Similar symptom patterns can also be found in the absence of demonstrable brain damage (Boder, 1968; Doehring et al., 1981; Gjessing, 1953; Johnson & Myklebust, 1967). The descriptions and classifications of the symptoms are remarkably similar across not only languages but professions analyzing them, even though they may be interpreted differently. A Norwegian formulation of a variety of distinctly different symptom patterns is described in the following, with examples in conjunction with the Gjessing dyslexia model.

The Dyslexia Model Studied

The dyslexia model that was studied in the Bergen Project was first presented in an educational journal in 1953 (Gjessing, 1953) and later in a medical journal (Gjessing, 1958b). The model had, however, been used for several years in the practice of school psychology to diagnose children with learning disabilities and to prescribe individualized instruction and treatment. The model had, from the very beginning, the following subcategories:

Auditory dyslexia
Visual dyslexia
Audiovisual dyslexia
Emotional dyslexia
Educational dyslexia
Other, rare forms of dyslexia

Also developed at that time was a differential reading instructional method that corresponded to the diagnostic system. The primary goal was to deal directly with the basic nature of the disability, while at the same time making optimal use of compensatory skills. The diagnostic system and its attendant remedial methodology have been used for a number of years by Norwegian school psychologists and special educators (Hagtvedt Vik, 1976).

The following are salient features of this model:

1. It is polythetic. Individuals are grouped on the basis of having a large number of traits and characteristics in common, without rigid rules regarding group membership. (In a monothetic approach, group membership is determined by the presence of a unique and invariant set of characteristics.)

2. It is hypothetical descriptive. The hypothetical basis is primarily the result of practical-clinical experiences and systematic analysis of reading and writing behavior. This does not, of course, preclude support from clinical neurology and cognitive theories and models.

3. The description of symptoms and the categorization of literacy behavior are based on principles that have been described here as interaction analysis and function analysis. This simply means that the meaning of single errors and of specific types of errors during the reading and writing process can be determined and understood only when viewed within the total context and in interaction with all other behaviors. In addition, literacy skills products and behavior must also be viewed within the larger interactive context where nonreading variables are taken into consideration. By nonreading variables we consider such things as sensory, linguistic, neurological, and social variables.

With this much background information we can now return to the basic model and its typology. The first three categories—auditory, visual, and audiovisual—are based on certain hypotheses regarding the relationship between different types of perceptocognitive modality problems and the development of reading and writing difficulties.

Dyslexia could be the result of an overdeveloped one-sided modality or sensory channel, of inadequate neurological integration between the modalities, or possibly of insufficient conversion of perceptocognitive perceptions. These kinds of impairment would tend to interfere with the linguistic-cognitive processes necessary for the development of abstract and symbolic processing at the level required for the attainment of literacy skills.

The first three types of dyslexia, then, could collectively be thought of as *modality-related* reading and writing difficulties. Their common feature is that the difficulties can be documented systematically, albeit at times somewhat equivocally, through observation of reading and writing behavior. Direct observation of the dyslexic's approach and error pattern during reading and writing, with a subsequent systematic, qualitative analysis of these behaviors, is generally the surest approach to diagnosis.

In contrast to the first three types, emotional and educational dyslexia are not modality related. But a systematic analysis of reading and writing behavior is also carried out in these cases. The reactions and the error patterns in these cases are more haphazard and inconsistent, and they do not support the hypothesis that the

difficulties are of neurological nature. There is reason to believe that psychological factors such as anxiety and lack of motivation, general immaturity, and unfortunate educational experiences are primary causative factors.

Other rare forms of dyslexia, the last category, is simply an indication that the
first five categories are insufficient. Of the problems in this category that are
fairly unique, and for which diagnosis and special treatment should be provided,
one can mention bilingualism or foreign speaking and some functional visual
problems in conjunction with problems of bilateral vision.

A more detailed description of the various subcategories is given in the following section. An even more comprehensive discussion can be found in the basic
text by Gjessing (1977).

Auditory Dyslexia

In auditory dyslexia the following characteristics are the most persistent and
representative:

1. Limited ability to perceive differences between phonologically similar letter
sounds (phonemes), such as the voiced and unvoiced consonant pairs *d-t*, *b-p*,
and *k-g*, as well as certain vowel sounds, like *e-i* (*pen–pin*), and the so-called *r*-
controlled vowel sounds (*fur, for, far*). Many other letter combinations also cause
problems for the reading disabled because of phonological similarities.

After some reading and spelling instruction it appears that many children overcome their auditory discrimination problems with regard to the sounds
represented by single letters. But the problem appears to persist when several
phonemes must be combined (blended) into words. The confusion now seems to
reappear, as in *dime–time*, *sit–set*.

2. Difficulty with phonetic synthesis. In the more serious cases of auditory
dyslexia, even very short and phonetically "regular" words of three or four letters
can cause enormous problems. Even though the letters are "sounded out" correctly and quickly in the proper sequence, the auditory dyslexic has a hard time
determining what word these sounds represent. Among the various symptoms of
problems with phonetic synthesis relating to this impaired auditory sequencing
are incomplete or partial reversals, where one or more letters within a word
switch position, as in *stop–spot*, *form–from*, *split–spilt*.

Another common symptom of difficulty with phonetic synthesis is the omission of letters in phonetically rather uncomplicated words. The words may be
phonetically regular or consistent, but have a high consonant/vowel ratio. Take
for example the word *black*, which contains four consonants and one vowel letter,
or *string*, with a consonant/vowel ratio of 5:1. In the first example an omission
could result in *back*; the second example could become *sting*, *sing*, *ring* or some
meaningless word. The type of error committed depends on the degree of impairment of phonological processing.

These errors have typically been referred to as "omissions" in the reading literature, but we prefer the more descriptive term *simplification*. And as mentioned

earlier, these simplifications are concrete expressions of the learner's inability to function adequately with respect to phonics.

The different errors in phonological processing can be most concretely illustrated by having the child spell. The experienced reading diagnostician is also able to observe these symptoms of dysfunction by having the dyslexic read orally. But correctly diagnosing reading behavior is more difficult than diagnosing writing behavior, if for no other reason than that writing does result in a product.

Whether one records reading errors while the pupil is reading or from tape recordings, one needs a record-keeping system that is as systematic and simple as possible. But at the same time the record-keeping system must capture all that has diagnostic utility. Function analysis was described a system that not only keeps track of errors or writing samples but also emphasizes many of the qualitative aspects of oral reading behavior, such as stress and tone of voice. This system is described elsewhere in this report (Chapter 9).

One might question the need for this detailed word-for-word record keeping. Is it not sufficient to make note of general impressions of the child's approach to reading, as is often done with other psychodiagnostic tests? The reasons why this system is necessary are as follows:

The use of the record-keeping system in function analysis makes possible a study of the reader's skills approach as well as general reading behavior not only with respect to individual words but also in the context of the material read.

This record-keeping system makes possible a concrete study of changes in reading behavior when there are changes in the reading conditions or in the degree of difficulty of the material, as well as technical and semantic changes.

The system provides a permanent record over time, enabling the diagnostician to go back and reanalyze and compare current records with the past.

Finally, it provides a concrete basis for discussion reading characteristics and reading problems with the dyslexic student. Even though reading is a very complex act, the recording system was developed to be simple enough to be understood and discussed with the students themselves.

So far we have discussed some of the main symptoms of auditory dyslexia as they are revealed in reading and writing behavior. But the children showing this behavior appear to have compensating qualities, notably average or even higher ability to read and spell whole words as configurations.

Some nonreading characteristics have also been found associated with this dysphonetic pattern of reading and spelling problems. Many children with auditory dyslexia exhibit delayed speech development and problems of articulation up to age 6 or even older. Another rather unexpected characteristic is an inability to reproduce a melody by singing or humming. Melody reproductions vary from out of tune but recognizable to an almost undifferentiated monotone.

There is a particular high incidence of boys in this dyslexia subgroup. One often finds a marked incidence of speech problems as well as reading and writing difficulties among the male relatives of either or both parent.

Visual Dyslexia

Some of the more prominent characteristics of children with visual dyslexia are:

1. Extreme dependence on phonetic analysis and synthesis with a tendency to want to sound out every word, behavior sometimes referred to in the American literature as "overanalytical." This is probably the most predominant feature of their reading and writing behavior. They will often persist in detailed phonetic analysis of words they have encountered innumerable times, and if the same word appears several times in a row they will laboriously decode that word each time. For many of these children, identifying even the most frequently occurring words as whole word configurations appears almost impossible.

2. Poor response to the teaching of whole words, even high-frequency, phonetically quite regular words. The problem is particularly noticeable with words that are meaningful if read from left to right or right to left, for example, *on–no*, *was–saw*, *top–pot*. This particular error is generally referred to as a *complete reversal*.

3. A tendency to spell phonetically irregular words phonetically. *Answer* is spelled *anser*, *any* is spelled *eny*, *guest* is *gest*, and so on. These errors must be differentiated from the homophone problem, which is a major spelling problem in English (e.g., *principal* spelled *principle*, *gait–gate*, *minor–miner*, etc.)

4. An inability to detect and correct the spelling of phonetically irregular words that have been spelled regularly; that is, the homophone problems just described. On the other hand, these children often show excellent ability to detect misspellings when a phonetically regular word is spelled incorrectly. This strong phonetic ability is also often revealed in excellent ability to sound out the phonemes in a word and to blend the sounds into the correct word. But this particular strength eventually becomes a liability because the children become excessively dependent on this skill. They become overanalytical, to the detriment of their sight vocabulary.

In reading and writing, visual dyslexics depend almost exclusively on letter-by-letter sounding (as in *a-f-t-e-r*). This approach persists over time, and after years of practice may still be used. The person can become so proficient that it takes an experienced examiner to detect that he or she is still sounding out most words.

This pronounced tendency and overdependence on phonics could be an overcompensation for a deficiency in the orthographic storage system in the inner lexicon. There could be other explanations as well. For example, Baron (1979) ascribed this tendency to a child's particular learning style, field dependence, conformity, and rigidity. The child spells phonetically irregular words phonetically in order to comply with the main rules of phonics.

With respect to the nonreading variables associated with visual dyslexia, we have not been able to identify correlates that are statistically consistent and reliable. There does, however, appear to be a somewhat higher incidence of lefthandedness and mixed dominance among visual dyslexics, along with some degree of hyperactivity in more extreme cases. On the other hand, we have practically never encountered delayed speech development or problems with articulation or oral expression in this group. Only rarely do we find problems with melody reproduction, which is so typical of auditory dyslexics. The sex ratio is also much more even in visual dyslexia than in auditory dyslexia (Gjessing, 1976).

In summary, one can say that when comparing children with auditory dyslexia with those with visual dyslexia, the main conclusion might be that the areas in which one group does relatively well the other group does poorly. Referring again to Figure 8.1, one can see that in the decoding process the auditory dyslexic has problems and interferences with respect to the phonological, or indirect, route, while the visual dyslexic has problems functioning along the orthographic, or direct, route. The normal reader will use both approaches to the lexicon in a more harmonious interaction; a one-sided imbalance between the two avenues is more characteristic of the two main types of modality-related dyslexia. This is discussed in more detail in Gjessing (1977). In the English language literature one can refer to Aaron (1982) and his imbalance hypothesis.

To better understand this functional interaction, one must go beyond the traditional categorization of errors such as omissions and reversals. Such categorization is too broad, since the same error may represent different functional characteristics. For example, omission of silent letters is most often symptomatic of weakness in the orthographic store, while omission of letters within a consonant cluster is typically a sign of problems with the phonological system.

Along this same vein, partial reversals are often an indication of difficulties in phonological sequencing, while complete reversals tend to indicate visuospatial problems. The letters *b* and *d* can be used to illustrate this point. These consonants are closely related in sound as well as in shape. They are confused in both auditory and visual dyslexia, but their confusion can only be interpreted within the total situation. It is only by seeing the context in which errors are made and relating the errors to all other symptoms that one can arrive at a conclusive message. This gets us back to function analysis, which will be discussed again later on.

Audiovisual Dyslexia

The third dyslexia type in our model, audiovisual dyslexia, is characterized by modality problems in the phonological path as well as the orthographic path to the inner lexicon. This is a very serious condition. Children with this problem will as a rule be so seriously disabled in the literacy skills as to be categorized functional illiterates.

A word of caution is in order here. Just because a child exhibits a mixture of phonological and visuospatial errors while reading and writing does not necessarily mean that the child has audiovisual dyslexia. The symptoms must be considered within the context of the methods and materials used to teach the child to read.

Norwegian children are typically taught reading with a phonetic approach, reflecting the fact that their written language is highly phonetic. Children who have particular problems with phonetic processing would not get much compensatory help from a whole-word approach. Such children would probably reveal symptoms in both areas, while the basic problem may be phonetic, that is, auditory dyslexia. This situation would also occur in American schools that use a phonetic (linguistic) approach to the teaching of reading. The opposite situation may quite likely occur where the methodology is more word-configuration and context oriented, such as a language arts, total language, or psycholinguistic approach. The basal-reader approach places emphasis on the development of a sight vocabulary as well as on systematic decoding instruction, so that a child with one of the modality-related problems would acquire some compensatory skills and therefore be less likely to be misdiagnosed as having audiovisual dyslexia.

By viewing all the various symptoms within the context of the instructional methodology used, one will generally find that what initially may appear as a mixed pattern is usually either auditory or visual dyslexia. The audiovisual pattern is, fortunately, relatively rare.

Emotional and Educational Dyslexia

With respect to the last two types of dyslexia in our model, emotional and educational dyslexia, one will not find any systematic and persistent patterns in reading or writing behavior. This in itself differentiates these patterns from the previous three.

The most predominant characteristic of emotional dyslexia is what can often be observed as a phobialike attitude toward reading. During oral reading one will hear a rather pedantic letter-by-letter sounding out. This behavior appears to be the result of anxiety about guessing, about taking chances. It does not differ much from the emphasis on minutia that is particularly characteristic of younger children with visual dyslexia. But as emotional dyslexics get older, they often switch to the opposite behavior; they rush through the reading material with highly unrealistic guessing, mumbling the words they are reading to cover up the errors they know they are committing.

Although this development is quite typical in emotional dyslexia, it also occurs at times with older students with reading disabilities. A problem as serious as dyslexia will almost always, sooner or later, result in emotional problems. Wild guessing and accelerated reading speed are common symptoms of compensatory reactions. By giving the learning disabled an understanding of the problem and some insight regarding its various characteristics, one can prevent or at least reduce a very unfortunate and emotionally loaded reaction to a learning problem.

In practical treatment as well as in research, it is very important to differentiate between the illogical guessing and the excessive speed. One is causative in dyslexia and the other is the effect of this disability. One must admit, however, that this differentiation is not always easily made in practice.

Among the first three types of dyslexia in our model — auditory, visual, and audiovisual — one will almost always find problems with reading as well as spelling. In contrast, in cases of emotional dyslexia one will often find no particular spelling problems. In cases where spelling performance is much better than reading, the diagnosis of emotional dyslexia would be a distinct possibility.

The last type of dyslexia listed, educational dyslexia, shows very little commonality in error patterns. What these children have learned and not learned appears to be rather haphazard. So far we have been unable to detect any systematic and stable error patterns along the lines described for the first three groups. Quite to the contrary, this haphazardness and inconsistency from one child to another seems to be the main criterion for identifying this group. It is not at all unusual to find that the problems are the result of instruction that has been inadequate in view of the children's needs and of other influences either at home or at school. Children in this group are often found to have been poorly prepared or lacking in school readiness at the beginning of their schooling. They therefore did not acquire the basic skills necessary to progress in reading and spelling, even though these skills were taught at the time when children would ordinarily acquire them.

Caveats About Our Classification

In the preceding presentation of our system for classifying dyslexia types, many interesting details have been left out to keep the discussion brief. These details would help in our subsequent discussion of function analysis. On the other hand, these details may not be particularly important. They would differ quite a bit from one language to another (and in Norway from one dialect to another) and they would also be influenced by the particular instructional methods used.

We also accept the fact that our model will undergo changes as additional clinical experiences and systematic research data accumulate. The same will also be the case with respect to the terminology used. "Auditory," "visual," and "audiovisual" are not really adequate since, among other things, they suggest a rather traditional definition that focuses on a sensory deficit. What is denoted by a certain label is, of course, primarily a question of how the concept is operationally defined. The labels "auditory" and "visual" have been given a broad definition here by including the sensory channels and the main qualities involved in the ideation and conceptualization process. Many other labels can be found in the professional literature, for example, dysphonetic, audiophonetic, anterior, dyseidetic, visuospatial, and posterior (Aaron & Baker, 1982; Boder, 1968; Ingram et al., 1970).

Some attempts to assign hemispheres to these two main categories of dyslexia are now emerging. The left, dominant hemisphere disabilities are referred to as phonetic, sequential-type dyslexia (our visual dyslexia), and the right hemisphere disabilities are referred to as configurational, dissociative dyslexia (auditory dyslexia). Bakker (1979) has been a major proponent of this view. He described a dyslexia type I person as someone who has skipped the spatioperceptual stage in reading acquisition and who is overly dependent upon syntactic-semantic strategies, depending primarily on word configurations for decoding. This reading behavior coincides with our auditory type; the person reads rapidly but inaccurately. The dyslexia type II person is overly dependent on spatioperceptual skills and phonics for decoding; his or her reading is overanalytical, labored, and slow, but accurate. This describes also our visual type. Bakker also claimed that in the case of type I dyslexia, speech is mediated by the left hemisphere, while type II dyslexia depends on the right hemisphere. Others refer to visual dyslexics as right brain readers and to auditory dyslexics as left brain readers, emphasizing what these people can do rather than their disabilities (Tzeng & Wang, 1985). There is currently a great deal of interest in this hemisphere specialization theory, primarily because it is supported by many hard data, not only from experimental psychology but also from neurology (Sasanuma, 1974). Interesting as this topic is, space limitations prevent further elaboration. If this theory turns out to be essentially correct, it would enhance the importance of the present research project because of the obvious overlap in dyslexia typology.

A differentiation has been made here between modality-related types of dyslexia (auditory, visual, and audiovisual) and the non-modality-related types (emotional, educational). The auditory and visual types are commonly classified as such in the international literature, although under a variety of labels. One rarely, however, finds the subcategories emotional and educational dyslexia in the professional literature.

The reasons why the non-modality-related types are rarely mentioned will vary a great deal. Some researchers do not view children with these reading disabilities as true dyslexics, even though they reveal a very sizeable discrepancy between school ability (IQ) and achievement in the literacy skills. The reason for such exclusion generally relates to etiology, especially if the researcher is working from a medical perspective. Other researchers overlook these types because their identity and special characteristics cannot be determined until they have gone through several years of schooling. It is also quite often necessary to maintain contact with them over a long period of time before a relatively reliable differential diagnosis can be made.

Some Practical Consequences

A central issue regarding our dyslexia model is, of course, its value in practice, for diagnosis as well as treatment. The question is often raised if the overlap between groups is a serious problem when the model is applied. The problem is undoubtedly there; it is one of the reasons why the model has been referred to as polythetic. But the problem is minimized by the use of function analysis, which is based on a qualitative understanding of the total pattern of literacy behaviors. Admittedly some cases simply do not fit the model. This is the reason for the final, sixth type, other, rare forms.

Another major question relates to the necessity for extensive analysis of all literacy behaviors and products in a function analysis. Could not the whole problem be solved by judicious use of a good, varied remedial instructional program based on a multisensory philosophy (Tarver & Dawson, 1978), thus eliminating the necessity for detailed diagnosis? Such a treatment would result in all learning-disabled children being given the same program; such a program would entail all so-called good principles of preventive and remedial instruction.

The multisensory approach makes use of all sensory channels, which would appear to be a sound principle. But this method is of little help to many children with learning disabilities. It may even be detrimental! This blunt and provocative statement may need an explanation.

First, self-insight and understanding of one's situation is in no way facilitated by a multisensory approach. It is not enough to tell the children that they make a variety of errors and to explain how each one can be rectified. The error patterns must be seen within the total context and be given a meaningful explanation. One can often observe the relief expressed by dyslexics once they receive an explanation of their own functioning and resultant error patterns in reading and writing behavior. An interpretation of the function analysis is generally well understood, often coinciding with their own diffuse perception of the problem. The importance of insight into one's own problems and the background in which they exist is well supported by research (Black, 1974; Rosenthal, 1973).

Second, the multisensory approach does not enhance motivation. Basic self-insight often has a motivational effect. By systematically dealing with various symptoms and symptom configurations, and by discussing these frankly with dyslexics, it is possible, as already mentioned, to provide the person with the necessary perceptions of what has happened and what improvements are taking place.

Finally, by using all sensory channels simultaneously there is always a danger of input overload. There is also the danger that such an approach will reinforce inappropriate or erroneous reactions rather than extinguish them. It is, of course, convenient to use a "tried and true" method, which usually means that one does things the way they have always been done and the way one happened to learn it.

In this connection it would seem useful to again mention the basic differences between auditory and visual dyslexia with regard to learning behavior and lack of achievement. The auditory group needs to develop linguistic awareness and the ability to perceive and apply phonetic principles, while at the same time trying to reduced the exclusive use of a look-see, whole-word approach to decoding. Reading that depends solely on sight vocabulary and context is not sufficient; many new words will have to be decoded, using the skills of phonetic and structural analysis. The visual dyslexic, on the other hand, must always be encouraged to memorize configurations as sight words and at times be stimulated to guess entire words from context. The problem here is to reduce the excessive use of phonics with every single word.

If these rather opposite needs are not taken into consideration, one is likely to give the learning disabled "stones for bread." Instead of the situation being improved through special or remedial education, it may be made worse. An acceptance of the whole function analysis approach must inevitably lead to giving up one's faith in the old, well-established ideas regarding universally good principles of instruction. One is led to the contrary opinion that what may be beneficial for one group of learners may be detrimental to another group (Hansen, 1979; Mathewson, 1979; Rosenshine & Berliner, 1978; Soar & Soar, 1977).

CHAPTER 9

Function Analysis of Literacy Behavior

H.-J. Gjessing

Principles and Application of Function Analysis

The term *function analysis* as used here denotes a certain approach to the analysis of children's reading and spelling behavior. It is a way of analyzing oral and silent reading, spelling characteristics, and behavior during the reading and spelling process. Diagnosis of literacy disorders has traditionally been concerned primarily with the *product* of reading and spelling errors, which results in fairly general statements regarding problems with these skills. In contrast, function analysis attempts to understand underlying *functions* as expressed in the products of reading and spelling and to interpret *behaviors* during reading and spelling. Integration of all of these areas results in a comprehensive diagnosis.

The term *function* is used in a great many contexts with a great many meanings. In mathematics a function is an entity that relates to another entity in such a way that any change in the numerical value of one results in a change in the other. In the analysis of reading and spelling difficulties, function is viewed as an interaction involving a series of elements whose value, significance, and meaning vary depending on the total context in which they occur (Gjessing, 1980a). Such a viewpoint makes it meaningless simply to categorize and count specific reading and spelling errors (products) without seeing them in some functional or interactional context.

One must differentiate between interpersonal and intrapersonal interaction. Function, as defined here, places particular emphasis on intrapersonal interaction, the interplay among each individual's unique internal traits.

Interest in a function-oriented, interactional, holistic approach is not particularly recent. Already in the 1950s, Gjessing (1958a) drew the following conclusions with respect to the status of dyslexia research at that time:

No specific causes can be found in all cases of dyslexia. The incidence of a variety of factors has revealed significant group differences between dyslexics and normals, but the differentiating factors do occur in both groups.

Despite the presence of a particular trait considered causative in dyslexia, some children acquire well developed literacy skills, while, on the other hand, some children who do not possess this trait become dyslexic.

It is likely, therefore, that dyslexia is the result of a set of inhibiting factors rather than one special factor, and that dyslexia will emerge in those cases where the frequency and/or the strength of the causative factors are greater than those factors which have a positive effect on the development of the literacy skills.

These conclusions, and similar conclusions drawn even earlier by Monroe (1932), have been supported by subsequent research. Nevertheless, much research has been carried out as if there was a reasonable basis for a single-factor theory of dyslexia, or at least as if similar factors had an almost constant influence on different people in different settings.

A variety of systems for tabulating and categorizing errors in reading and orthography have been developed. These error classification systems will not be described in detail here (Goodman & Gollasch, 1980; Liberman, Shankweiler, Orlando, Harris, & Berti, 1971; Marshall & Newcombe, 1973; Miles & Ellis, 1981; Richards, 1974; Weber, 1968). These systems can be classified variously as *selective*, *quantitative*, or *functional analytical*.

The *selective* approach concerns itself with specific errors, for example, reversals, and focuses almost exclusively on these. This approach was quite common in the early phase of dyslexia research. It is still in use today, particularly in medicine and in conjunction with the study of neuropathological aspects of dyslexia, especially acquired dyslexia or alexia.

The *quantitative* method classifies all errors on the basis of surface-type categories such as substitutions, deletions, and reversals. Deletions of letters within words, such as *sand* (for *stand*), *Mach* (for *March*), *wat* (for *what*), and *figer* (for *finger*), are all registered as identical errors. On the surface they are identical, of course, but they differ functionally.

Letter substitutions are also subsumed under the same rubric. Errors such as *stanp* (for *stamp*), *nay* (for *may*), *prefur* (for *prefer*), and *penut* (for *peanut*) are, on the surface, letter substitutions, but they may represent different types of orthographic processing.

A third category of spelling error is reversals, such as *gril* (for *girl*), *form* (for *from*), *pot* (for *top*), and *meat* (for *team*). The first two examples represent partial reversals, while the last two represent full reversals. These two error types generally have different significance.

The *function analytical* approach utilizes a more specific categorization of errors. It is not based on surface-type spelling errors; rather, it is founded on hypotheses relating to various problems of processing print, hypotheses based on theoretical models and clinical observations. The difference between the quantitative and the function analytical method is illustrated in Table 9.1. This table lists common spelling errors in the middle column, categorized according to the quantitative approach in the left-hand column and the function analytical approach in the right-hand column.

The rationale for this approach and theories relating to the functional processing context of specific spelling errors will not be detailed here. The topic was covered briefly in Chapter 8 and more exhaustively elsewhere (Gjessing, 1977).

TABLE 9.1. Classification of orthographic errors by quantitative and function analytical methods

Quantitative category	Example: error (word)	Function analysis category
Letter substitutions	end (and) stanp (stamp) nay (may)	Phonologically based substitutions
	tost (toast) prefur (prefer) penut (peanut)	Visuoorthographic based substitutions
Letter deletions	sand (stand) Mach (March) figer (finger)	Phonologically based deletions
	wat (what) suprise (surprise) thum (thumb)	Visuoorthographic based deletions
Reversals	form (from) gril (girl) slove (solve)	Partial reversals (usually phonological weakness)
	was (saw) pot (top) meat (team)	Total reversals (usually visuospatial weakness)

Let us return briefly to Table 9.1. A few comments may be helpful. Under the "reversals" category, the two types of reversals have been categorized with the reservation "usually." This reservation is particularly appropriate for reversals, but could also be so for the other function analysis errors. Children with dyslexia are simply not consistent in their response to print or in their writing, which makes completely reliable error classifications virtually impossible.

Single reading and spelling errors must be evaluated in light of the functional totality in which these errors occur. The same pupil may confuse the /k/ sound with /g/ and the /d/ sound with /t/, but not always. Error may be caused by confusion regarding the voiced and unvoiced consonant sounds; it may occur in a semantically unfamiliar context or in phonologically "irregular" words.

Reversal errors also deserve some special mention because of the emphasis placed on these in the dyslexia literature. Except for such common reversals as was–saw and on–no, the so-called reversible words tend to reverse only one way, from an unknown to a known word. A child who can recognize not instantly may pronounce the unknown word ton, for not. But it is extremely rare to hear not pronounced ton; such an error would suggest neuropathology, perhaps, not merely a visuospatial weakness.

Reading and spelling errors that are inconsistent and not explainable on this basis may be situationally determined. One would then have to look for environmental factors that could influence literacy performance, such as classroom disturbances and distractions, individual versus group work settings, availability of a quiet place to do home assignments, and so on.

Without our going into any further detail, it should be clear that an understanding of these premises for function and dysfunction is essential for diagnosis, instructional planning, and individually prescribed instruction. This is all part of function analysis. The various literacy skills errors are assumed to indicate certain symptoms of faulty processing within the underlying dyslexia theory. Some errors may indicate a certain type of disability rather unequivocally, while others are difficult to associate with a particular type of dyslexia unless they are seen within the context of an entire configuration of symptoms. This is true not only of the direct symptoms—reading and writing behavior and reading and spelling errors—but also of various indirect symptoms as well, such as delayed language development, mixed dominance, and familial incidences.

A couple of examples, using direct symptoms, may help clarify this point. The two letters *b* and *d* have phonological as well as orthographic (visual) similarities. This is also true of such letter pairs as *m* and *n* and *p* and *b*. These letters are often confused with each other because of these two similarities. Such confusions must, therefore, be viewed within the framework of the total symptomatology. (In the English language, however, the letters that young children find most difficult to discriminate are *b* and *d* and *p* and *q*, mainly because of the visual similarity.)

Perhaps an even better example relates to reversal errors. When a child is attempting to read a word like *pots*, the full reversal, *stop*, is visuospatial in nature, while such partial reversals as *tops* or *spot* are typically of a phonological nature. But this may not always be the case. There are two ways of clarifying this problem. One is the approach suggested above, interpretation of the specific error in light of the total clinical picture. The other is through direct observation of the reading or writing behavior. If a considerable amount of sounding out is going on, all three mistakes may be phonological in nature. But if it appears that the child is trying to read the word as a sight word, it is more likely a visuospatial processing problem. One must also, of course, make note of the extent to which the child pays attention to the *context* in which the word appears.

The approach labeled "function analysis" requires rather careful study of process as well as product. Analysis of the misspelling or the mispronunciation of the word *pots* is a good example of the need for careful study of reading and spelling behavior. This requires careful note taking of the child's behavior, which is discussed below. It also requires an objective diagnostician whose interpretation of questionable symptoms goes beyond self-fulfilling prophesies.

Materials Used for Reading Assessment

A large amount of material was developed for the Bergen Project, not only for reading assessment but for instruction as well. Much of it was an extension of earlier research by Gjessing (1977)—his dyslexia model and its practical applications. This model has thus been described previously.

Since we are talking about several types of dyslexia from the standpoint of testing as well as remediation, it becomes essential to have tests that differentially identify these types. The following is a brief discussion of these tests. Instructional materials are discussed in the next section.

Gjessing's Diagnostic Test for the Analysis of Reading and Writing Difficulties (Dia-Gjessing)

This test is based on the theoretical model discussed earlier in this book. It is a large battery of relatively short tests designed to yield a differential diagnosis of the main types of dyslexia and to assist in designing an individual instructional program. With all subtests it takes 2 to 3 hours to administer.

The test material consists of the following:

1. The test manual.
2. A set of reusable stimulus materials.
3. The answer document (a 36-page booklet in which the child responds to questions and performs a variety of writing tasks).
4. The examiner's recording booklet (a 32-page booklet in which the examiner keeps track of the child's responses and behavior during the test; one such booklet and one answer document are needed for each child).
5. An error analysis key (a card that explains the symbols used to record the errors made during oral reading).

In addition, the examiner needs pencils, crayons, stopwatch, and cassette recorder.

There are, altogether, 21 sub-tests—10 main tests (H-1 to H-10) and 11 supplementary tests (S-1 to S-11). While the main tests are administered to everybody, the supplementary tests are used when appropriate for a particular child, according to the clinical judgment of the examiner. All of these subtests were administered in the Bergen Project.

H-1, Copying Sentences

The child is asked to copy a three-sentenced paragraph, each sentence containing five words. Two of the 15 words contain only two syllables, the rest are monosyllabic. The time limit is sufficiently generous to allow all but the slowest children to finish.

This test reveals the child's approach to writing, whether letter by letter, by word parts or entire words, or by sentences. It is the first test because it is a relatively easy task for practically all children, a calming and reassuring way of establishing rapport.

H-2, Writing Letters

A series of letters is dictated, one at a time, for the child to pronounce and then to write. This test indicates how the child approaches the basic elements of the written language. It is also used to test the child's ability to pronounce the dictated letters, chosen so as to cover the main sounds of the Norwegian language represented by single letters.

H-3, Writing Dictated Words

The task here is to write words dictated by the examiner. The child is asked to pronounce the word, pronounce each phoneme in the proper sequence, and then write the word.

The child's ability in phonics is tested here by the choice of stimulus words, which range from phonetically simple (FE) to phonetically of medium difficulty (FM), phonetically complex (FK), and phonetically irregular (IF). All but the last would be considered phonetically regular, but the words vary in length and in blends (clusters) and digraphs. Examples are *in* (FE), *ever* (FM), *blast* (FK), and *right* (IF). The words are arranged in order of difficulty.

H-4, Listening Comprehension

The examiner reads a story consisting of 10 sentences of about 10 words each. There are 26 specific details in the story. As the child retells the story, the examiner keeps track of the specific details recalled. After the spontaneous recall, the examiner asks five comprehension questions. This test is used to assess language competence in the auditory mode, as well as the individual's recall of a story.

H-5, Reading Letters

The child is asked to read individual letters in lower case (LC) and upper case (UC) presented in random order. This test gives information not only about knowledge of letter names but also about the efficiency (rate) at which this relatively easy reading task is performed.

H-6, Reading Words Orally

The test words here are the same words used in H-3, presented in a different order. Each word is presented tachistoscopically; if the child fails this presentation, each word is presented again without a time limit. The purpose of this test is to determine the ability to read or decode words of increasing phonetic complexity and to analyze strengths and weaknesses in this area.

H-7, Learning Efficiency

The words used in this test are eight words from H-3 that the child failed to spell correctly. Half the words are the first misspelled words from categories FE, FM, and FK, while the remaining four are the first four misspelled words from category IF. The examiner goes over the child's mistakes and then allows the child a specified amount of time to practice writing the eight words. The child is then asked to write the words again from dictation. During the second testing session (the next day or later), the child is again asked to write each word.

Test H-7 gives the examiner an opportunity to observe closely the child's approach to a school learning task, as well as the effect of practice. (This subtest has not been standardized.)

H-8, Writing Dictated Sentences

Eight unrelated sentences of increasing difficulty are dictated. The words sampled in these sentences have been classified by phonetic complexity according to the system used in H-3.

This test gives additional information about how the child writes certain words and how context is used in the writing process. The results are compared with the performance on H-3.

H-9, Silent Reading Comprehension

The test material here is a story consisting of 11 sentences. The last word in each sentence is on a separate line along with three distractors. The child must choose the one word out of four that fits. The child has 5 minutes to read this story, which has a readability level of about second grade. In this test the examiner observes how the child tackles a silent reading task and what the degree of comprehension is.

H-10, Oral Reading

The oral reading material consists of a continuous story. Ten sentences are arranged in four paragraphs of increasing difficulty. The test is timed. The examiner keeps careful track of all errors. Six comprehension questions are asked orally after the child has finished, including questions relating to predicting the outcome of the story.

The main purpose here is to determine the child's special strengths and weaknesses in oral reading, in decoding, and in ability to read with expression and understanding.

S-1, Auditory Discrimination of Sounds

The child is given a certain letter sound and must determine if that sound occurs in a word pronounced by the examiner. If the correct answer is given, the child is also asked to determine if the sound appears in the beginning, middle, or end of the word.

This test indicates the child's ability to identify certain phonemes independent of printed cues. It is used when the child has shown severe problems with phonics in the main tests and when a significant visual difficulty is suspected. Children with no such problems will have little difficulty with S-1.

S-2, Auditory Blending

The examiner pronounces the phonemes of a word in sequence but as individual sounds (e.g., /s/-/a/-/t/) and the child must identify the word. The 10 test words are taken from H-3, sampling words of increasing degree of phonetic complexity. The objective here is to determine the child's ability to blend sounds presented orally, a kind of phonemic synthesis.

S-3, Auditory Syllabication

Words are pronounced by the examiner. The child is asked to pronounce each word, syllable by syllable. This test not only gives insight into the child's ability to perceive syllables, but also reveals the child's sensitivity to the natural rhythm of the language.

S-4, Writing Numerals

The child is asked to write numerals from dictation. The first four items are single digits and the remaining eight are two-digit numerals. This supplementary test is usually given to children who have difficulty writing letters (H-2) and to children who have indicated reversal tendencies.

S-5, Single/Double Consonants

This test assesses an essential decoding skill in the Norwegian language, the ability to used the proper vowel sound when the vowel letter is followed by a single or double consonant, as in the Norwegian words *sin* (pronounced *seen*) and *sinn* (pronounced *sin*). The parallel problem in the English language would be the addition of final *-e*, which changes a previous vowel sound from short (unglided) to long (glided), as in *fin* and *fine*. The task in S-5 is for the child to pronounce a word where the doubling of one consonant alters the preceding vowel sound. Both single and double consonant words are used. Since the grade level at which this skill is taught varies considerably, the test is not normed.

S-6, Spelling Nonsense Words

The task here is to write synthetic or nonsense words that follow common phonetic principles. The words have been constructed to represent the different degrees of phonetic regularity, as in test H-3, although the phonetically irregular (IF) category is not used. The purpose of the test is to determine phonetic encoding (spelling) ability without the aid of previous learning of specific word configurations. Performance is compared with the results of H-3.

S-7, Speed of Letter Recognition

The child is shown a page of individual letters arranged in random order and is asked to circle every one of a certain letter as quickly as possible. This test reveals the extent to which a child can quickly identify letters visually.

S-8, Speed of Consonant Blend Recognition

The child is shown a page of individual words and is asked to circle every word that contains a certain consonant blend as quickly as possible. The test covers such blends (clusters) as *bl* and *fr*; there are no variations in spelling. The results are interpreted along with the results of S-7.

S-9, Word Reversals

The child is asked to read words that are "reversible." These are words that are meaningful if read from left to right or right to left, as *was–saw*, *on–no*, and *pot–top*. The test reveals directional and reversal tendencies in reading.

S-10, Reading Nonsense Words

The words used in this test are the same as those in S-6, representing different degrees of phonetic regularity. The reading of nonsense words is done to minimize the effects of previous learning and to provide a more "pure" evaluation of the child's decoding ability. The results of S-10 are compared with those of H-6.

S-11, Identifying Irregular Spelling

This is essentially a proofreading test. The child is asked to identify phonetically irregular words that have been spelled phonetically. The incorrect spellings do not alter the meaning of the sentence in which a word occurs. (Example: *guess* and *gone* in the sentence "I gess they are all gon.") The misspelled words are selected from the IF words in H-3 and H-8. The test is used to evaluate visual memory and spelling ability.

Observational Guide and Checklist

To do a function analysis, a process that is described later in this chapter in some detail, it is important to keep track of a variety of behavioral characteristics during the reading and writing process, not just the error patterns. A recording system thus was worked out to include all aspects of reading and spelling behavior.

Literacy functions are extremely complex, and any systematic approach to the study of these is also bound to be complex. Precise and reliable observation schemes had to be developed and then described in sufficient detail to be replicable in other research projects. The system is described briefly here.

The record of writing behavior deals with 25 categories. These include such writing characteristics as switching or omitting letters; replacing a word with another word with similar meaning or with similar configuration or simply an entirely different word; assimilating; making partial or total reversals; confusing double and single consonants; adding or deleting letters or words; dividing or combining words; capitalizing; reversing letters and numerals; and using encoding skills inappropriately.

The record of oral reading behavior is divided into two parts: the record of oral reading errors (products) and the observations made during the reading process (functions). For the examiner to be able to keep track of all these characteristics during the examination, considerable effort was expended to develop as simple a system as possible. It is recommended, however, that the child's oral reading be tape-recorded during the examination.

The classification of oral reading errors was limited to five categories: omissions, additions, reversals, vowel errors, and other errors. The vowel errors here relate to a characteristic of the Norwegian language discussed earlier, where the duration of the vowel sound, determined by whether the following consonant is single or double, determines the meaning of a word, for example, *filer* (pronounced *feeler*) and *filler* (pronounced *filler*). It is similar to, but not identical with, the differentiation between long and short vowels in English.

Test Development and Standardization

The development of a test of this magnitude is time consuming and difficult. The theory on which the test is based was developed after extensive clinical work with dyslexic children and experimental tryouts of a large variety of tasks related to the four language functions of talking, listening, reading, and writing. The first version of the test was produced in early 1977. After experimental tryouts with primary grade children, the test went through two slight revisions before the standardization edition was completed.

The norming process was carried out with the help of special educators and school psychologists in Bergen. The norms were based on the testing of 130 second graders (around 8 years of age) during the months of November and December 1977. The schools and classrooms from which the norming sample was drawn were chosen randomly, but the choice of pupil to be tested in any one grade was left to the teacher's judgment. The type of pupil wanted was specified for each teacher, who made the choice based on the pupil's past achievement in reading and writing. The pupils were chosen so as to represent different levels of achievement. Additional details are found in the test manual (Gjessing, 1979).

A study of the test's concurrent validity was done by comparing the test results with the teacher evaluations described previously. The correlations between the teachers' judgments and the main scores on *Dia-Gjessing* were oral reading, .66; silent reading, .69; and spelling, .68. The total of these three subscores correlated .75 with the teacher evaluation, which was interpreted to mean that the test was of satisfactory validity.

Differential Diagnosis of Dyslexia With the Test

The various subtests were designed and developed to serve two specific objectives. First, each subtest should indicate the level of functioning in the specific skill for which the test was designed. Second, the entire set of subtests should portray accurately each pupil's sensory channels and modalities with respect to the visual and auditory skills involved in the literacy functions. The pupils could show impairments in the auditory or visual channel, in both, or in neither.

To get a better sense of the validity of the various subtests as they relate to the two major objectives mentioned above, a thorough clinical examination was made of those pupils in the standardization sample who scored at the extreme low end of the scale. From this study, 10 pupils were identified as clearly having auditory dyslexia syndrome, 8 as having visual dyslexia, and an additional 10 who showed a mixed pattern of deviating in both sensory channels. The last 10 children had what has been referred to as educational or emotional dyslexia. Additional details regarding the test's ability to differentiate among the dyslexia types will be given later in this chapter.

Observational Checklist of Behaviors During Individual Testing

Three major types of observations were made by the diagnosticians during the individual assessment. The first were *general impressions* of the child's reading and writing behavior. These observations covered such areas as decoding techniques (e.g., use of letter names or letter sounds), tendencies toward audible sounding out of words during silent reading, kinds of structural analysis techniques employed, work tempo, voice quality, volume and pitch during oral reading, and unique or special characteristics such as finger pointing, head tilting, and distance from the eyes to the print.

The second type of observation dealt with *oral language*, relating to such factors as the children's ability to express themselves, the quality of their oral language, articulation problems, speed of talking, pitch and volume during conversation (compared with voice quality during oral reading), and special speech difficulties such as stuttering, articulation problems, mixed-up word order, and anomia (inability to find the right word).

The third type of observation dealt with observed *behavior* and *attitudes* during the assessment process. The types of behaviors emphasized here related to reaction speed (plodding vs. excessive speed), degree of self-confidence, social contact, perseverance, attitude toward school work, self-appraisal, ability to concentrate, and attentiveness. Finally, certain physical characteristics were observed, such as muscular tension, ability to relax, squinting, tics, and handedness.

Materials Used for Instruction

A set of instructional materials was developed to deal with the types of dyslexia described in this book. This material was designed to provide a total and integrated program of diagnosis and treatment, involving a coordinated effort among teachers, specialized personnel, and parents. Emphasis was heavy on involving the child in the whole process, as well as the teacher and the parents. The material consists of four components.

Teacher's Guide

This 70-page easy-to-read book was given to every teacher involved in the Bergen Project. It contains a simplified summary of Gjessing's (1977) basic text on dyslexia along with an expanded discussion of the practical solutions. It covers reading and writing problems, reading instruction, principles of good teaching, readability, and instructional methodologies. There are also concrete suggestions on how to deal with reading-disabled children in the regular classroom as well as cooperation with the home. The book has a professional bibliography.

Orientation for Parents

This 18-page booklet presents pivotal points from the *Teacher's Guide* simply and briefly. Some trial editions of this booklet were used with parents of children not involved in the Bergen Project prior to the publication of the final version. *The Orientation for Parents* was given to every parent who had a child with learning difficulties and who participated in the Bergen Project.

Guide for Individual Planning

This booklet contains 50 sets of detailed instructional techniques and suggestions for teaching dyslexic children. The appropriate instructional plans for each child were selected from this guide on the basis of the results of the diagnostic assessment. After the individualized instructional exercises had been selected and checked off in this guide, copies of the guide with the prescribed exercises marked were given to the parents, the teacher, and the participating special educator. The purpose was to establish and maintain a concrete and systematic pattern of cooperation between the school and the home and between the two educators who were responsible for dealing with the child's learning disabilities. The *Guide* has four sections:

1. The first section deals with basic principles of educational psychology, with emphasis on developing insight into the problems associated with learning difficulties, such as adjusting reading material to the child's level, developing motivation and self-concept, giving assignments of appropriate length and level of difficulty, and interacting with the child with regard to school learning.
2. The second section covers prereading and enriching activities such as concept enrichment, listening activities, sharpening of visual perception, attention span, relaxation, and coordination activities.
3. Basic concepts of reading and writing instruction are covered in the third section, which deals with developing a sight vocabulary, decoding skills, auditory and visual syllabication, and phonics and various other specific decoding-related activities.
4. Finally, a section is devoted to the development of comprehension. It emphasizes understanding and application of the material read and the use of syntax and context to enhance comprehension.

Instructional Material

This relates back to the specifics of the *Guide for Individual Planning* and deals with the techniques and materials to be used to teach each child. The material consists of 325 detailed worksheets in the form of reproducible blackline masters, pages of exercises that can be photocopied by the schools without violating copyright regulations. Included in this material are pictorial stimulus tasks, sight words to be taught, a variety of games, text for use with reading and writing activities, and other appropriate exercises for an individualized plan. Teachers and parents can provide additional appropriate activities from the material such as games and homework assignments, depending on individual needs. School-home cooperation is greatly facilitated with the use of such concrete materials.

If the parents expressed a desire to do more with their own children, they were given additional materials to work with at home, after a professional educator had explained the nature and purpose of the activity to them.

A main reason for the development of all these individual exercises was to facilitate a coordinated and cooperative program by the school and the home. Large textbooks and workbooks do not work well in this situation because they lack specificity for individualized instruction. Using pages and sections from textbooks and workbooks selectively would be too cumbersome and expensive.

Results of Factor Analysis of the Diagnostic Reading and Spelling Tests

Assumptions Underlying the Analyses

The diagnostic test battery was constructed on the basis of our extensive practical clinical experience and theoretical background. Factor analysis was not carried out initially, although that process could have validated and possibly shortened the test. A diagnostic test battery should include nuances and skills that may be of interest for only a few children with reading disabilities; these may not be drawn out of an item pool. Theoretical-practical insight seemed the more appropriate approach initially.

The factor analysis was done a posteriori in order to validate the test, and the results of the factor analysis should be viewed against this background. The data that were analyzed were the responses of the dyslexic pupils in this study, not those of the normative cohort.

The clinical interpretation of reading and spelling errors was based on the assumption, mentioned previously, that there are systematic differences among dyslexic pupils in their errors and literacy behaviors which differences form relatively unique and distinct patterns. This approach has much in common with statistically based analyses of correlations and interactions. An analysis of the intercorrelations among the variables identified by the diagnostic tests should result in sets of variables with distinct patterns of internal correlations. A study of these patterns should then make it possible to explain what specific skill areas were identified by each factor.

The variables studied all came out of the diagnostic test battery. The factor analysis involved direct variables from the literacy skills tests and all error types noted in the reading and writing behavior, altogether 74 variables. A close inspection of the various frequency distributions showed that most variables had enough spread to differentiate among groups of varying levels of achievement. The intercorrelations also showed a great deal of variability in magnitude, and there were positive as well as negative correlation coefficients.

Grouping of Variables on the Basis of the Factor Analysis

There was a great deal of variability among the intercorrelations. A principal component analysis (PCA) resulted in 11 factors that contained constellations of variables that made a meaningful interpretation possible. Another approach, a principal factor analysis (PFA), yielded about the same results. Orthogonal and oblique rotations also yielded nearly identical results, which confirmed the validity of the defined factors (Dixon et al., 1983).

The first two factors were quite comprehensive, encompassing 20 and 13 variables respectively. These two factors combined represented about 40% of the common variance. As one might expect, not all variables were singularly related to one factor; some had loadings on several.

On the basis of the dyslexia model, the factors were arranged in a certain numerical order. The factors numbered first were those that were presumed to differentiate most sharply between pupils with auditory and those with visual dyslexia (those with auditory dyslexia scored low while those with visual dyslexia obtained relatively high scores). The factors assigned the highest numbers were those on which the auditory dyslexics were presumed to do quite a bit better than the visual dyslexics. The factors numbered in the middle were those presumed not to differentiate particularly between auditory and visual dyslexia, at least not this early in school. The factors are given in numerical order below, along with a brief description of the data base for each. (The Roman numerals in parentheses show the original sequence in which the factors emerged from the factor analysis.)

Factor 1: Complex Phonological Functions (I)

The major aspects of this factor involve those aspects of reading and writing behavior that according to the theory underlying the tests, assess audiolinguistic functioning. The specific skills involve knowledge of phoneme-grapheme correspondences, phonetic analysis and synthesis, decoding of synthetic (nonsense) words in which configuration is of no help, and some more complex reading and writing outcomes, which, at this early stage of literacy skills development, were presumed to be phonetic in nature.

Factor 2: Phonological Cluster Functions (VI)

This factor is closely related to factor I. It is dominated by phonological problems, such as the tendency to simplify consonant clusters, to make short repetitions, and to make incomplete reversals.

Factor 3: Phonological Assimilation (X)

The dimensions of this factor should, according to our dyslexia theory, belong among the phonological factors. This factor involves functions that reveal particular problems with the long and short vowel sounds and with mixing up related phonemes.

Factor 4: Orthographic Error Detection (IX)

This factor is associated with specific dimensions of the reading assessment, particularly spontaneous self-correction during oral reading. It is difficult to place this factor along the auditory-visual continuum; it appears to be quite neutral with respect to these processes.

Factor 5: Severe Reading Problems (XI)

The functions represented in this factor are serious and quite complex, characterized by choppy oral reading with long pauses, a great deal of difficulty with single words, audible sounding out during silent reading, and long repetitions. These behaviors are considered symptomatic of auditory dyslexia, but some aspects of visual dyslexia are also detectible at this early stage of literacy development, notably the long repetitions.

Factor 6: Semantic Literacy Functions (V)

This factor relates primarily to reading comprehension and word meaning. Particular strengths and weaknesses are both involved. This factor can express itself as the use of alternative words which may be semantically correct, contextually meaningful, or completely erroneous. A tendency to add words during oral reading is also present. Strength or weakness in this factor is not particularly associated with the auditory or visual dyslexia dimension.

Factor 7: Reversals (VIII)

Full reversals in oral reading are the main component of this factor. This problem is associated with visual dyslexia in our theory, although the link is not particularly strong at the early stages of literacy skills development. This issue was discussed earlier in this chapter.

Factor 8: Attentiveness (VII)

This factor is associated with such characteristics as speed of visuosensory identification of graphemes and grapheme combinations, typically as assessed by tests S-7 and S-8 in the diagnostic battery. But the factor is not singularly tied to the visual, graphemic skills; it is also related to the ability to retell a story that has been read orally. (See test H-4 in the diagnostic battery.) It is assumed, therefore, that this factor has a strong attentiveness element in it. Problems in this area are assumed to be associated with visual dyslexia in our dyslexia theory.

Factor 9: Orthographic Speed (III)

Subsumed under this factor are such behaviors as speed of literacy functions, including spelling, copying a paragraph, and letter identification. Slow reactions in these areas have been associated with visual dyslexia in the underlying theory.

Factor 10: Phonological Dependence (IV)

The functions encompassed by this factor are basically characterized by excessive dependence on phonetic and structural analysis, letter reversals, and the addition of words during oral reading. The underlying theory assumes these characteristics to be symptomatic of visual dyslexia.

Factor 11: Complex Orthographic Functions (II)

As is the case with factor 1, this final factor also entails a large number of variables. It therefore has to be considered a rather complex variable. The assessed characteristics involve relatively global literacy behaviors, more so than factor 1. They include the amount of time required for a variety of reading tasks, the ability to detect spelling errors in words spelled phonetically correctly but misspelled, and the ability to spell phonetically irregular words. This is a collective factor, representing a variety of behaviors dependent on phonetic as well as orthographic skills. Some of its dimensions are also part of factor 1, although most of its aspects relate to functions which, when impaired, are for the most part characteristic of visual dyslexia.

A General Evaluation of the Factor Analysis

As can be gathered from the previous discussion, two very broad and complex factors emerged (I and II, the first and last factors on the list). Literacy activity represents complex and integrating processes, and the fact that a very broad, complex phonological factor came out, representing phonological processing at the levels of phonemes, morphemes, and larger words, was certainly no big surprise. In addition to the complex phonological factor I, two more specific phonological factors emerged. One (VI) showed a clear connection with the ability to deal with consonant clusters (blends), while the other (X) dealt with phonological differentiation. Since factors that dealt with phonological processes were placed first, these three factors were labeled 1, 2, and 3 above.

The other broad and complex factor was factor II. It represented the more global reading and spelling characteristics, which were more closely tied to the orthographic skills than factor I. As such, it also encompassed phonological functions. This was confirmed by the fact that it also contained some small loadings on factor I. But factor II was considered most representative of visuoorthographic processing, so it was placed last, as factor II.

Other factors that were most closely associated with factor II were VIII, VII, III, and IV. Those factors all seemed to represent more specific and circumscribed visuoorthographic functions. They were therefore assigned numbers 7, 8, 9, and 10 in our system. The middle numbers (4–6) in this system were assigned to those factors which, according to our dyslexia theory, at least this early in literacy skills development, had no particular differential diagnostic value with respect to phonological processing or visuoorthographic processing. Problems in the former area were assumed to indicate auditory dyslexia, while difficulties with the latter-type processing were assumed to indicate visual dyslexia.

The overall impression regarding the various factors within the factor matrix was that most of the dimensions of the diagnostic test were represented quite unifactorially. The exceptions were, as suggested above, factors I and II, which overlapped to a considerable degree. The relatively insignificant overlap among the other factors suggests that the diagnostic test could differentiate among the many specific literacy skills.

Another question of interest was whether the various subtests and skills identified in the diagnostic test battery clustered the same way as in the factor analysis. The answer to this question was pretty much affirmative. Even though there were some relatively unimportant items in the diagnostic battery that did not fit the theory, the correspondence between the dyslexia theory and the factor analysis was excellent. Our overall impression from the statistical analysis is that the diagnostic test battery has considerable validity.

Profile Analyses of the Clinical Groups

The 4 factors that emerged could be viewed as a new set of literacy skills variables. Each pupil's factor scores could then be seen as a literacy skills achievement profile. Since this approach conceivably has general applicability, scores on these new variables were obtained by combining the standard scores for those variables that were represented within each factor. The combined scores were then converted to ordinary z scores (mean = 0, standard deviation, s, = 1). Each pupil's z score on each of the 11 factors represented that pupil's literacy achievement.

The mean achievement profiles for the four dyslexia groups were drawn and analyzed. The clinical analyses of the dyslexia cases had resulted in four dyslexia types—auditory, visual, audiovisual, and other types of dyslexia. (This part of the study is described in detail in Chap. 13.)

Because of the practical need for early diagnosis and a desire to start systematic remedial instruction as soon as possible, the diagnostic workup was done in the early part of second grade. From a research point of view, this was probably too early an age. The basic reading instruction in Norway places very strong emphasis on phonetic decoding techniques (Hagtvedt Vik, 1976). Difficulties with phonological processing thus emerge very early in school. Difficulties with orthographic processing, however, will be present only at a later stage, probably toward the end of second grade or early in third grade (Gjessing, 1977). The non-modality-related problems (other types of dyslexia) emerge much later in school.

At the time the diagnostic assessment took place, the non-modality-related types of dyslexia could not be readily identified and differentiated. These types were therefore combined into one category.

At the outset, each of the four categories of dyslexia was divided in two, the relatively "pure" types and the more "complex" types. This division was dropped later, since the number of cases in some of the eight categories became so small as to make relevant statistical analyses too ambiguous.

The four dyslexia groups were compared across the 11 factors that had emerged from the factor analysis. This would determine if the statistically based variables would yield achievement profiles consistent with the results predicted from the clinical analyses. Positive findings here would have to be interpreted as a mutual validation of the clinically and statistically based combining of variables. It would also confirm that a clinically based analysis could be used to categorize pupils with specific learning disabilities into subgroups with different profiles, based on the proposed dyslexia theory.

The four dyslexia groups varied with respect to mean scores on the test of general mental ability. The test used was the Norwegian edition of Wechster Intelligence Scale for Children–Revised edition (WISC-R). The mean total IQs on WISC-R were 94.5, 98.3, 99.3, and 95.2, respectively, for the groups auditory, audiovisual, visual, and other types of dyslexia. These differences in mean IQ could conceivably influence the means on the 11 factors; the degree of this influence would, of course, vary with the extent to which the factor scores correlated with IQ. Except for factors V, VII, IX, and X, the factor scores did correlate significantly with the WISC-R IQs as well as with the group test for scholastic aptitude. The profile scores were therefore corrected for differences in IQ.

Figure 9.1 shows the profiles of the corrected means. The results are plotted as profiles for each of the four dyslexia groups across the 11 factor variables. The values along the abscissa show the mean z scores. The 11 variables are arranged along the vertical axis in the rank order described previously in this chapter. The variables with which the children with auditory dyslexia presumably would have the greatest amount of difficulty were listed on top, the variables that the visual dyslexics were presumed to have the most difficulty with were listed toward the bottom.

The grand mean for the total dyslexia sample is represented by the zero score ($z = 0$), the vertical solid midline. Since this dyslexia sample was drawn from the total cohort ($N = 3,090$), it was assumed that this zero score "profile" was a representative norm for pupils with specific learning disabilities.

One could safely assume that pupils who had been selected systematically on the basis of different criteria would have a profile that differed from the zero score straight-line profile. Figure 9.1 confirms that assumption. The group "other types" (the non-modality-related types) had, as expected, a relatively flat, unsystematic profile across the 11 variables. This group's weakest areas were attentiveness and orthographic speed. There was a relatively small amount of variability among the various means within this group.

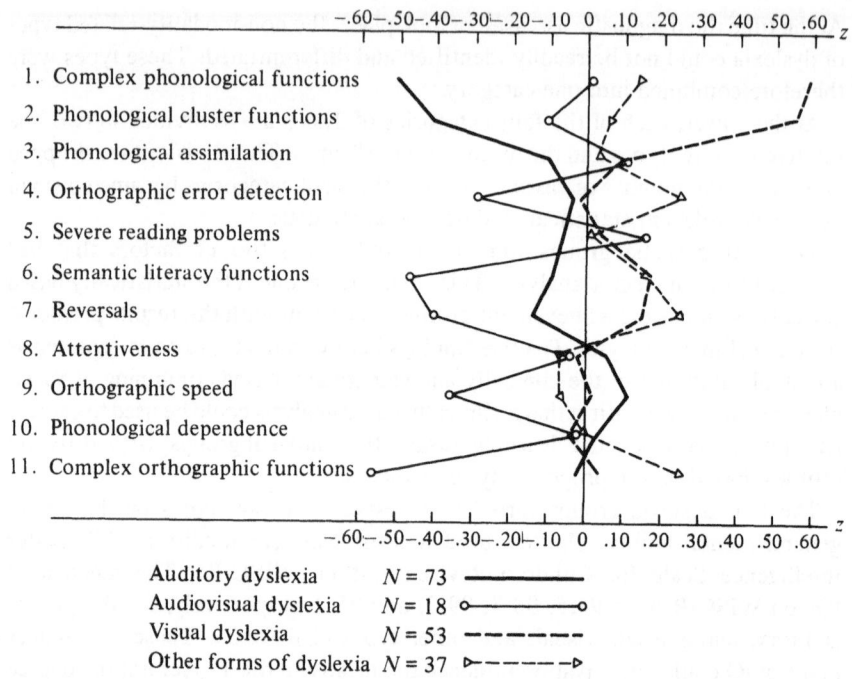

FIGURE 9.1. Profiles of the four dyslexia groups across the 11 factors for "direct variables," adjusted for differences in mean IQs (*n* = 181).

The remaining, modality-related groups, however, showed essentially different profiles, with a wide spread among the means within each group. The particular features of each one of these profiles were of most interest as they related to the underlying dyslexia model.

The two groups, visual dyslexia and auditory dyslexia, had profiles that pretty much mirrored each other around the zero score mean profile. The biggest profile differences related to the first two variables, complex phonological functions and phonological cluster functions, the auditory dyslexics scoring much below average and the visual dyslexics scoring way above average. Accompanying these extreme mean scores were profiles in which the auditory dyslexics showed a gradual increase in means from the top of the profile to the bottom, where the means approximated the grand means for the total dyslexia sample. The visual dyslexics showed the opposite pattern, with relatively high means on top of the profiles to scores near or below the zero means on the bottom. Variables that most clearly represented audiolinguistic functioning differentiated the most between the auditory and the visual dyslexics. But the differences were statistically significant for only the first (top) two variables (*p* < .01). Even though the remaining differences between these two groups were not statistically significant, they did help demonstrate the unique features of each profile. There was clearly an interactional relationship between these two profiles.

The variables listed in the middle and lower portions of the profile also helped demonstrate a unique and specific profile for the audiovisual dyslexics. Within this group the lowest means were for the five variables orthographic error detection, semantic literacy functions, reversals, orthographic speed, and complex orthographic functions. This group had mean scores for the remaining variables which were close to the total dyslexia sample mean of zero ($z = 0$). This group's weaknesses related, for the most part, to functions of particular importance to reading achievement. These functions involved comprehension, reading rate, proofreading ability, tendency to sound out during silent reading, self-corrections, problems with sight words, letter-naming speed, and problems with spelling of phonetically irregular words. These areas of difficulty were also considered characteristic of pupils with visual dyslexia, according to the Gjessing model. But the audiovisual dyslexics had significantly lower means than the visual dyslexics on the first two variables as well as on three of the five variables just listed semantic literacy functions, reversals, and complex orthographic functions.

The children who, according to the clinical analysis, had been classified as audiovisual dyslexics had a profile in which the indicated weaknesses were also the weaknesses that were presumed to be characteristic of visual dyslexia. This might lead to a reconsideration of the differentiation among the modality-related dyslexias. The relationship between visual and audiovisual dyslexia would certainly deserve a reanalysis.

A Summary of the Profile Analyses

Data from the variables that related to direct reading and spelling functions were analyzed for the total dyslexia sample of 195 pupils. A factor analysis specified 11 factors that, according to the characteristics sampled, could be interpreted from the viewpoint of Gjessing's dyslexia theory. This study led to the conclusion that the diagnostic test battery yielded data that, on the basis of statistical analyses, could be combined into cluster scores. These scores in turn could be used to differentiate among dyslexic students along variables of central interest to the dyslexia theory.

The pupils had been divided into four dyslexia groups on the basis of clinical analyses. This classification was done on the basis of the same data that were subjected to factor analysis, but long before the factor analysis was carried out. The factor analysis resulted in 11 main factors, and the mean profiles of the four dyslexia groups were drawn across these 11 factors. The resultant four profiles were clearly different from each other and corresponded quite closely with the patterns that had been anticipated from the dyslexia theory.

The group, "other forms of dyslexia" had a relatively flat, undifferentiated profile. According to the specifications for this group, it was presumed to be quite heterogeneous, consisting of pupils with emotional, educational, and rare forms of dyslexia. The relatively flat profile was, therefore, not particularly surprising.

The two groups that had been classified as auditory dyslexia and visual dyslexia had mirror profiles. The biggest difference between them related primarily to areas of audiolinguistic functioning. But in areas in which it had been assumed that the visual dyslexics would do much more poorly than the auditory dyslexics, the two groups had fairly similar means. This was explained as being associated with the age at which the children were diagnosed, early second grade. According to the dyslexia theory, symptoms of auditory dyslexia can be identified by the end of first grade, while symptoms of visual dyslexia would begin to emerge later on in the second grade (Gjessing, 1977). The mean profile for the visual dyslexics showed, nevertheless, that the results of the most typical auditorially related functions were better than for the most typical visually related functions. The profiles for these two groups showed clearly an interactional relationship.

The last group, the audiovisual dyslexics, had a mean profile that deviated the most from the underlying theory. It indicated weaknesses in the areas for which the dyslexia theory predicted particularly low scores for the visual dyslexia group. In contrast, the audiovisual dyslexia group had mean scores fairly close to the total dyslexia averages in most of the typical audiolinguistic functions. These findings may initiate work on some further differentiation between visual and audiovisual dyslexia.

Part IV Results of the Study of Dyslexia and Dyslexia Types

CHAPTER 10

Descriptive Analysis of the Entire Dyslexia Group

H.-J. Gjessing and H.D. Nygaard

Purpose of the Analysis

From research done by others and our own observations and clinical experiences, it seems reasonable to accept the notion that "dyslexia" and other similar labels are terms that connote a variety of literacy dysfunctions of etiological or behavioral nature. The thrust of the Bergen Project was thus to study subgroupings of the total dyslexia sample chosen by typological classification and possibly statistical methods. The practical consequences of this thrust are found in the next chapter, where the total dyslexia sample has been subdivided and described on the basis of *clinical* and *statistical* tests. This chapter, however, follows the traditional research strategy of treating the data from the total dyslexia sample as one group. This analysis of the total sample was based on our desire to determine which indirect, nonreading variables from our enormous data base (tests, observations, etc.) showed general effects on the total sample. (The next chapter will analyze the relationships of the same variables to the various dyslexia subgroups.)

A second main purpose for the analysis of the total group was to draw comparisons and parallels with the results from norm groups and, of course, from the results of other major dyslexia research.

Data were gathered on the entire dyslexia sample. Because of scattered missing data on the central diagnostic variables, however, the sample size was 181 pupils in most of the analyses.

Variables Studied

The set of educational and psychological variables studied is given in Table 10.1. This table needs close study for understanding of the subsequent analyses and discussions. Two kinds of variables are listed in this intercorrelation table, direct and indirect.

By *direct variables* is meant here the literacy skills variables, which are the first four variables listed vertically as well as horizontally. These are as follows:

TABLE 10.1. Correlations among main educational and psychological variables studied in 181 dyslexic pupils[a]

Characteristics	Variables assessed	Literacy skills variables						WISC-R			Sex
		Dia-Spelling	Dia-Oral reading	Dia-Silent reading	Dia-Total	Group silent reading	Group spelling	Verbal	Performance	Total	
Direct											
Literacy skills	Dia-Spelling	—				.45[b]	.72[b]				.09
	Dia-Oral reading	.67[b]	—			.55[b]	.52[b]				.06
	Dia-Silent reading	.58[b]	.70[b]	—		.57[b]	.37[b]				-.02
	Dia-Total	.84[b]	.91[b]	.86[b]	—	.60[b]	.60[b]				.04
Indirect											
Scholastic aptitude	WISC-Verbal	.29[b]	.11	.22[b]	.22[b]	.23[b]	.25[b]				-.20[b]
	WISC-Performance	.28[b]	.18[c]	.17[c]	.23[b]	.33[b]	.29[b]	.48[b]			-.15[c]
	WISC-Total	.33[b]	.17[c]	.22[b]	.26[b]	.32[b]	.31[b]	.88[b]	.84[b]	—	-.20[b]
Perception and memory	Bender Gestalt[d]	.29[b]	.34[b]	.27[b]	.34[b]	.28[b]	.28[b]	.28[b]	.28[b]	.32[b]	-.10
	VADS Aural-Oral	.12	.02	.07	.08	.12	.15[c]	.31[b]	.16[c]	.29[b]	.12
	VADS Visual-Oral	.34[b]	.26[b]	.26[b]	.33[b]	.27[b]	.34[b]	.21[b]	.09	.18[c]	.02
	VADS Aural-Written	.31[b]	.17[c]	.16[c]	.24[b]	.23[b]	.41[b]	.23[b]	.10	.20[b]	.11
	VADS Visual-Written	.30[b]	.20[b]	.24[b]	.28[b]	.20[b]	.22[b]	.26[b]	.18[c]	.26[b]	.05
	VADS Total	.39[b]	.24[b]	.25[b]	.33[b]	.28[b]	.40[b]	.30[b]	.22[b]	.33[b]	.07
	VADS Aural-Input	.26[b]	.14	.14	.20[b]	.35[b]	.20[b]	.30[b]	.17[b]	.28[b]	.11
	VADS Visual-Input	.38[b]	.28[b]	.28[b]	.28[b]	.34[b]	.28[b]	.34[b]	.21[b]	.29[b]	.02
Oral language	Word pronunciation	.36[b]	.34[b]	.30[b]	.38[b]	.27[b]	.32[b]	.19[c]	.14	.19[c]	.01
	Melody reproduction	.11	.07	.02	.07	-.03	.10	-.03	.09	.04	.23[b]
	Auditory discrimination	.17[c]	.12	.11	.16[c]	.23[b]	.17[c]	.21[b]	.23[b]	.25[b]	-.20[b]
	Syntax	.27[b]	.28[b]	.19[b]	.30[b]	.19[c]	.25[b]	.08	.20[b]	.15[c]	.04
Laterality	Hand preference[e]	.04	-.06	-.05	-.05	-.10	-.09	.01	-.06	-.04	.03
	Hand asymmetry	.12	.16	.21[c]	.18[c]	.05	-.03	-.05	-.06	.00	.08
	Eye preference[e]	.03	-.01	-.03	-.02	.03	-.02	-.07	-.07	-.08	.04
Self-image	Self-concept	.06	.06	.02	.05	-.06	.13	.05	-.03	.00	-.07

		C1	C2	C3	C4	C5	C6	C7	C8	C9
Social factor	Parent occupation	.16	.21^c	.23^b	.27^b	.12	.28^b	.28^b	.33^b	-.08
Teachers' classroom observations	Oral language reception	.44^b	.27^b	.40^b	.29^b	.52^b	.33^b	.22^b	.36^b	-.07
	Oral language expression	.36^b	.17^b	.29^b	.18^c	.42^b	.31^b	.20^b	.36^b	-.05
	Behavior	.38^b	.22^b	.35^b	.32^b	.42^b	.32^b	.23^b	.34^b	-.05
	Motor development	.24^b	.19^b	.27^b	.26^b	.24^b	.09	.11	.15^c	-.06
Diagnosticians' observations during testing with Dia-Gjessing	Approach to reading^f	.42^b	.45^b	.53^b	.47^b	.40^b	.18^c	.05	.17^c	.05
	Sounding out^f	.35^b	.24^b	.32^b	.18^c	.30^b	-.01	.15	.09	.19^c
	Speech: quantity	.05	.08	.09	-.06	.02	.13	-.01	.05	.02
	Speech: quality	.41^b	.29^b	.39^b	.11	.33^b	.17	.16	.18^c	-.09
	Articulation	.27^b	.10	.23^b	.07	.24^b	.05	.11	.07	-.02
	Personal interaction	.29^b	.37^b	.41^b	.32^b	.21^c	.08	.15	.16	.04
	Achievement attitude	.40^b	.30^b	.40^b	.29^b	.44^b	.01	.18^c	.11	-.02
	Social contact	.23^b	.21^b	.22^b	.18^c	.15	.11	.03	.10	-.05
	Persistence	.44^b	.30^b	.40^b	.28^b	.38^b	.12	.09	.17^c	.10
	Work adjustment	.29^b	.15^c	.23^c	.17^c	.18^c	.03	.01	.10	.02
	Concentration	.40^b	.37^b	.40^b	.28^b	.31^b	.14	.15	.15	-.03
Parents' observations reported during case history	Age of talking^f	.20^b	.06	.16^c	.15	.27^b	.15	.08	.16^c	.06
	Headaches^f	.10	.13	.11^c	.17^c	.15	-.04	.06	.01	-.02
	Sleep disturbances^f	.06	-.03	.00	.05	.03	.03	.11	.08	-.11
	Restless sleep^f	.02	-.01	-.02	.01	.03	.05	.04	.09	-.16
	Poor appetite^f	.13	.15	.16	.02	.07	.04	-.02	.01	-.09
	Stomachaches^f	.10	.08	.09	.18^c	.01	.06	.10	.10	-.06
	Enuresis: nocturnal^f	.01	.00	-.01	.00	.01	.18^c	.25^b	.26^b	-.07
	Enuresis: diurnal^f	.03	.12	.03	.11	-.05	-.03	.00	.05	-.01

^{a} The total dyslexia group of 195 pupils has been reduced to 181 because of missing data on some of the variables.
^{b} Significant at .01 level.
^{c} Significant at .05 level.
^{d} The Bender scale has been inverted so that the higher the score, the better the performance.
^{e} Hand and eye dominance are dichotomized: 1 = right, 0 = left or ambivalent.
^{f} The scale runs in the positive direction, the higher the better.
WISC-R, Wechsler Intelligence Scale for Children–Revised Edition; VADS, Visual Aural Digit Span test.

Dia-Spelling. The total score for the main spelling test within the diagnostic reading and spelling test battery used, Dia-Gjessing (Gjessing, 1979).

Dia-Oral reading. The summary score from the main oral reading test within Dia-Gjessing.

Dia-Silent reading. The total score for all silent reading tasks in Dia-Gjessing.

Dia-Total. The sum of the three scores just described.

The *indirect variables* are the nonliteracy skills variables relating to such characteristics as school aptitude, perception, oral language, motor development, and socioemotional factors. They are divided into two groups in the table, depending on how the relevant information was obtained:

1. Indirectly *measured* variables.
2. Indirectly *observed* variables.

The various characteristics that were assessed are described in the first column under "Characteristics," and the specific attributes measured or observed are described briefly in the second column under "Variables." There are altogether 43 indirect variables. Space does not permit a detailed description of each of these; it is hoped that the brief descriptions given in the table are sufficient.

Correlations Between Direct and Indirect Variables

Table 10.1 gives the intercorrelations within the set of direct variables, as well as the correlations between the direct and the indirect variables. The WISC-R intercorrelations are included, as are the correlations between the WISC-R scores and the other indirect variables. The results of the group tests in reading and spelling, as well as the pupils' sex, are also given. The table is arranged to show how the remaining indirect variables correlated not only with the direct variables but also with the indirect variables of IQ, sex, and the group test results for reading and spelling.

Direct Variables

Intercorrelations among the Dia-Gjessing subscores for spelling, oral reading and silent reading were .67, .58, and .70 (Table 10.1). The correlations with the total scores were, of course, artificially elevated, since each subscore was part of the total.

The relative magnitude of these first intercorrelations were about what one might expect, the highest being between oral and silent reading and the lowest between spelling and silent reading. This is quite reasonable, since the processing involved in silent reading is substantially different from that involved in spelling. In silent reading, semantics plays an increasingly large role and phonetics diminishes in importance. Oral reading, however, demands a more accurate phonetic reproduction of the text, resulting in a somewhat higher correlation with spelling. Comparisons of the relative performances for these three skills is useful in diagnosis because each skill reveals a different process. This will be discussed later.

It is also of interest to analyze the relationships between the direct variables from Dia-Gjessing and the group achievement test scores in silent reading and spelling. The group tests were administered at the transition from grade 1 to 2. Correlations ranged from .72 to .37, being largest between the two spelling tests and lowest between Dia-Silent reading and the group spelling test. Again, these are consistent with expectations. The Dia-Total score correlated the same for the two group tests ($r = .60$), which indicates that Dia-Total represents reading and spelling functions about equally.

The purpose of these comparisons has not been to validate the tests. Within the diagnostic context, the highest possible correlation between subtests or between different reading and spelling tests is not particularly desirable. Relatively moderate correlations tend to indicate that the tests tap somewhat different but nevertheless related attributes. The degree of relationship found in this study was considered reasonable as well as desirable in relationship to the purposes of Dia-Gjessing. It is also worth noting that the correlations between these variables and sex were essentially zero. This suggested that there was no need for an analysis by sex for the literacy skills variables for the total dyslexia sample.

Indirect (Nonreading) Variables

We first discuss the relationships between the direct variables and the measured indirect variables, then the relationships between the direct variables and the observed indirect variables.

Direct and Measured Indirect Variables

Table 10.1 shows a range of correlations for the Dia-Gjessing scores and the measured indirect variables from $-.06$ to $+.39$. The correlations with Dia-Total are of about the same magnitude as those for the individual Dia scores (spelling, oral reading, and silent reading). These correlation coefficients tend to be highest for the variables related to scholastic aptitude (IQ), perception and memory, and some of the oral language variables. The tests of perception included the Bender Gestalt Test and the Visual Aural Digit Span Test (VADS).

The word pronunciation test (an articulation test) had the highest correlations of all measured indirect variables with three of the four Dia scores, Dia-Spelling being the exception. The Dia-Spelling correlation (.36) was slightly lower than the VADS-Total correlation (.39), but the spelling test probably contributes more to prediction because of the much higher correlations between VADS-Total and the WISC-R variables as compared to the WISC-R correlation with word pronunciation.

The correlations for the four subtests and the two combination input scores on VADS varied considerably. The Aural-Oral (verbal stimulus-oral response) had negligible correlations with the Dia scores, whereas Visual-Oral (written stimulus–oral response) had the highest correlations. Aural-Written (verbal stimulus–written response) and Visual-Written (written stimulus–written response) also showed moderately high, statistically significant correlations with most of the Dia scores. It is worth noting that the VADS subtest that functionally resembles oral reading the most (Visual-Oral) had the highest correlations with the Dia scores, and the test furthest removed from the literacy skills (Aural-Oral) had by far the lowest correlations with the Dia variables. These relationships are also reflected in the VADS combination input scores.

The laterality variables showed inconsequential correlations with the direct variables. The correlation (+.21) between Dia-Silent reading and hand asymmetry (difference in writing ability for the right and left hand) is worth noting. Even though this correlation is rather modest, observations based on reading and writing behavior suggest that this particular relationship is not spurious. Many signs suggest similarity in processing of silent reading and certain aspects of laterality. Silent reading tends to take place at a faster rate than other literacy activity, and it is not as "sequence dependent" as oral reading or spelling, both of which challenge the pupil's spatial orientation.

It is also worth noting that the correlations between the Dia-variables and self-concept are all virtually zero, a finding quite consistent with the socioemotional data presented earlier.

Before leaving this discussion of the measured indirect variables, a few findings deserve more detailed discussion. Of particular interest here are the inter-correlations among the measured indirect variables.

As can be seen from Table 10.1, there are significant negative correlations between the three WISC-R scores and sex. According to the way sex was tabulated, the negative correlations indicate that the girls in this sample obtained lower average WISC scores than the boys. This could suggest that among boys and girls at average or higher levels of intelligence, the boys are more likely to develop dyslexia. This will be discussed later in conjunction with other indirect variables.

The Bender Gestalt was found to correlate .32 with the WISC-R-Total IQ, which is quite a bit lower than the correlation of .48 that Koppitz reported for a group of 8-year-olds with learning and/or emotional problems (Koppitz, 1964).

The VADS, essentially a memory span test, had a significant positive correlation with all three WISC scores; the correlations with WISC-R-Verbal was higher than with WISC-R-Performance. Similar data have been reported in the American norm data for VADS (Koppitz, 1977).

Another finding of interest in conjunction with WISC-R and VADS is their correlation with parent occupation, a variable ordinarily used as an index of socioeconomic status. WISC-R-Total and VADS-Total had a significant correlation (.33), and each correlated positively with reading and spelling. Parent occupation correlated significantly with WISC-R-Total ($r = .33$) and with Dia-Total (.23), but not with VADS Total, which yielded a correlation coefficient of .02 (not shown in Table 10.1). VADS appears, then, to be independent of socioeconomic status as assessed here. This could mean that the memory factors represented by VADS are stable across levels of socioeconomic status, possibly being genetically determined.

The data relating to the oral language variables are also of interest. The test of word pronunciation had, as mentioned previously, the highest correlations with the direct variables of all measured variables. This test consisted of 25 simple items. A short sentence was read to the pupil, who was asked to repeat one specific word in the sentence. Various articulation problems were noted.

The syntax test had to do with the understanding of the linguistic-syntactic structure of sentences; it correlated highly with the direct variables. The remaining oral language test, melody reproduction (musical ability) and auditory discrimination (discriminating between similar sounds), had low correlations with the direct variables. Nevertheless, these data deserve some comment. Melody reproduction and auditory discrimination both correlated significantly with sex, but in opposite directions. The girls did much better in melody reproduction, a test that had no correlation with WISC. The girls also obtained lower average scores in auditory discrimination, a variable that correlated positively with WISC-R (on which the girls, as mentioned previously, performed more poorly). Melody reproduction appears to be related to sex but independent of scholastic ability. The sex differences obtained for auditory discrimination appear from these analyses to be the result of the sex differences observed with respect to scholastic aptitude.

Observed Indirect Variables

The variables involved in teachers' classroom observations were based on an observation form developed by H. R. Myklebust. The correlations between these variables and the direct (literacy skills) variables ranged from .17 to .44. The relatively high correlations in this group suggest that the teachers' systematic evaluations in the classroom are at least as good predictors of literacy skills achievement as any of the measured indirect variables. These results may surprise some, but they are not unique in the research literature (e.g., Myklebust, 1971; Myklebust & Boshes, 1969).

The next group of characteristics, diagnosticians' observations, dealt with a variety of observations of individual children with learning disabilities in individual contacts. These observations related to the children's functioning and reactions while responding to the diagnostic reading and spelling test (Dia-Gjessing). The correlations with the Dia-variables ranged from .05 to .53 – among the highest correlations with the direct variables except for the few low correlations. These findings suggest that detailed systematic observations carried out by specially trained psychoeducational diagnosticians are of considerable value.

For the last set of observed indirect variables, parents' observations reported during case history, the correlations with the direct variables are quite low, ranging from −.04 to +.20. The correlation relating to parents' judgment regarding the age of talking was the highest.

An analysis of the relationship between the indirect observed variables and sex revealed only one difference between the sexes, which was not related to scholastic ability: Sounding out, the tendency to sound out unknown words audibly while reading silently, was more prevalent among the boys. This suggests that despite their dyslexia, the girls had developed somewhat better decoding skills than the boys.

Brief Conclusions and Discussion of the Intercorrelations

The variability among the direct variables is interesting from the aspect of diagnosing verbal processing. The point of view developed here is that not enough emphasis has been placed on the analysis of interskill variability in the literacy skills by dyslexia researchers. This point will be discussed further in the section on analysis of subgroup data.

The intercorrelations between the direct and the indirect variables varied considerably, from $-.05$ to $+.53$. This may suggest that some of the indirect variables yield little useful information. But it must be emphasized that these correlations pertain to the total dyslexia sample. When this sample is divided by dyslexia type, some of these variables with low correlations may be of interest. Our clinical experiences suggest that even indirect variables that yield zero correlation with the direct variables for the total sample can provide useful information. This is especially true for the variable melody reproduction, which also should be considered by pupil sex. This brings to mind Cronbach's admonition regarding the significant–not significant decision. He warned researchers not to pour the data down the drain just because significance was not obtained, such data could still be valuable (Cronbach, 1975).

Another related situation also needs to be pointed out. Some indirect variables, although hardly correlating with the direct variables, can be of value if they also have low correlation with other indirect variables such as those measured by WISC-R. They may represent a specific factor that has not been picked up by any other variables and that may provide valuable information for certain subgroups and, maybe more importantly, for certain pupils. Table 10.1 suggests that such variables could be hand asymmetry, sounding out, articulation, and achievement attitude.

The sex variable and its relationship to the various correlations is also worth a closer look. As mentioned earlier, no sex differences were found for the correlations with the literacy skills variables, and this was also much the case with respect to the indirect variables. There was one exception to this general finding, however. The WISC-R variables revealed relatively substantial correlations with sex, since as a group, the girls performed significantly lower than the boys. The same trend was found for auditory discrimination.

Table 10.2 shows that girls tended to score higher than boys in literacy skills. This suggests that the girls were better able to compensate for their weaknesses in scholastic aptitude and auditory discrimination.

TABLE 10.2. Reading and spelling data by sex for 181 dyslexic pupils

	Boys		Girls			
Variable	$\bar{X}$	SD	$\bar{X}$	SD	F	p
Group silent reading test	−1.38	0.28	−1.38	0.30	0.00	.96
Group spelling test	−2.10	1.20	−1.83	0.97	2.86	.09
Dia-Spelling	2.87	1.17	3.20	1.10	3.64	.06
Dia-Oral reading	2.95	1.28	3.18	1.27	1.35	.24
Dia-Silent reading	3.04	1.37	3.12	1.27	0.14	.71
Dia-Total	2.96	1.15	3.16	1.03	1.38	.24

Comparing the Total Dyslexia Sample With Normative Data and Other Research Findings

This section deals with the indirect (nonreading) variables listed in Table 10.1. Each characteristic will be viewed in light of normative data and other dyslexia research. The comparisons with other dyslexia research will be kept to a minimum, because of lack of comparability for certain definitions, selection criteria, and sampling (representative vs. referral); of variability in ages across and within samples; and of the great diversity of assessment tools and techniques for the school subjects and nonreading variables.

As is well known, an overwhelming volume of reports relate to conditions that could be causes of reading and writing disabilities. The older literature in particular contains extensive and detailed documentation with careful comparisons. The more recent literature shows increasing awareness of the lack of common premises for such comparisons. One now finds more general verbal and qualitative discussion. Works that exemplify this trend include those of Monroe (1932), Robinson (1946), Malmquist (1969), Klasen (1972), Gjessing (1977), Vellutino (1979), Harris and Sipay (1985), Lundberg (1983).

A variety of correlational data from the Bergen Project was presented earlier in this chapter. That information is useful but not sufficient. This section will supplement the correlational data with summary statistics that relate the indirect variables within our data bank to boys and girls separately as well as to the total group, comparing the data with available normative data and other research.

The normative data used for WISC-R come from a relatively new Norwegian edition (Undheim, 1978). For most of the other variables, the normative data used are those obtained during the Bergen Project, in our "own norm group." This group consisted of 40 pupils, evenly divided by sex, selected from the pupils in the total cohort of about 3,000 who had average scores in the school subjects of reading, spelling, and math as well as in scholastic aptitude measured by a group IQ test. "Our own norm group" should therefore be quite representative of average pupils, even though it was a relatively small group. It would have been desirable to have a larger group with whom to compare the dyslexics. It should also be kept in mind that our norm group is not a normative group, because of lack of variability.

Scholastic Aptitude Variables

The WISC-R data are reported by sex and for the total dyslexia sample in Table 10.3. The mean WISC-Verbal for the entire sample was 94.63, or about 5 IQ points below the Norwegian norm. The WISC-Performance mean IQ of 99.13 was just about at the norm, and the mean WISC-Total IQ of 96.38 was slightly below the Norwegian norm of 100.

There were consistent sex differences in mean IQ for the dyslexia group across all three scales, the difference favoring boys consistently by 4 to 6 points. The boys mean WISC-Performance IQ was the same as the national norm, and their mean total IQ was just barely below the norm. The girls in this dyslexia sample did particularly poorly on WISC-Verbal, with a mean IQ of 91.03.

Variability is also indicated in Table 10.3. The various standard deviations were slightly below the norm of 15, but only by a couple of points; they were all about the same across the various IQs and across the sexes. The girls showed less variability, as shown by the range. Even though the range of scores varied little for the three WISC-R IQ scores and for the sexes, they are nevertheless interesting. For WISC-Total the range was 69 IQ points.

The data pertaining to standard deviations and ranges within this dyslexia sample indicate that the entire IQ range was represented, with possibly the exception of above-average IQ girls. To get a closer look at this situation the students were classified by three IQ levels: the below-average group with IQ of 90 or less, the average group within the IQ interval of 91 to 110, and an above-average group with IQ 111 or higher. (The normative or expected incidence percentages for these three groups are 25%, 50%, and 25%.) These data are presented in Table 10.4 As can be seen, the boys are fairly well represented at all three IQ levels, but the girls are grossly underrepresented in the above-average IQ category. This tendency is most pronounced for WISC-Verbal. Of the total dyslexia sample, about one third scored IQ 90 or lower.

It is common practice in international dyslexia research to exclude children with learning disabilities who also have low IQ scores. Such a lower limit was not employed in this project, for reasons discussed in Chapter 7. But the criterion of a significant discrepancy between IQ and achievement in the literacy skills was maintained at all times. This means that all the dyslexics in this sample were at least 1 standard deviation poorer in reading and/or 1½ standard deviations poorer in spelling than predicted from the results of the group school ability test.

What has been described so far are the summary statistics for WISC-R and the distribution of WISC-R scores at three different IQ levels. These data show quite clearly that there are clear differences in mean Verbal and mean Performance IQ for the dyslexia sample. The Verbal-Performance difference, its magnitude and direction, has been a central topic in much dyslexia research (e.g., Hynd & Cohen, 1983). Our own data are summarized in Table 10.5. This table presents

TABLE 10.3. Means and standard deviations by sex for WISC-R variables in 181 dyslexic children.

WISC-R variable	Boys		Girls		Boys + Girls		Range			F	p
	$\bar{X}$	SD	$\bar{X}$	SD	$\bar{X}$	SD	Girls	Boys	B+G		
Verbal	96.75	13.25	91.03	11.88	94.63	13.06	58–118	59–126	58–126	8.71	<.01
Performance	100.72	13.40	96.48	12.81	99.13	13.34	65–128	65–136	65–136	4.30	<.05
Total	98.52	13.07	92.82	11.97	96.38	12.96	66–112	61–130	61–130	8.61	<.01

WISC-R, Wechsler Intelligence Scales for Children–Revised Edition.

TABLE 10.4. Percentages of 181 dyslexic children scoring below average (<90), average (91–110), and above average (111+), by sex, on WISC-R IQ variables.

WISC-R IQ	Norm data	Verbal IQ			Performance IQ			Total IQ		
		Boys	Girls	B+G	Boys	Girls	B+G	Boys	Girls	B+G
<90	25	27.7	42.4	33.1	24.6	36.4	29.1	27.3	40.9	32.4
91–110	50	57.1	54.6	56.3	53.6	50.0	52.2	51.7	53.0	52.2
111+	25	15.1	3.0	10.7	21.8	13.7	18.1	20.9	6.1	15.3
	100	100.0	99.9	100.1	100.0	100.1	100.1	99.9	100.0	99.9

WISC-R, Wechsler Intelligence Scales for Children–Revised Edition.

TABLE 10.5. Differences between WISC-R-Verbal IQs and -Performance IQs in 181
dyslexic children

Group	Verbal IQ		minus	Performance IQ
	$\bar{X}$	SD		Range
Boys	−3.96	13.95		−40.00–32.00
Girls	−5.45	13.12		−33.00–27.00
Boys + Girls	−4.53	13.66		−40.00–32.00

WISC-R, Wechsler Intelligence Scales for Children–Revised Edition.

the mean differences between the Verbal and Performance IQs based on the
difference for each child. A negative number indicates that the verbal score was
lower. These mean differences varied from about 4 IQ points for the boys to about
5½ points for the girls. For the total group the difference amounted to 4½ points,
all in favor of the Performance IQ. The range of differences is quite sizeable, the
deviations from zero being of almost the same large magnitude in both directions.

How do these WISC-R data for the total dyslexia sample compare with data
from other studies, with the subtest analyses being limited to WISC-Verbal and
WISC-Performance? Such comparisons are, as mentioned earlier, quite
problematic. Nevertheless, some of the relevant studies will be discussed.

Our total dyslexia group had a mean WISC-Total IQ of 96.4 (Table 10.3). This
is relatively low in comparison with other studies. On the basis of 13 studies, Belmont and Birch (1966) reported mean WISC-Total IQs from 91.8 to 109.8.
Klasen (1972) reported on nine studies in which the Total mean IQs ranged from
96.0 to 109.7. In his own research on 488 dyslexics, the mean Total IQ was 106.0.

We found the three WISC IQs to represent a wide range of abilities, although
the lower levels were clearly overrepresented. This latter trend was most prominent for girls. The range for WISC-Total for both sexes combined was more than
5 standard deviations. This is slightly less variability than reported by Klasen
(1972), who found an almost perfect normal distribution with respect to standard
deviation as well as range. She found dyslexics who scored +3 standard deviations, her standard deviation being just under the normative 15 points, while ours
was about 13 points.

As mentioned above, boys and girls and the total group all revealed lower mean
WISC-Verbal IQs than mean WISC-Performance IQs. This finding is quite con-
sistent with the results from most of the comparable research (e.g., Belmont &
Birch, 1966; Hunter & Johnson, 1971; Levine & Fuller, 1972; Vellutino, 1979;
Vernon, 1971; Warrington, 1967). But as was true of the Bergen data, many
report that a significant number of cases had Verbal IQs that were higher than
Performance IQs. In a summary of 20 studies, Huelsman (1970) found that 40%
of the cases with reading disabilities had a higher Verbal than Performance IQ.
By using tests of significance, Klasen (1972) determined that 22.3% of her cases
scored significantly higher on the verbal scale, while 18.9 scored significantly
higher on the performance scale.

In a study of 53 boys and girls with severe reading disabilities, Karlsen (1954) compared the WISC IQ patterns of the 15 "nongainers" and the 15 "good gainers" in an intensive remedial program, finding no significant differences in the patterns. The mean Performance IQ was 2 points higher than the Verbal IQ for the good gainers, the difference for the nongainers was 1 IQ point, none of it significant. Lytton (1972) also compared WISC IQ patterns of 12 pupils with reading disabilities who had shown a great deal of improvement in a special instructional program with those of 12 pupils who, despite special instruction, had shown very little improvement. The two groups were equivalent with respect to chronological age and WISC-Performance IQ. To control for the effect of sex, data for the eight boys in each of the two groups were compared. The comparison revealed no significant difference between the two groups on WISC-Total, but the group that showed good improvement had a higher mean WISC-Verbal IQ than the other.

The data from these two studies were inconclusive, but they deal with an issue that has been almost ignored, that is, the differential prognostic value of WISC IQ patterns seen in relationship to age and sex. There were sex differences in WISC IQ patterns in the Bergen data. Klasen (1972) also revealed findings along this line. There is reason to believe that an analysis of sex differences within a multivariate design may reveal some significant relationships.

The WISC-R IQ patterns have been discussed in some detail here; the subtest patterns will be discussed in the next chapter. The reason for our close attention to the WISC IQ patterns here is not based on a conviction that they have special significance as a diagnostic tool for children with learning disabilities. Most studies have found that these patterns show very modest relationships with school achievement, from a diagnostic as well as prognostic point of view (Harris & Sipay, 1985).

We have several reasons for our preoccupation with the WISC-R data. The results of the WISC-R demonstrate that there are dyslexics — meaning underachievers in reading and spelling — at all levels of intellectual ability. It is important to document this as well as the fact that here are dyslexics with low measured intelligence who need to be given consideration in research and in remedial instruction.

It may now even be necessay to dispel the notion that dyslexics are intellectually gifted persons. Reported mean IQs for dyslexics in the IQ range from 105 to 110 may stimulate such a notion. (See, for example, the review by Klasen, 1972.) It should be quite apparent by now that such findings result from the method of sample selection; that is, most of the samples studied are clinical referral samples that commonly exclude anyone below IQ 90. A certain amount of overrepresentation of the lower ability levels would be a more reasonable expectancy, since it cannot be denied that all linguistic skills are to some extent associated with general mental ability as measured by the WISC.

There are some sex differences in the WISC results among dyslexics. One cannot, therefore, exclude the possibility that the WISC IQ pattern may have diagnostic and/or prognostic utility, particularly when working on the basis for multivariate and typological principles. The sex differences found suggest that boys are more vulnerable with respect to school learning disabilities.

A final point with respect to our special interest in the WISC data: WISC has been used very extensively in dyslexia research, but most of the studies reported used the English (American) version of the test. Data from an entirely different language and environment have considerable comparative value.

Perception and Memory Variables

Included in this group of variables are the Bender Gestalt and the VADS tests. Data from these two tests are summarized in Table 10.6. This table illuminates a variety of relationships. For the dyslexia sample one can compare the data for boys and girls, as well as the total sample. The right side of the table shows results for dyslexia versus normal for boys and girls separately and for the combined groups. The outcomes of these comparisons are indicated by outcomes of the various tests of significance.

Bender Gestalt Results

The Bender Gestalt test resulted in very small and nonsignificant differences. The test appears to provide no differentiation between dyslexics and normals, although the dyslexia mean was the lower of the two. Comparisons by sex revealed no appreciable differences either.

How do these results compare with the data reported in other research studies? A great many different tests are utilized in dyslexia research to study visual perception and visual-motor abilities. The two best known are probably the Frostig Developmental Test of Visual Perception (Frostig, 1961) and the Bender Gestalt test (Bender, 1938). Very extensive research literature relates to both of these tests, especially as results relate to diagnosis and prognosis for children with learning disabilities.

The Bender Gestalt test was chosen for the Bergen Project. There are good reviews of the literature pertaining to this test by Keogh (1969), Bender (1970), and Vellutino (1979), among others. The analysis by Vellutino is particularly exhaustive, relating to the test's theoretical foundation, psychometric qualities, and a large diversity of research findings.

The research data are so varied and ambiguous as to defy general conclusions. Several studies have found that the differences revealed by the Bender Gestalt test between normal and disabled readers often disappear when one corrects for differences in intelligence between the two groups (Ackerman, Peters, & Dykman, 1971; Giebink & Birk, 1970; Obrzut, 1972). These results are quite consistent with ours. The total dyslexia group did not differ significantly from the normal sample. We will, however, continue the discussion of this test in the next chapter, where the test's ability to differentiate between dyslexia types will be analyzed.

VADS Results

This test of immediate memory attempts to tap different kinds of memory by using varied types and combinations of stimuli and responses—verbal, visual, and written. The summary data for the VADS variables are given in Table 10.6.

TABLE 10.6. Means and significance data for the dyslexia group ($n = 181$) and the normal comparison group ($n = 40$) by sex

Characteristics	Variables	Dyslexia group			Normal group			Significance test[a]				
		Boys	Girls	B+G	Boys	Girls	B+G	1	2	3	4	5
Perception and memory variables	Bender Gestalt test	5.06	4.90	5.01	5.29	5.67	5.47	—	—	—	—	—
	VADS Aural-Oral	4.46	4.70	4.55	4.48	4.65	4.58	—	$p<.05$	—	—	—
	VADS Visual-Oral	4.82	4.93	4.86	5.15	4.93	5.05	—	—	—	—	—
	VADS Aural-Written	4.09	4.32	4.17	4.11	4.36	4.24	—	$p=.05$	—	—	—
	VADS Visual-Written	4.60	4.73	4.65	4.98	5.11	5.05	$p<.05$	—	—	—	—
	VADS Total	17.97	18.68	18.23	18.72	19.04	18.91	—	$p=.05$	—	—	—
	VADS Aural-Input	8.60	9.07	8.76	8.77	9.10	8.96	—	$p<.05$	—	—	—
	VADS Visual-Input	9.45	9.66	9.52	10.13	10.29	10.22	$p<.01$	$p<.05$	—	—	—
Oral language	Word pronunciation	8.80	9.03	8.88	10.57	11.18	10.88	$p<.001$	$p<.001$	—	—	—
	Melody reproduction	3.92	4.41	4.09	3.72	4.19	3.98	—	—	—	—	—
	Auditory discrimination	36.93	36.24	36.69	36.51	37.17	36.81	—	$p<.001$	—	—	—
	Syntax	12.00	12.19	12.07	12.84	12.90	12.88	$p<.01$	—	—	$p<.05$	—
Self-image	Self-concept	38.61	37.84	38.34	43.00	44.61	43.77	$p<.01$	—	—	—	$p<.05$
Social factors	Parent occupation	1.95	2.05	1.98	2.10	2.63	2.40	—	—	—	—	—
Teachers' classroom observations	Oral language reception	10.67	10.79	10.71	11.53	11.80	11.67	$p<.05$	—	—	$p<.05$	—
	Oral language expression	13.48	13.75	13.58	14.30	15.29	14.81	$p<.05$	—	—	$p<.05$	—
	Behavior	16.76	16.68	16.74	17.41	18.80	18.10	$p<.01$	—	—	$p<.05$	$p<.01$
	Motor development	5.86	5.79	5.83	5.88	5.99	5.92	—	—	—	—	—

[a] Significance test results from group comparitons between:
1. Total dyslexia group versus total normal group.
2. Dyslexia group versus total normal group.
3. Normal boys versus normal girls.
4. Dyslexic boys versus normal boys.
5. Dyslexic girls versus normal girls.

The sharpest differentiation between the dyslexia and the normal group was found for the combination score Visual-Input, where the dyslexia group scored significantly lower. Significant differences in the same direction were also found for the subtest Visual-Written. These results are not surprising—they are consistent with our previously stated generalization that these two variables are most nearly analogous to literacy functions. The other scores did not differentiate between these two major groups.

When the boys and girls within the dyslexia group were compared, several differences turned out to be significant at the .05 level, the boys' average being consistently lower. It is worth noticing that these sex differences pertained to variables that were further removed from the literacy skills than the two variables discussed in the previous paragraph; also, that no such sex differences were found for the normal sample.

Memory functions have been of major concern in dyslexia research as well as in clinical work. There has been interest in short-term and long-term memory, rote memory and meaningful memory. The main research finding seems to indicate that dyslexics have particular problems with memory for a series of digits, letters, or words (Aaron, 1982; Lundberg, 1983; Miles & Ellis, 1981).

In recent years cognition psychology has been preoccupied with information retrieval, and memory functions have been studied from a variety of angles. There has been interest in the very shortest memory span, where sensory inputs last just a fraction of a second before they are extinguished, commonly referred to as iconic memory or iconic store (Höien, 1980; Neisser, 1967; Riding & Pugh, 1977; Sperling, 1960). And, of course, a lot of attention has been paid to short-term memory (lasting a few seconds) and long-term memory, which is usually meaningful, information-transmitting "lexical" memory. The nature and function of the memory process are still being clarified.

Two dimensions of memory will be dealt with here: The relation of memory to concentration and attention, and the degree to which the memory functions are modality specific.

It has long been assumed that memory is more or less modality bound, and a variety of tests and subtests have been developed to measure auditory and visual memory, such as Benton Visual Retention Test, Illinois Test of Psycholinguistic Abilities (ITPA), and WISC-R. These tests all treat the modality inputs independently. When VADS was developed, Koppitz constructed, within the same test battery, comparable tests across the modalities, and by means of combination scores tried to assess the extent and degree of integration across the modalities. Many findings and observations suggest that a lack of cross-sensory integration may be a significant etiological factor in the development of dyslexia (Aaron, 1982; Gjessing, 1977). It was the capability of VADS discussed here that led to its selection for use in the Bergen Project.

Koppitz (1964, 1975) has done extensive work with the test's construction and underlying theory and has carried out several studies, comparing normal readers and groups with a variety of problems, including reading disabilities (Koppitz, 1970, 1981). She and other researchers have also run comparison studies between VADS and other tests (Koppitz, 1975; Uhler, 1977). Aside from the work by its author, the test has had limited use in dyslexia research (Coff, 1978; Gouge, 1976; Hooper & Hynd, 1985).

Koppitz has reported considerable predictive and diagnostic value of VADS. Its greatest usefulness in this regard may relate to various subtypes of dyslexia, which is the main topic of the next chapter. No comparable data have been published, but it is hoped that the VADS will contribute to our understanding of the dyslexia types.

Oral Language Variables

Certain specific aspects of oral language are hard to delineate, such as the distinction between expressive and receptive language, the distinction between language problems and speech problems, delayed language development versus manifest language, and articulation difficulties. Definitions and delimitations are often nebulous from a theoretical as well as a psychometric point of view. Our research in this area was limited to several survey-type tests.

We found some distinct group differences for several of the oral language tests used, the most pronounced difference being for the word pronunciation test, a relatively simple articulation test. It differentiated quite sharply ($p < .001$) between the two main groups, dyslexics and normals, as well as between the dyslexic boys and girls. The dyslexia group was, as expected, the lower scoring group, as was true of the dyslexic boys. It would seem appropriate to mention at this point that a problem with articulation appears to be one of the more significant correlates of dyslexia (e.g., Harris & Sipay, 1985; Vellutino, 1979).

The melody reproduction test did not distinguish between the two main groups, dyslexics and normals, nor between boys and girls in the normal sample. But it did distinguish quite sharply ($p < .001$) between the dyslexic boys and girls; again, the boys obtained the lower mean score. As may be recalled from the data presented in Table 10.1, we found a significant correlation between performance on this test and sex, but insignificant correlations with all Dia variables. It is our clinical impression that melody reproduction has considerable diagnostic value. This test will be discussed again in the next chapter, which will give additional very interesting data regarding its role in the study of dyslexia types.

The auditory discrimination test revealed no significant group mean differences for the various group constellations. We can simply assert here that this test did not elicit any group differences, at least when the dyslexics were studied as a group or by sex without typological subdivisions.

The last oral language variable studied, syntax, differentiated clearly between the dyslexic and normal boys ($p < .05$), the difference favoring the normals.

These oral language tests turned out to produce some of the sharpest group differences of all the indirect measured variables. The articulation test word pronunciation differentiated clearly between dyslexic and normal boys, as well as between the two major groups. The dyslexic boys also scored significantly lower than the dyslexic girls. The results for the syntax test were in the same direction.

The importance of oral language for the acquisition of literacy skills is gaining in attention, even in English-speaking countries where the connection between oral and printed phonetics is not quite as self-evident as in countries with more phonetically regular printed languages (e.g., Ingram, 1969; Lyle, 1970). Many studies have now revealed oral language and linguistic characteristics as major correlates, if not causative factors, in dyslexia (Gjessing, 1976; Johnson & Myk-lebust, 1967; Klasen, 1972; Lundberg, 1983; Vellutino, 1979). On the other hand, many dyslexic children have no oral language difficulties (Gjessing, 1976; Harris & Sipay, 1985).

There were significant sex differences in the Bergen data, but the dyslexic girls did not differ significantly from the normal girls. Many studies have not reported data separately for boys and girls; those that have show data similar to the Bergen findings. Klasen (1972), who differentiated between sexes and age groups in his clinical samples, found the boys clearly at a disadvantage with respect to oral lan-guage, especially at the elementary school level (ages 6–13).

Self-Concept

The self-concept test was designed to assess how dyslexic children perceive them-selves, particuarly in a school situation. The pupils were asked to react to a vari-ety of statements presented verbally by the examiner. The statements dealt with how each student thought he or she was perceived by the other students.

The results of the self-concept test showed virtually no correlation with the Dia variables, nor did it differentiate between the sexes. The dyslexia sample's aver-age was significantly below the average for the normal sample, a difference caused by the much lower mean for the dyslexic girls than for the normal girls; there was no difference between the two groups of boys.

With regard to the connection between self-concept and learning disabilities, highly varied and equivocal results have been reported in the research literature. Some of the better controlled studies suggest that the average learning disability child will score significantly below the norm with respect to self-concept. Our data also suggest that there is a connection between these two factors. These data are discussed in much detail in Chapter 5.

Parent Occupation

Socioeconomic status (SES) is a factor that is generally considered in behavioral research, including studies of dyslexia. A variety of indices and scales have been developed to study this factor. But family background is a very complex area in which a large variety of economic, social, and cultural factors interact. Among the many facets that have been studied are home milieu, parents' education and occupation, family structure (two- or one-parent families, siblings, birth order, etc.), and more psychological aspects of the family situation such as the parents' attitude toward school, domineering or rejecting parents, and parental aspira-tions for their children.

Many of these issues were explored in the Bergen Project, but the discussion here will be limited to only one index of SES, parental occupation, about which the schools had good information. A rating scale was developed within this project, rating occupations from 1, unskilled labor, to 5, professions requiring a college education and degree.

As can be seen from Table 10.6, there were no significant differences between the two major groups with respect to SES, nor were any differences revealed by comparing the sexes separately. This finding is surprising and of considerable significance, since SES is such a potent factor in school achievement in the United States that it must be controlled for when norming tests. Lack of success in school is commonly associated with low SES (Deutsch, 1965; Lundman, 1979; Svendsen, 1979). One would expect that the same relationship would hold for children with dyslexia.

It is hard to find comparable studies of professional quality. Parental occupation and/or educational level has been the most commonly used relevant index of SES for comparison purposes. A number of studies have found data similar to ours; no appreciable differences in SES characteristics can be found between dyslexics and normal readers. This finding is perhaps least ambiguous for the Scandinavian countries and for the European countries with Germanic languages (Gjessing, 1958a; Linder, 1961; Lundberg & Olofsson, 1981; Malmquist, 1958; Schenk-Danziger, 1968). Although there are exceptions to this general trend (e.g., Robinson, 1946), most of the American research appears to yield similar results (Klasen, 1972; Smith & Dechant, 1961; Vellutino, 1979).

The possibility exists, of course, that the lack of difference in SES is the result of sampling. Clinic samples tend to be of relatively high SES because of the fact that clinics tend to charge fairly substantial fees. Some researchers have compensated for this by controlling for SES in the selection of a matched normal sample (Karlsen, 1954).

A Swedish study examined the SES factor in dyslexia quite thoroughly. The 46 dyslexia cases in the Umeå Project were compared with a control group, matched by grade in school, sex, and IQ but without reading disabilities. The analysis of these data, including the results of home visitation, revealed no appreciable differences with respect to the parents' occupation, education, or income (Lundberg & Olofsson, 1981).

It is our conclusion that dyslexia is fairly evenly represented across all levels of SES (Klasen, 1972), and that most studies have been unable to demonstrate significant group differences between dyslexics and normal readers with respect to this particular characteristic.

The question has been raised, and with good reason, why we do not find an overrepresentation of low SES among dyslexics, since this is generally the case with respect to other forms of school failure. This appears to be a particularly complex issue; it will not be discussed at length here, beyond reporting this extremely significant finding. Our data lend support to the hypothesis that dyslexia, more than any other school learning disability, is a genotypic deviation, and that problems with the acquisition of literacy skills are more related to individual than to environmental characteristics (Gjessing, 1977; Hallgren, 1950; Hermann, 1969; Lundberg, 1983; Vellutino, 1979).

Observations

Teachers' Classroom Observations

The teachers were asked to fill out a pupil rating scale for each of the children, the dyslexics as well as the normal control group. The scale used was based on the principles underlying the "Pupil Rating Scale" by Myklebust (1971), but developed for Norwegian conditions by Solheim and Nygaard (1984b). The scale covered the following areas: oral language reception (comprehension), oral language expression, behavior, and motor development.

As can be seen in Table 10.1, there were very substantial correlations between the teachers' ratings and the Dia scores. The highest correlations related to oral language reception, the lowest ones to motor development. The WISC-Total correlated higher with the teachers' classroom observations than with any other set of characteristics studied. Myklebust concluded that his "Pupil Rating Scale" could identify pupils with learning disabilities with considerable accuracy (Myklebust, 1971; Myklebust & Boshes, 1969). The Bergen data supported that conclusion, since it differentiated significantly between the dyslexics and the normal controls, except for the variable Motor development. The oral language expression and the behavior variables also differentiated at the group level between the dyslexic and the normal control girls in the expected direction. (See Table 10.6.)

It is our conclusion that the "Pupil Rating Scale" can be a useful tool for identifying pupils with dyslexia.

Observations by Diagnosticians and Parents

There were no data in these areas pertaining to the normal control group, making any comparisons between the two major groups impossible. In the dyslexia group there were very minor within-group differences between the sexes, the girls scoring slightly higher in one category, sounding out.

Familial Incidences

The incidence of learning disabilities among relatives has been of much interest in dyslexia research. This interest is not surprising, since from the beginning of the study of dyslexia, around the turn of the century, there has been speculation whether we are dealing with a genetically or an environmentally determined syndrome. The fact that something occurs in certain families does not necessarily mean that it is genetic. The issue is much more complex and equivocal when it comes to dyslexia. The issue will not be dealt with in great detail here; the reader is referred to such sources as DeFries and Decker (1982) and Klasen (1972). The very thorough Colorado study by DeFries and Decker demonstrates how complex and unclear the hereditary issue is with regard to dyslexia.

The studies of Hallgren (1950), Norri (1954), and Walker and Cole (1965) support the notion of a strong hereditary factor in dyslexia. Our own clinical data as well as others' indicate that there is a tendency for this condition to occur in certain families (Gjessing, 1976; Smith, 1970). Random sampling, however, has not produced very convincing evidence that this is the case. (Clark, 1970; DeHirsch et al., 1966).

We tend to agree with Harris and Sipay (1985) that much of the discrepancy between the clinical and the statistical data can be ascribed to sample selection and size. Clinical sampling typically has a large bias of unknown magnitude and even direction, and such samples are often too small to warrant statistical tests of significance.

Information regarding the family situations of the Bergen sample was in almost every case provided by the mother as part of the case study interviews by the school psychologists. The interview dealt with such issues as living conditions, siblings, relatives (including parents), and any unique problems or characteristics relating to reading, writing, language development, and laterality in the family.

With regard to the family situation, specifically the number of siblings, it was found that 6.9% of the dyslexics were only children, 37.3% had one sibling, 34.5% had two siblings, 14.4% had three, and 6.8% came from families with five or more children. The corresponding numbers for the entire Bergen cohort ($n \approx$ 3,000) were 8.8%, 45.6%, 30.9%, 10.4%, and 4.3%. The average number of children in the cohort was 2.6, whereas the average for the dyslexic group was 2.8. The slight difference between the two groups can probably be attributed to sampling.

An issue of considerably more interest is the incidence of learning disabilities within the families of the dyslexics. Data were gathered on relatives, the core family as well as more distant relatives. The data on the distant relatives were so scattered, unreliable, and insufficient that it was decided to limit the statistical analysis to the core family—mother, father, and siblings.

The mothers of all the dyslexics provided information pertaining to how many had or had had difficulties with reading and/or spelling. They reported that they thought 14.4% of the fathers had or had had such problems, and 21.6% reported that they had or had had such problems themselves. These incidence figures are certainly peculiar; past research and clinical experience would lead one to expect a much higher incidence for the fathers. Maybe all that the data tell us is that secondhand information of this sort is highly unreliable. The mothers either did not know that their husbands had or had had any learning problems, or they were unwilling to report it. A tendency to cover up information of this sort has been reported by other researchers (e.g., Lory, 1966).

Regarding the incidence of reading and spelling problems among the siblings, the mothers reported that 45.2% of the dyslexics had at least one sibling with such problems. This incidence figure is based on those 102 dyslexia cases whose siblings had received reading instruction. Although this frequency did not appear unreasonable, the fact that the siblings were evenly split between boys and girls was a bit surprising. On the basis of clinical experience and available research, a much higher incidence for male siblings was anticipated (e.g., Bannatyne, 1971; Gjessing, 1976; Klasen, 1972). This unexpected incidence was probably not the result of mothers giving out erroneous information so much as it was related to how the school was communicating with the parents. There were almost as many girls as boys in our own dyslexia sample (see Chapter 12). This issue will be discussed later on in this book.

The confusion surrounding the heritability of dyslexia has already been mentioned. The data and their interpretation are far from unambiguous. It is even difficult to arrive at some sort of consensus with regard to this issue. Klasen's (1972) extensive review of the related literature reports familial incidence figures ranging from 11 to 70%, but 40% appears to be a fairly common figure. As just suggested, this may be primarily the result of variability in the quality and size of the material. In addition, there is considerable variation in how the data are collected. It is quite common practice to determine the percentage of core families that have one or more members with learning disabilities, rather than the number of individuals. This information is often supplemented by data of varying reliability regarding more distant relatives.

The existing research seems to suggest that about 40% of the members of the immediate families of dyslexics have reading and/or spelling difficulties. This is fairly consistent with the Bergen data, which showed that 45% of the siblings and 22% of the mothers had difficulties. The incidence figures obtained for the fathers were too unreliable to be taken into account. Generally speaking, our data suggest that there is a relatively high incidence of dyslexia in the dyslexics' immediate families.

Summary Remarks

This chapter contains the main descriptive material of the nonmedical aspects of dyslexia pertaining to the Bergen dyslexia sample. The only subdivision of this sample was limited to sex differences. The next chapter deals with the subdivisions of this sample based on clinical and statistical approaches.

The variables studied were categorized as "direct" (measures of various literacy skills) and "indirect" (nonreading variables). The intercorrelations within and between these two sets of variables were studied; the variables were also compared with the data from a normal comparison group (Table 10.6).

Throughout, the Bergen data have been compared with the findings of other researchers. For the most part, our data were consistent with other relevant research, and they were consistent with expectancies. The most unexpected data related to familial incidence. It was anticipated that there would be a preponderance of males among the family members with dyslexia. This finding was explored further and will be discussed in more detail later on.

The analyses and comparisons among the direct (reading and spelling) variables yielded results that have significance for our understanding of literacy skills processing. These variables involved individual diagnostic tests (Dia-Gjessing) and group reading and spelling tests. Dia-Gjessing involved various aspects of spelling an oral and silent reading.

The correlations between the various direct and indirect variables covered a wide range. The highest correlations related to the measured indirect variables and the direct variables pertaining to perception and memory variables, along with certain oral language variables. But the very highest correlations obtained were between the direct variables and some of the observational variables based on teachers' and diagnosticians' impressions. Such observations appear to be at least as good predictors of dyslexia as many of the elaborate tests used, such as VADS and the Bender Gestalt test.

Table 10.6 presents the results for the total dyslexia group, for the normal comparison group, and for both groups by sex. Some of the differences here were revealing. The difference between the sexes on the oral language variable word pronunciation was particularly significant. This variable also differentiated rather sharply between the dyslexics and the normals. The variable melody reproduction also differentiated sharply ($p < .001$) between the dyslexic boys and girls, while at the same time showing virtually no correlation with the literacy skills variables.

A rather persistent trend with respect to the results of the main indirect variables was the sex differences within the dyslexia samples, with the boys outscoring the girls. This was particularly true of scholastic ability (IQ). On the other hand, the girls tended to excel with respect to the literacy skills. Generally speaking, there was a larger discrepancy between scholastic aptitude and achievement for the dyslexic boys than the girls, and there was a much higher percentage of boys among the dyslexics with high scholastic aptitude, suggesting that boys are more vulnerable to learning disabilities.

Of major concern in this project has been the determination of how different indirect variables, independent of each other, can contribute to the prediction of achievement in the literacy skills for a large group of pupils with dyslexia. There has also been some concern about the intercorrelations among the indirect variables. On the other hand, there has been little interest in the multiple correlations of these variables with literacy skills achievement, the reason being that the main thrust in this project has been the study of dyslexia subgroups. Some regression analyses have been undertaken nevertheless, but mainly to get a feeling for the predictability of the variables studied, and to determine the relative contributions of these variables within this context.

A stepwise selection regression analysis was carried out, using the score for Dia-Total (the sum score for reading and spelling) as the criterion variable. The predictor variables used were, first, the oral language variables word pronunciation and syntax. These two combined accounted for 20% of the variance in Dia-Total. The other two oral language tests, auditory discrimination and melody reproduction, made insignificant additional contributions. The Bender Gestalt test added 7.7%, VADS an additional 3.3%, and hand asymmetry 4.6%. Five of these seven variables appeared to have predictive value, explaining a total of 35%

of the variance in Dia-Total. Adding the rather time-consuming WISC variables behind the seven variables just mentioned added only 0.2%. (If the WISC results had been entered first they would have explained 6.8% of the variance.)

Some of the observational variables that the earlier correlation analysis had identified as particularly significant were also entered into the regression analysis. They contributed significantly, even though they were entered into the regression equation behind the seven language variables and the WISC variables. The observational variables that contributed most significantly were approach to reading, sounding out, concentration, achievement attitude, and personal interaction. These variables together added 22% to the explained variance. The addition of these variables to the regression equation resulted in a total of 63% of the explained variance, or a multiple correlation of $r = .79$ between these variables and Dia-Total.

These analyses suggest that the oral language tests combined with the direct observations of reading and spelling behavior are very strong predictors of achievement in a group of pupils with dyslexia. This conclusion is supported by the correlational data presented in Table 10.1. If the purpose is to study a group of pupils, relatively simple assessments of certain indirect variables may be as helpful as the more comprehensive tests, such as WISC.

CHAPTER 11

Multivariate Analyses of Clinical and Statistical Groupings

H.-J. Gjessing and H.D. Nygaard

Premises of the Analyses

The similarity between clinical and statistical methods for the grouping of reading and writing characteristics of children was discussed earlier in conjunction with the description of *Dia-Gjessing* and its factor analysis. There are also similarities between clinical and statistical methods when classifying people. Dyslexics can be grouped on the basis of practical clinical experiences and theory according to certain patterns of behavior and test profiles. Various statistical methods also group people by similarities in data profiles. The two methods used in the Bergen Project were Q-factor analysis, which employs correlational techniques, and cluster analysis, which utilizes euclidian distances. Only the results of the Q-factor analysis will be described here.

The background for the clinical analyses carried out in the Bergen Project was covered in Chapters 8 and 9: test profiles based on data from *Dia-Gjessing* for the four dyslexia types covering 11 variables (Chapter 8) were identified by means of a factor analysis (Chapter 9). The clinical analyses will be elaborated on here, and some data will be presented showing the extent of agreement among clinicians (interscorer reliability).

Subgrouping by Clinical Methods

The Subgrouping

The 259 pupils selected for detailed diagnostic workup included all of the learning disabled children – 195 with specific learning disabilities (dyslexics) and 64 with general learning disabilities (retarded). (The retarded students were included for comparison purposes only.) The dyslexic children were classified by a team of examiners form the office of school psychology according to the dyslexia model by Gjessing (1977), from their test results. The Gjessing model has six categories – auditory, visual, audiovisual, emotional, educational, and other. The same data were then subjected to blind analysis by two researchers (HJG and HDN). They included in their considerations notes taken by the examiners, which included records of reading and spelling errors. The large number of variables involved made it imperative that the clinical analysis have a theoretical rationale as to which variables indicated similar types and how the different tests revealed functioning in the literacy skills.

This second analysis resulted in even further differentiation of dyslexia types, as additional symptoms and characteristics were identified. This was particularly true for the case of the modality-related types—auditory, visual, audiovisual. Handwriting problem was the most frequently noted additional problem. Another very common complicating factor was emotional or school adjustment difficulties.

Only a few pupils were categorized as having emotional or educational dyslexia. This may be related to the fact that analysis was done at a fairly early age. As mentioned earlier, these two types are hard to identify until after several years of schooling.

The final outcome of the clinical analysis was a subdivision of each of the modality-related dyslexias into two categories each, one relatively pure type and one more complex type with additional problems. The other three types were combined into one, but this one group was split the way the others were, one fairly clear-cut type and one with complications. Many of the analyses were carried out for these final eight categories.

The 195 dyslexic students were classified into the following four categories:

1. *Auditory dyslexia* ($n = 79$). The predominant problem here was severe impairment of auditory discrimination; some children in this group had additional problems, especially in the area of motor coordination, but none of these appeared modality related.
2. *Audiovisual dyslexia* ($n = 20$). The main difficulty in this group was related to both the auditory and the visual modalities. Some pupils had additional but unrelated problems.
3. *Visual dyslexia* ($n = 55$). The main problem related to certain aspects of visual perception and retention; some children had additional, unrelated difficulties.
4. *Other types of dyslexia* ($n = 41$). Children in this group appeared to have neither auditory nor visual perception problems.

The frequencies of these four types are shown by sex in Table 11.1. As can be seen, auditory dyslexia was the most common (40.5%), audiovisual the least common (10.3%). These figures are quite similar to the data in a previous study (Gjessing, 1976). Other researchers who have used similar classifications have also found a predominance of cases with auditory language perception difficulties (e.g., Bannatyne, 1971; Boder, 1973). Boys are particularly vulnerable to auditory language perception problems, the ratio being 57:22, or 2.6 boys for each girl. Bannatyne suggested that this ratio may be as high as 10:1. Our data for visual dyslexia show a 30:25 ratio, that is, 1.2 boys for each girl. A correction for the difference in total numbers of boys and girls would change these ratios to 1.5 and 0.67, respectively. The incidences of audiovisual and other types of dyslexia show virtually identical percentages for the two sexes.

TABLE 11.1. Dyslexia sample ($n = 195$) categorized by dyslexia type and sex

Sex		Auditory dyslexia N (%)	Audiovisual dyslexia N (%)	Visual dyslexia N (%)	Other forms of dyslexia N (%)	Total N (%)
Boys	N	57 (45.6)	13 (10.4)	30 (24.0)	25 (20.0)	125 (100)
	(%)	(72.2)	(65.0)	(54.5)	(60.1)	(64.1)
Girls	N	22 (31.4)	7 (10.0)	25 (35.7)	16 (22.9)	70 (100)
	(%)	(27.8)	(35.0)	(45.5)	(39.1)	(35.9)
Total	N	79 (40.5)	20 (10.3)	55 (28.2)	41 (21.0)	195 (100)
	(%)	(100)	(100)	(100)	(100)	(100)

Interrater Agreement

The professionals engaged in the classification work were all highly familiar with *Dia-Gjessing* and the attendant dyslexia theory. The team consisted of school psychologists and special education staff with training and experience in diagnosing reading and writing difficulties.

Evaluation of interrater agreement was done by each of the two researchers independent of each other and of the school psychology team (SPT). They compared their classifications with those of the team. In other words, there were three categorization judgments for each child.

The percentages of overlap for the two researchers (HJG and HDN) and the school psychology team (SPT) were as follows: HJG $\times$ HDN = 93.4%, HJG $\times$ SPT = 62.1%, HDN $\times$ SPT = 62.1%, and HJG $\times$ HDN $\times$ SPT = 59.1%. This degree of correspondence seemed relatively good, especially in light of the kinds of differences that occurred, which consisted mostly of one using the category audiovisual while another used either auditory or visual. This correspondence was also analyzed statistically: The Chi-square test was applied to the three resultant 4×4 matrices, resulting in contingency coefficients C of .84 for HJG $\times$ HDN, .65 for HJG $\times$ SPT, and .66 for HDN $\times$ SPT. These three values were converted to estimated correlation coefficients of .97, .75, and .76, respectively, using $C_{max} = .866$.

These interrater agreements are quite satisfactory. They do, however, reveal some of the problem areas in differential diagnosis. One of these is the presence of symptoms of both auditory and visual dyslexia. According to Gjessing, such a case would be classified as auditory dyslexia because the symptoms of visual dyslexia are typically the result of extremely low achievement in reading and spelling and tend to disappear with improvements in the literacy skills. This particular phenomenon resulted in the two researchers making more use of the auditory dyslexia category than the SPT.

Another feature of the Gjessing dyslexia theory is that there is considerable overlap between the symptoms of visual and emotional dyslexia, especially in the area of oral reading characteristics. The SPT had better background information on the children studied than we did, since they had contacts with the teachers, the parents, and even the children themselves, the result was more children being classified as having emotional dyslexia by SPT and as having visual dyslexia by HJG and HDN.

The focus of this analysis was, of course, the interrater reliability of the diagnostic test battery. The data showed that it is possible, by means of this assessment, to uncover systematic patterns and differences among the pupils to the extent that they could be categorized with a fair degree of reliability. This approach is not the only one, and it may not even be the best. A statistical approach to the classification problem will be described later on in this chapter. First, we will look at the indirect variables described in the previous chapter and what they indicate about the dyslexia groups that were identified clinically.

Results of Indirect Variables and Diagnostic Test Scores
for the Four Dyslexia Groups

Individual Variables

The analyses described in the previous chapter were based on the total dyslexia sample of 195 children. The fact that some indirect variables were good predictors of reading and spelling scores does not necessarily mean that they would differentiate among the dyslexia types. Conversely, the fact that some indirect variables showed no significant correlation with literacy skills achievement does not preclude their being helpful in differentiating among dyslexia types.

The first step in this analysis was review the summary statistics for each indirect variable by dyslexia type, as shown in Table 11.2. The summary data from Dia-Gjessing are also included in this table, as are the data for 35 retarded pupils, for comparison purposes. The right column in Table 11.2 shows the results of tests of significance for pairs.

The variables were all quantified in such a way that a high score could be interpreted as better than a low score. Table 11.2 shows that, as a general trend, the lowest average scores were attained by either the auditory or the audiovisual dyslexics. The auditory and visual dyslexics differed significantly on three of the four Dia-Gjessing scores—spelling, oral reading, and total—as indicated by the 2 in the last column. Most of the differences related to audiolinguistic characteristics, which is, of course, consistent with the theory. However, most of the other variables also showed a difference between these two dyslexia types, although the differences were not always significant.

Two main factors appear to have influenced these group differences. First, the groups differed in mean total IQ, the auditory group's mean being 94.5 whereas the visual group's mean was 99.3. Second, the sex ratios for the two groups differed, the auditory group having a much higher percentage of boys. An analysis of covariance with WISC-Total IQ as covariate revealed that some of the differences changed somewhat when the effect of IQ was eliminated, but the differences that were significant to begin with were still there after the analysis of covariance. In this connection it is also illuminating to compare the dyslexia groups' data with those for the retarded children. Even though the auditory dyslexics had a much higher mean IQ, their mean word pronunciation score of 8.31 was significantly lower than the retarded mean of 8.82 ($p < .01$). This fact contributes to the notion that some of the variability among the dyslexia groups is of rather specific nature within the broader area of audiolinguistic functioning.

A stepwise discriminant analysis was carried out to determine which of the indirect variables discriminated most sharply between the groups with auditory and visual dyslexia (Dixon, 1983). Four such variables were found: melody reproduction, VADS Aural-Input, word pronunciation, and sounding out. All of these variables place heavy demands on audiolinguistic functioning.

TABLE 11.2. Summary data for direct and indirect variables for the four dyslexia groups and the general learning disability group (n = 181)

Characteristics	Variable	Type of dyslexia				Retarded group (n = 35)	Tests of significance[a]
		Auditory	Audiovisual	Visual	Other		
Direct							
Literacy skills	Dia-Spelling	2.30	2.88	3.89	3.14	3.09	2^b 3^b 4^b 5^b 8^c 9^b
	Dia-Oral reading	2.73	2.73	3.50	3.32	3.35	2^b
	Dia-Silent reading	3.07	2.54	3.25	3.37	3.20	
	Dia-Total	2.71	2.68	3.55	3.29	3.20	2^b 5^b
Indirect							
Scholastic aptitude	WISC-Verbal	92.70	96.50	97.30	93.20	84.30	4^c 7^b 9^b 10^c
	WISC-Performance	97.80	100.60	101.60	98.50	78.30	4^b 7^b 9^b 10^b
	WISC-Total	94.50	98.30	99.30	95.20	79.10	4^b 7^b 9^b 10^b
Perception and memory	Bender Gestalt[d]	4.60	4.90	4.90	5.20	3.06	4^b 7^c 9^b 10^b
	VADS Aural-Input	8.40	8.30	9.20	8.70	8.30	2^b 9^c
	VADS Visual-Input	9.20	9.70	9.80	9.30	8.90	0
	VADS Total	17.60	17.90	19.10	18.00	17.15	2^c 9^b
Oral language	Word pronunciation	8.31	7.85	9.58	9.18	8.82	2^b
	Melody reproduction	3.74	4.00	4.40	4.32	4.00	2^b 3^c
	Auditory discrimination	36.26	36.40	37.21	36.40	33.67	4^b 7^b 9^b 10^b
	Syntax	11.85	11.60	12.24	12.23	10.66	9^b 10^b
Laterality	Hand preference[e]	1.77	1.60	1.65	1.78	1.64	0
	Hand asymmetry	9.20	6.90	9.50	10.40	7.11	0
	Eye preference[e]	1.45	1.68	1.36	1.38	1.35	0
Self-image	Self-concept	37.40	38.80	39.30	38.93	37.67	0
Social factor	Parent occupation[f]	2.10	1.60	1.80	2.10	1.54	0
Teachers' classroom observations	Oral language reception	10.08	10.20	11.27	10.76	9.03	2^c 9^b
	Oral language expression	12.96	12.60	14.09	13.66	11.94	9^b
	Behavior	16.01	16.05	17.11	17.00	14.94	9^c
	Motor development	5.70	5.30	5.98	5.83	5.29	0

Diagnosticians' observations during testing with Dia-Gjessing	Approach to reading	2.55	2.44	3.20	3.13	2.73	0
	Sounding out	3.54	3.06	4.13	4.14	3.80	5[c]
	Speech: quantity	2.94	2.73	3.07	2.91	3.00	0
	Speech: quality	2.81	2.83	3.06	3.00	2.90	2[c]
	Articulation	2.73	3.06	2.98	3.06	2.84	2[b] 3[b]
	Personal interaction	2.07	1.61	2.05	1.88	2.07	0
	Achievement attitude	2.45	2.56	2.82	2.44	2.50	0
	Social contact	3.17	3.06	3.38	3.38	3.07	0
	Persistence	2.88	2.79	3.38	2.97	2.78	2[c] 9[b]
	Work adjustment	3.41	3.31	3.64	3.58	3.23	0
	Concentration	3.03	2.81	3.19	3.00	2.70	9[c]
Parents' observations reported during case history	Age of talking	2.58	2.94	3.06	3.03	2.87	2[b] 3[c]
	Headaches	2.81	2.80	2.73	2.77	2.77	0
	Sleep disturbances	2.73	2.80	2.70	2.81	2.85	0
	Restless sleep	2.90	3.00	2.90	2.84	2.78	0
	Poor appetite	2.79	2.73	2.82	2.90	2.81	0
	Stomachaches	2.81	2.87	2.70	2.81	2.89	0
	Enuresis: nocturnal	2.73	2.73	2.79	2.75	2.82	0
	Enuresis: diurnal	2.91	2.87	2.97	2.94	2.92	0

[a] The numerals indicate statistically significant differences between the following pairs of means:
1. Auditory dyslexia versus audiovisual dyslexia.
2. Auditory dyslexia versus visual dyslexia.
3. Auditory dyslexia versus rare forms of dyslexia.
4. Auditory dyslexia versus general learning disabilities.
5. Audiovisual dyslexia versus visual dyslexia.
6. Audiovisual dyslexia versus rare forms of dyslexia.
7. Audiovisual dyslexia versus general learning disabilities.
8. Visual dyslexia versus rare forms of dyslexia.
9. Visual dyslexia versus general learning disabilities.
10. Rare forms of dyslexia versus general learning disabilities.
[b] Significant at .01 level.
[c] Significant at .05 level.
[d] The numerical scale runs in the positive direction, so that a high score is better than a low score. The Bender scale goes from 0 to 8; 8 is a deviation score of 0.
[e] The hand and eye preference scale has three values: 0 = uncertain, 1 = leftsided, 2 = rightsided.
[f] Parent occupation was established at the beginning of schooling.

The difference in sex ratio between the two dyslexia groups would affect results for those variables that correlate with sex. These variables are WISC-Total ($r = -.20$), melody reproduction ($r = +.23$), auditory discrimination ($r = -.20$), and sounding out ($r = +.19$) (Table 10.1) (negative correlations mean that the boys obtained the higher scores). The sex differences were taken into consideration in the statistical analyses.

Interaction Among Variables

Some type of interaction analysis is implicit in any kind of clinical study in which one wants to determine if a child's unique strengths and weaknesses are symptomatic of a specific underlying deficit. Interaction analyses also play a central role in the statistical analyses of dyslexia.

The concept of interaction, as used in this study, is exemplified by the differences in sex ratio in auditory and visual dyslexia, a relatively uncomplicated phenomenon. The phenomenon becomes more complex as one views the relationship between sex ratio, type of dyslexia, and other variables, such as melody reproduction. The interaction between melody reproduction and certain dyslexia types is different for the two sexes. Another variant of this problem comes into play as one takes variables that are highly correlated into account. Is, for example, the correlation between reading and spelling the same for auditory dyslexia and visual dyslexia? Different correlations would indicate an interaction between dyslexia type and literacy skills. Some of these relationships are discussed in the next section.

Interaction Between Dyslexia Types and Sex for Some Indirect Variables

The auditory dyslexia group's mean auditory discrimination score was lower than the score for the visual dyslexia group. The girls scored lower than the boys on the same variable. This was also true of the WISC-R results. A two-way analysis of covariance with WISC-R as covariate revealed no significant difference between these two dyslexia groups, nor between boys and girls. Further, there was no interaction between sex and dyslexia type. In other words, the group differences with respect to auditory discrimination could be accounted for by the initial differences in WISC-R IQs.

The variable melody reproduction differentiated between the two dyslexia groups, the auditory dyslexia mean being the lower one, but the results were independent of sex. Nor was there any correlation with scholastic aptitude (WISC-R, Table 10.1). Table 11.3 summarizes the statistics by sex. Although there was a significant difference between boys and girls ($p < .05$) and between dyslexia groups ($p < .01$), there was no interaction (two-way analysis of variance). The visual dyslexia mean was higher than the auditory mean for both sexes, and the differences in both cases were larger for the boys than for the girls. There was, then, a slight sex difference between the two dyslexia groups with respect to melody reproduction, but the interaction was not significant. Melody

TABLE 11.3. Summary data for melody reproduction and sounding out for the auditory and visual dyslexia groups by sex ($n = 181$)

Variable	Sex	Auditory $\bar{X}$	Auditory SD	Visual $\bar{X}$	Visual SD	Statistical significance, p
Melody reproduction	Boys	3.59	1.08	4.25	0.68	Sex, < .05
						Dyslexia group, < .01
	Girls	4.11	0.88	4.59	0.50	Interaction, n.s.
	Boys	3.46 (3.45)[a]	1.33	4.05 (4.02)	1.36	Sex, n.s.
Sounding out						Dyslexia group, < .05
	Girls	3.74 (3.78)	1.28	4.32 (4.32)	0.89	Interaction, n.s.

[a] Means after correction for differences in scholastic aptitude (IQ).

reproduction does differentiate between auditory and visual dyslexia, especially for boys, but is independent of general ability (IQ).

The girls did better than the boys on the variable sounding out, a tendency to sound out words audibly during silent reading (Table 11.3). (A low value indicates much audible phonetization during silent reading.) The average for the visual dyslexics of both sexes was also significantly higher than the auditory average. There was, however, no significant interaction between type of dyslexia and sex.

These findings are quite consistent with our dyslexia theory. Difficulties or uncertainties with phonetic processing result in labored, excessive repetitions of sounds and word parts. In some cases this tendency is quite pronounced and loud (Gjessing, 1977).

Interaction Between Dyslexia Types and Literacy Skills

Table 11.2 shows that the auditory and audiovisual dyslexia groups obtained mean Dia scores below 3.0, whereas the other two dyslexia groups and the retarded group obtained averages above 3.0. The scholastic aptitude mean scores also varied, the auditory dyslexia group attaining the lowest average (WISC-R-Total = 94.5).

Table 10.1 showed rather high positive correlations between the Dia scores and results on the WISC-R for the total dyslexia sample. But relatively high Dia scores for the retarded group were interpreted to mean that low Dia scores suggest *specific* literacy skills disabilities rather than low scholastic aptitude. This conclusion was maintained even after correcting for differences in scholastic aptitude.

The Dia-Gjessing data for the four dyslexia groups, after correction for differences in mean IQ (WISC-R), are presented in Figure 11.1 The vertical scale shows the means on Dia-Gjessing. For all four dyslexia groups, but especially for

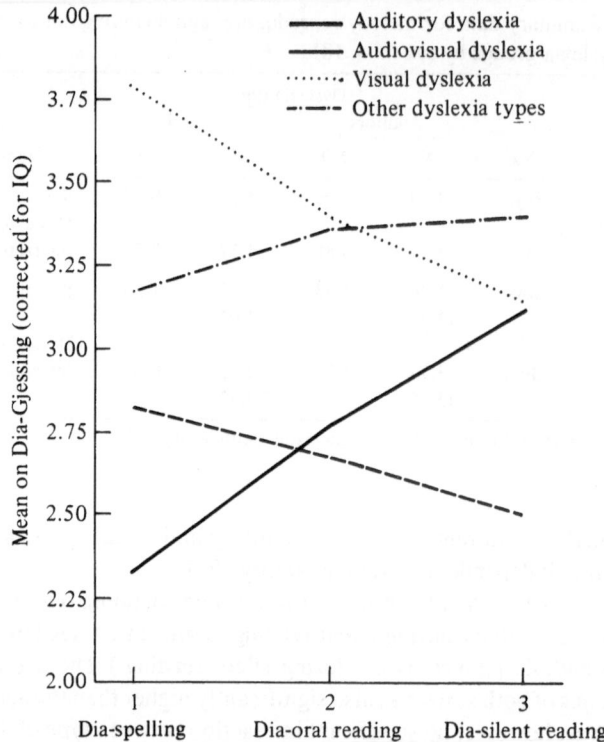

FIGURE 11.1. Mean achievement test profiles for the four dyslexia groups, corrected for differences in mean WISC (Wechsler Intelligence Scale for Children) IQs.

the three modality-related ones, there is a bigger difference between the scores for spelling and oral reading than between spelling and silent reading. The fourth group, other forms of dyslexia, has a much flatter profile, with only a slight difference between oral and silent reading.

The differences in level of achievement for spelling and reading are in opposite directions for auditory and visual dyslexia. This is quite consistent with the underlying theory. Two-way analyses of variance for repeated measures showed the interactions between the auditory and visual dyslexia groups to be significant. The auditory dyslexia group had lower scores in spelling than in silent reading, whereas the opposite pattern was true of the visual dyslexia group. There was also a significant interaction between the data for the auditory dyslexia group and those for the audiovisual group.

The total dyslexia sample showed no variability among the three Dia scores. But when the group was divided into subtypes, differences were clear-cut. An awareness of this tendency contributes much to an understanding of literacy skills processing and has considerable utility for diagnostic practice.

TABLE 11.4. WISC-R Verbal (VIQ) and Performance (PIQ) discrepancies for the four clinical dislexia groups

| | | Dyslexia group | | | | |
| | | Auditory | Audiovisual | Visual | Others | Total |
Discrepancy						
VIQ < PIQ	N	44	11	38	23	116
	%	62.0	61.1	71.7	65.7	65.5
VIQ > PIQ	N	27	7	15	12	61
	%	38.0	38.9	28.3	34.3	34.5
Total	N	71	18	53	35	177
	%	100	100	100	100	100

Interaction Between Dyslexia Types and WISC-R

For the total dyslexia sample, the mean WISC-Verbal IQ was lower than the mean Performance IQ (discrepancy 4.5 IQ points). The mean Verbal minus mean Performance IQ for each of the four dyslexia groups was as follows: auditory, -5.1; audiovisual, -4.1; visual, -4.3; other forms, -5.3, (Table 11.2). These differences are quite similar, and they are all in the same direction. A two-way analysis of variance for correlated (repeated) measures showed no significant interaction between dyslexia types and WISC IQ scores. Although the trend was for the mean Verbal IQ to be lower than the mean Performance IQ, about one third (34.5%) of the pupils had a higher verbal IQ, as shown in Table 11.4.

It has been suggested that a preponderance of pupils with auditory dyslexia should have lower verbal IQ than Performance IQ, while the opposite should hold true for visual dyslexia (Hynd & Cohen, 1983). This may be a reasonable speculation, but we need to test it in a representative sample of dyslexics. This notion is not supported by the Bergen data: about two thirds of the pupils in all four dyslexia groups had higher performance IQs. In fact, this tendency was even more pronounced among visual dyslexics—71.7% had a higher performance IQ. Additional analyses, counting only pupils with a discrepancy between the two IQs of at least 10 points, yielded essentially the same results.

Bannatyne (1971) has suggested that the WISC subtests should be grouped into three categories for the study of children with learning disabilities:

Spatial: Block design, object assembly, and picture completion.
Conceptual: Vocabulary, similarities, and comprehension.
Sequential: Digit span, coding, and picture arrangement.

Bannatyne claimed that children with what he called "genetic dyslexia" obtain the highest scores in the spatial area and the lowest in the sequential tests.

Table 11.5 shows the means for the four dyslexia groups in each of these three sets of WISC subtests. We subjected Bannatyne's approach to considerable statistical analysis, which will not be detailed here. Suffice it to say that his pro-

TABLE 11.5. Summary data for the three-way split of the WISC subtests for the four clinical dyslexia groups ($n = 181$)

	WISC category					
Dyslexia group	Spatial		Conceptual		Sequential	
	$\bar{X}$	s	$\bar{X}$	s	$\bar{X}$	s
Auditory	9.82	2.13	9.36	2.74	9.02	1.92
Audiovisual	10.19	1.94	9.72	1.60	8.59	1.49
Visual	10.45	1.82	9.83	2.14	9.60	2.15
Other	9.91	2.28	8.98	1.83	9.35	2.02
Total	10.05	2.08	9.45	2.33	9.20	2.00

file for genetic dyslexics appears to be common to all four dyslexia types. Similar findings are also reported by Rugel (1974a).

Interaction Between Dyslexia Types and Bender Gestalt and VADS Variables

The summary statistics for the four dyslexia groups on the Bender Gestalt test and VADS are shown in Table 11.2. The slight variation in the Bender Gestalt test means virtually disappeared when the means were corrected for differences in WICS-Total IQ.

The auditory dyslexia mean for VADS was significantly lower than the visual dyslexia mean on the subscores Aural-Input and VADS Total (Table 11.2). These differences were primarily the result of the large difference between these two groups on the subtest Aural-Written. But the American as well as the Norwegian normative data show the subtest Aural-Written to be the most difficult.

Further analysis of the Bergen VADS data showed that any summary score that contained the Aural-Written subtest differentiated among the dyslexia groups. The data for the four dyslexia groups are plotted in Figure 11.2.

Table 11.2 shows that the auditory dyslexia average was lower than the visual dyslexia average for Aural-Input and Visual-Input. A two-way analysis of variance for correlated measures, using WISC-Total IQ as covariate, showed no interaction. We concluded that the division of the VADS scores into Aural-Input and Visual-Input had no value for the differential diagnosis of auditory and visual dyslexia as defined in the Bergen model.

Dyslexia and Laterality

Probably no nonreading characteristic has been subjected to more study in learning disabilities than laterality. At first the research dealt with handedness, then eyedness, then mixed dominance, then footedness and earedness and all the different combinations. In recent years there has been a renewed interest in earedness with the development of dichotic listening tests. No attempts will be

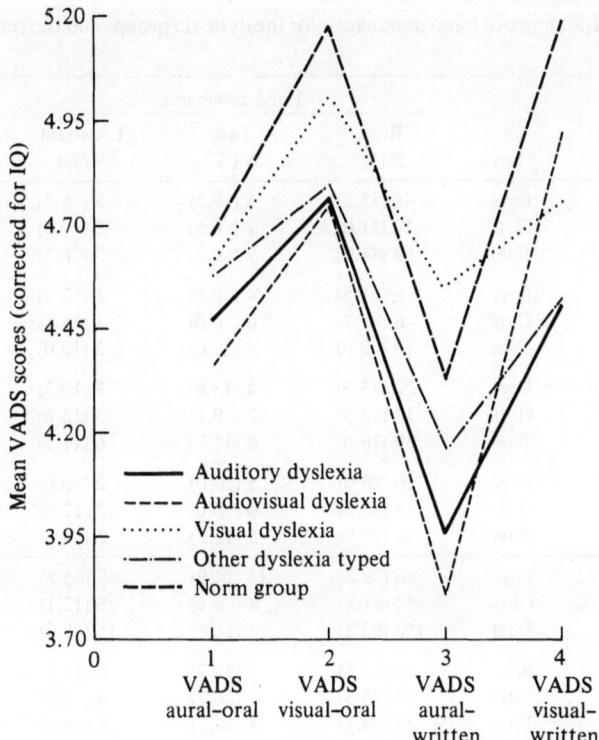

FIGURE 11.2. Mean VADS (Visual Aural Digit Span Test) profiles for the four dyslexia groups and the norm group.

made here to review this enormous literature. Since some researchers (Geschwind, 1983; Klasen, 1972; Malmquist, 1969) had reported higher incidences of left-handedness and mixed eye-hand dominance in reading disability cases, and since left-handedness and mixed dominance were presumed by Gjessing (1977) to be related to visual dyslexia, data were collected in the Bergen Project on these characteristics.

The handedness data are presented in Table 11.6. The incidence of left-handedness in visual dyslexia (11.7%) was slightly above that of auditory dyslexia (9.3%). The difference was even more pronounced for boys, which was also true for the entire dyslexia sample. The incidence of left-handedness for the retarded children (24.2%) was, however, twice that for the dyslexia group (11.8%).

Mixed eye-hand dominance was also analyzed in considerable detail (Table 11.7). In the visual dyslexia group, 48% of the cases had the same laterality for hand and eye, while this percentage was over 50% for each of the other three dyslexia groups. There appears, then, to be a somewhat higher incidence of mixed and unclear eye-hand laterality in visual dyslexia.

TABLE 11.6. Incidence of hand dominance for the dyslexia groups and the retarded, by sex (n ½ 220)

| Group | Sex | Hand dominance | | | Total |
		Right N (%)	Left N (%)	Uncertain N (%)	N (%)
Auditory	Boys	46 (85.2)	5 (9.3)	3 (5.5)	54 (100.0)
dyslexia	Girls	17 (81.0)	2 (9.5)	2 (9.5)	21 (100.0)
	Total	63 (84.0)	7 (9.3)	5 (6.7)	75 (100.0)
Audiovisual	Boys	8 (61.5)	4 (30.8)	1 (7.7)	13 (100.0)
dyslexia	Girls	6 (85.7)	0 (0.0)	1 (14.3)	7 (100.0)
	Total	14 (70.0)	4 (20.0)	2 (10.0)	20 (100.0)
Visual dyslexia	Boys	22 (75.9)	4 (13.8)	3 (10.3)	29 (100.0)
	Girls	17 (77.3)	2 (9.1)	3 (13.6)	22 (100.0)
	Total	39 (76.6)	6 (11.7)	6 (11.7)	51 (100.0)
Other types of	Boys	20 (80.0)	5 (20.0)	0 (0.0)	25 (100.0)
dyslexia	Girls	14 (87.5)	0 (0.0)	2 (12.5)	16 (100.0)
	Total	34 (82.9)	5 (12.2)	2 (4.9)	41 (100.0)
Total dyslexia	Boys	96 (79.3)	18 (14.9)	7 (5.8)	121 (100.0)
sample	Girls	54 (81.8)	4 (6.1)	8 (12.1)	66 (100.0)
	Total	150 (80.2)	22 (11.8)	15 (8.0)	187 (100.0)
Retarded	Boys	12 (66.7)	4 (22.2)	2 (11.1)	18 (100.0)
group	Girls	11 (73.3)	4 (26.7)	0 (0.0)	15 (100.0)
	Total	23 (69.7)	8 (24.2)	2 (6.1)	33 (100.0)

Summary of the Clinical Group Data

Analyses of the data so far in this chapter have dealt with dyslexia subgroups divided on the basis of clinical analyses and classifications and sometimes also according to sex. The interactions among literacy skills variables and nonreading variables have been of particular interest. These interactions did not appear in the analysis of data for the total dyslexia sample.

The first issue studied related to the reliability with which dyslexic children could be classified by independent raters. The interrater overlap ranged from 62 to 93%, depending on who did the categorizing.

The summary statistics for the four dyslexia groups were then compared across a number of direct and indirect variables. In the areas of spelling and oral reading, the visual dyslexia group outscored the auditory and the audiovisual groups. There was also a significant interaction between spelling and oral reading for the two auditory and visual dyslexia groups. The visual group did better in spelling than in silent reading, whereas the auditory group did the opposite. An understanding of relationships such as these is of importance to our understanding of literacy skills processing as well as to the diagnosis of reading and spelling difficulties.

TABLE 11.7. Mixed dominance: hand and eye dominance of the dyslexia groups and the retarded group (n = 215)

Laterality		Dyslexia Group				Retarded	Total
Hand	Eye	Auditory N (%)	Audiovisual N (%)	Visual N (%)	Other N (%)	N (%)	N (%)
Right	Right	39 (53.4)	10 (52.5)	20 (40.0)	20 (50.0)	13 (39.4)	102 (47.4)
	Left	15 (20.5)	3 (15.8)	17 (34.0)	6 (15.0)	8 (24.2)	49 (22.8)
	Uncertain	7 (9.6)	1 (5.3)	1 (20.0)	7 (17.5)	2 (6.1)	18 (8.4)
Left	Right	2 (2.7)	2 (10.5)	0 (0.0)	2 (5.0)	1 (3.0)	7 (3.3)
	Left	3 (4.1)	1 (5.3)	4 (8.0)	2 (5.0)	6 (18.2)	16 (7.4)
	Uncertain	2 (2.7)	0 (0.0)	2 (4.0)	1 (2.5)	1 (3.0)	6 (2.8)
Uncertain	Right	1 (1.4)	2 (10.6)	3 (6.0)	1 (2.5)	1 (3.0)	8 (3.7)
	Left	4 (5.5)	0 (5.5)	1 (2.0)	1 (2.5)	1 (3.0)	7 (3.3)
	Uncertain	0 (0.0)	0 (0.0)	2 (4.0)	0 (0.0)	0 (0.0)	2 (0.9)
Total		73 (100.0)	19 (100.0)	50 (100.0)	40 (100.0)	33 (100.0)	215 (100.0)

For the indirect variables, one finding was of particular interest: musical ability is of diagnostic significance. The test of melody reproduction was included because clinical experience with auditory dyslexics has shown that they have extreme difficulties with such a task (Gjessing, 1977). Further analysis of these data (Table 11.3) showed this to be particularly true of boys. This finding was independent of IQ. Children with auditory dyslexia also had greater problems than those with visual dyslexia with respect to several linguistic-phonological variables, such as word pronunciation, oral language reception, speech quality, and articulation (Table 11.2).

Dyslexia researchers around the world have been preoccupied with the analysis of WISC data. Our interest was in exploring the patterns of the three WISC IQ variables for the various dyslexia types and in studying Bannatyne's three-way classification of the WISC subtests. Although all dyslexia groups had mean verbal IQs that were 4 to 5 IQ points below the mean performance IQ, no group had a unique pattern for these mean IQs. This finding was contrary to expectations. The Bannatyne three-way categorization of subtests into conceptual, spatial, and sequential assessments did not yield any differential data for the dyslexia group as a whole or for the various dyslexia types.

Koppitz (1977) has raised considerable expectations for the differential diagnostic value of the VADS test. But only one of the VADS scores appeared to have some diagnostic utility—the Aural-Written test, on which the auditory dyslexia mean was significantly lower than the mean for visual dyslexia.

Laterality patterns were also explored, since it has often been assumed that left-handedness and mixed eye-hand dominance are associated with dyslexia to some extent; also, that left-handedness is particularly prevalent among dyslexic boys. These trends were found in the Bergen data, although they were not particularly strong. Mixed and uncertain dominance occurred slightly more often in visual dyslexia than in the other groups. There was a higher incidence of left-handedness, mixed, and uncertain dominance among the visual dyslexics compared with the auditory group, consistent with the underlying theory, but this was not a particularly strong tendency.

There was a very high incidence (24%) of left-handedness among the children with general learning disabilities. This is consistent with past research in mental retardation.

Subgrouping by Statistical Methods

Clinical Versus Statistical Grouping

As mentioned earlier, there are many similarities between clinical and statistical approaches to the systematic grouping of psychological variables or of people. Clinical analyses depend on hypotheses relating to the relationships among various human functions, hypotheses that are often based on practical clinical experiences in interpreting certain behaviors, symptoms, and signs.

Our own clinical analyses assumed that each diagnostician would be able to diagnose each pupil according to Gjessing's guidelines. The investigators had had enough clinical experience to be able to identify certain signs and symptoms and to see these in the total context of the individual child.

Whereas the clinical analysis made no reference to the total dyslexia sample, the statistical analysis used the total dyslexia group as the point of reference for each pupil. Since this sample consisted of every dyslexic child in an entire cohort, the cohort itself served as a norm group, and the entire dyslexia group served as a basic reference group.

The Basis for the Statistical Analyses

The statistically based subgrouping could be done by a Q-factor analysis or by cluster analysis. Mathematically, these approaches are identical to traditional factor analysis (R-factor analysis), which was used to analyze the diagnostic test (Dia-Gjessing). Traditional factor analysis uses correlations among variables within a group of people to determine which *variables* can be grouped together. Q-factor analysis uses correlations among people across a set of variables to determine which *people* can be grouped together.

A major problem with Q-factor analysis is the selection of variables. For dyslexic children the method demands, first, that the variables consist of a representative selection of the total set of variables that can contribute to differentiation among the children. Second, the number of variables should exceed the number of people involved (Gorsuch, 1983; Nunally, 1967). These demands are hard to comply with. We decided that meaningful results could be obtained even though the data base did not fulfill these demands. Other dyslexia studies have made the same assumption (e.g., Doehring & Hoshko, 1977; Lundberg, 1983).

The cluster technique used was based on euclidian distance (Dixon et al., 1983). This method appeared suitable for the analysis of profile similarities (Nunally, 1967). The possibilities of fitting individual pupil profiles into a certain pupil group will generally increase as the number of variables increases. Within the context of cluster analysis, this means that the number of geometric dimensions increases. One, two, or three variables correspond to one-, two-, or three-dimensional space. Although this is hard to visualize, it causes no problems mathematically.

Q-factor analysis and cluster analysis could both affect the *number* of pupil groups that get formed. In this respect there is similarity to the clinical approach, which ordinarily starts with a predetermined number of groups.

Some Preliminary Statistical Analyses

Some rather extensive preliminary statistical analyses were carried out to evaluate how these two statistical methods related to the clinical analyses with respect to the clinical groups that were formed. Space limitations prevent going into these analyses in detail; they will be summarized briefly.

By keeping the number of factors (groups) in the Q-factor analysis to three, we found that each factor represented two "mirror groups"; that is, each group consisted of children with plus loading and children with minus loading. The three factors, therefore, represented six pupil groups. In addition, a seventh group of pupils turned out to have very low loadings in either direction on all factors.

The cluster analysis used (Engleman & Harligan, 1983) necessitated the formation of 11 separate groups, in order to keep any group size from being excessively large.

The preliminary analyses showed, first, that the two statistical grouping methods, Q-factor analysis and cluster analysis, resulted in groups that overlapped to an appreciable degree. Second, the statistically based groups also overlapped with the clinically selected groups. Further, the preponderance of pupils in each of the statistical groups belonged to either the auditory or the visual clinical groups. The statistically based groups appeared to consist of children whose main learning disability could be described as auditory or visual dyslexia. In comparison with the clinical analysis, the two statistical approaches yielded fairly similar results.

The Final Statistical Grouping

After various preliminary statistics had been carried out, a final analysis was done of the 74 variables that had been taken into consideration in the clinical analyses.

Because of the magnitude of the data base and space limitations here, the results of the cluster analysis will not be reported, only the comparison between the clinical grouping and the Q-factor analysis. This seems reasonable, since the preliminary data indicated that the two factor analyses yielded fairly similar results.

Three factors were defined in the final Q-factor analysis. As mentioned, each represented two contrasting groups, a plus-loading and a minus-loading group. These, then, accounted for six pupil groups.

Around 40 children showed loadings on two or more factors; in some cases the difference between the loadings was quite small. Taking a cue from the emphasis on polythetic principles from the clinical groupings, we interpreted this to mean that these children had one set of characteristics in common with one group and another set in common with another group. The children were placed in the group for which they had the highest loading. Children whose factor loadings were below .20 on all six factors were separated out as a seventh group of 30 children.

The sizes of the groups were as follows:

Factor I: 26 and 40
Factor II: 22 and 25
Factor III: 13 and 25
Seventh group: 30 Total: 181
(Fourteen of the original sample of 195 were left out because of missing data.)

TABLE 11.8. Summary data of scholastic aptitude scores (group IQ) in grade 1+2 for the seven groups identified by the Q-factor analysis ($n = 181$)

Q-factor group (loading)	Mean, z	Standard deviation, r	N
I-minus	−1.01	0.75	26
I-plus	−0.04	0.69	40
II-minus	−0.44	0.80	22
II-plus	−0.38	0.88	25
III-minus	−0.69	0.86	13
III-plus	−0.43	0.74	25
Residual	−0.38	0.72	30
Total	−0.43	0.81	181

To provide some descriptive information about these seven groups, their mean ability test results were calculated using the entire cohort of over 3,000 as the norm group, which had a mean of $z = 0$ and a standard deviation (SD) of 1.0. These summary statistics for the seven groups are given in Table 11.8.

Group 1 (factor I-minus) had the lowest mean of −1.01, while group 2 (factor I-plus) had the highest mean, −0.04, a difference that was significant ($p < .01$ from one-way analysis of variance). The remaining groups had means that varied somewhat, from −0.38 to −0.69. As can be seen from the relatively small standard deviations, each group was fairly homogeneous.

The school ability test results were not utilized in the Q-factor analysis, so they did not influence group membership. But all subsequent analyses entailed variables that correlated to varying degrees with school ability. The differences in school ability among these seven groups were therefore corrected, so that no group differences could be attributed to the differences in IQ.

The Q-Factor Groups: Characteristics on the Direct and Indirect Variables

Once the seven Q-factor groups had been identified, it was possible to describe them in relation to the indirect variables, to the factor analysis results described in Chapter 9, to the clinical groupings, and of course to the dyslexia model. There were thus detailed descriptions of each group, descriptions that made it possible to clarify some of the nuances of the various dyslexia types and even refine the clinical typology. The sex ratios for the various groups are also reported, since they varied quite a bit.

Q-Factor I

Figure 11.3 shows the profiles of the two groups identified by the first factor in the Q-factor analysis. This figure was drawn on the basis of the same principles

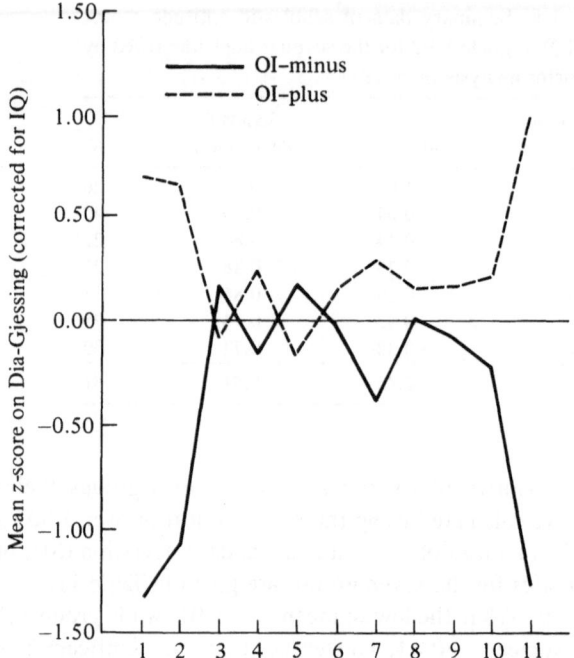

1. Complex phonological functions   7. Reversals
2. Phonological cluster functions   8. Attentiveness
3. Phonological assimilation   9. Orthographic speed
4. Orthographic error detection   10. Phonological dependence
5. Severe reading problems   11. Complex orthographic functions
6. Semantic literacy functions

FIGURE 11.3. Direct variables profiles for the Q-factor groups I-minus and II-minus.

used in Figure 9.2. The variables that related most strongly to the phonological (analytical) functions were placed on the left side, while the factors relating most strongly to the orthographic (configurational) functions are on the far right side of the figure. The means for the total dyslexia sample on these 11 variables are represented by the horizontal zero line ($z = 0$). These two profiles appear to mirror each other around this line. But tests of significance revealed that of the 11 variables, the groups differed significantly on only four: 1, complex phonological functions; 2, phonological cluster functions, 7, reversals, and 11, complex orthographic functions.

Group QI-Minus

The group whose profile is drawn with a solid line in Figure 11.3 consists of the pupils with a minus loading on Q-factor I. This group is characterized by extremely low scores on variables 1, 2, and 11, which represent factors I, VI, and

II in the R-factor analysis described in Chapter 9. These relate to some very central reading and spelling functions in both the phonological and the orthographic areas. Variable 11 was placed last because it represents orthographic (visual) functions very strongly. But the functions tapped by this variable are quite complex for the grade level at which these data were obtained. This notion is supported by the fact that it also has a loading in the phonological area, although to a lesser degree. Variable 11 appears to represent a more global function that relates to phonological as well as orthographic abilities.

Extreme weaknesses at both ends of this profile would most likely suggest audiovisual dyslexia, but a closer look at the data and their interrelationships suggests a different interpretation. In the primary grades one often finds pupils who have difficulties in both of these main areas without having audiovisual dyslexia. The symptoms are more likely the result of lack of experience in reading and writing. It has been our experience that over time the visual, configurational difficulties disappear while the audiophonetic problems persist. Such a pattern, then, suggests auditory dyslexia. A variety of relationships supports this conclusion. Low scholastic aptitude contributes little to reading experiences or the development of reading interests. The mean aptitude (IQ) score for this group was the lowest for all seven groups, being about 1 standard deviation ($z = -1.01$) below the cohort mean, which is extremely low. (See Table 11.8.)

Table 11.9 gives the results of the standardized reading and spelling group tests for the seven groups. This table shows that the QI-minus group also obtained the lowest mean scores on these two tests. In other words, the QI-minus group deviated quite markedly below the remaining dyslexia groups with respect to ability as well as achievement.

The sex ratios for the Q-factor groups are shown in Table 11.10. Again, they varied among the different groups. Since the boy/girl ratio was 1.7:1 in the total dyslexia sample, the ratios in Table 11.10 were corrected by this amount, to be able to compare the sex ratios for the various Q-factor groups with those for the total sample. The corrected QI-minus group's ratio was 1.3:1, a higher proportion of boys than in the total sample.

TABLE 11.9. Mean achievement test scores in reading and spelling for grades 1+2 for the seven groups identified by the Q-factor analysis ($n = 181$)

Q-factor group	$\bar{z}$: Reading	$\bar{z}$: Spelling
I-minus	−1.65 (−1.58*)	−3.43 (−3.22)[a]
I-plus	−1.21 (−1.26)	−1.13 (−1.27)
II-minus	−1.15 (−1.15)	−2.35 (−2.34)
II-plus	−1.45 (−1.45)	−1.45 (−1.46)
III-minus	−1.43 (−1.42)	−1.99 (−1.94)
III-plus	−1.39 (−1.39)	−1.87 (−1.86)
Residual	−1.42 (−1.43)	−2.22 (−2.23)

[a] Means after correction for differences in scholastic aptitude (IQ).

TABLE 11.10. Distribution of the dyslexia sample by Q-factor group and sex (n = 181)

Sex	Q-I		Q-II		Q-III			Total
	Minus N (%)	Plus N (%)	Minus N (%)	Plus N (%)	Minus N (%)	Plus N (%)	Residual N (%)	N (%)
Boys	18 (15.8)	24 (21.1)	12 (10.5)	12 (10.5)	10 (8.8)	17 (14.9)	21 (18.4)	114 (100)
Girls	8 (11.9)	16 (23.9)	10 (14.9)	13 (19.4)	3 (4.5)	8 (11.9)	9 (13.4)	67 (100)
Total	26	40	22	25	13	25	30	181
B/G ratio	2.3:1	1.5:1	1.2:1	0.9:1	3.3:1	2.1:1	2.3:1	1.7:1
(Corrected[a])	(1.3:1)	(0.9:1)	(0.7:1)	(0.54:1)	(2.0:1)	(1.2:1)	(1.4:1)	(1.00:1)

[a] Corrected for the uneven distribution by sex in the total sample.

TABLE 11.11. Summary data for indirect variables for the seven Q-factor groups covering the main indirect variables ($n = 181$).

Characteristics	Variable	Q-factor group													Test of significance[a]
		I-minus		I-plus		II-minus		II-plus		III-minus		III-plus		Residual		
		X	SD	X	SD	X	SD	X	SD	X	SD	X	SD	X	SD	
Direct	Dia-Spelling	1.51	0.31	4.24	0.74	2.59	0.80	3.52	0.81	2.69	1.29	2.86	0.70	2.71	0.85	1-3,5-12,18
		(1.69)		(4.11)		(2.60)		(3.51)		(2.84)		(2.87)		(2.71)		
Literacy skills	Dia-Oral reading	1.36	0.46	4.34	0.56	3.51	1.29	2.46	0.84	2.70	1.41	3.08	0.67	3.00	1.05	1-3,5-6, 8-11
		(1.44)		(4.29)		(3.52)		(2.46)		(2.86)		(3.08)		(3.00)		
	Dia-Silent reading	1.81	0.48	4.60	0.88	3.97	1.20	2.13	0.45	2.80	1.34	2.73	0.81	2.66	0.99	1-2,5-6,8- 12,14-15
		(1.94)		(4.52)		(3.98)		(2.12)		(2.94)		(2.73)		(2.65)		
	Dia-Total	1.53	0.31	4.38	0.46	3.32	0.97	2.70	0.56	2.76	1.31	2.91	0.57	2.84	0.76	1-3,5-11
		(1.66)		(4.30)		(3.33)		(2.70)		(2.92)		(2.91)		(2.84)		
Indirect Perception and memory	Bender Gestalt	4.0	1.88	5.7	1.69	4.7	2.15	4.4	2.17	4.6	2.11	4.8	2.35	5.0	1.52	1
		(4.42)		(5.48)		(6.69)		(4.22)		(4.78)		(4.76)		(4.97)		
	VADS Aural-Input	8.3	1.38	9.0	1.41	8.5	1.26	9.4	1.37	8.8	1.09	8.5	1.30	8.2	1.16	18
		(8.62)		(8.84)		(8.51)		(9.35)		(8.88)		(8.52)		(8.13)		
	VADS Visual-Input	8.3	1.38	10.2	1.52	9.1	1.21	9.7	1.61	9.9	1.32	9.2	1.20	9.5	1.28	1,4
		(8.58)		(10.10)		(9.14)		(9.72)		(10.03)		(9.24)		(9.45)		
	VADS-Total	16.7	2.51	19.2	2.51	17.6	1.94	19.1	2.76	18.7	2.06	17.7	2.11	17.7	1.92	1
		(17.20)		(18.93)		(17.65)		(19.06)		(18.91)		(17.76)		(17.58)		
	Word pronunciation	7.56	2.58	9.65	1.90	8.43	2.42	9.29	1.71	9.00	2.65	8.64	1.38	8.35	2.79	1
		(8.08)		(9.34)		(8.39)		(9.27)		(9.23)		(8.66)		(8.24)		
Oral language	Melody reproduction	4.08	1.06	4.14	1.03	3.90	0.97	4.38	0.67	4.17	0.84	4.04	0.93	4.04	1.02	0
		(4.13)		(4.11)		(3.90)		(4.38)		(4.19)		(4.04)		(4.03)		
	Auditory discrimination	35.72	2.54	36.88	3.01	35.64	3.06	37.39	2.39	37.18	1.66	37.04	2.09	36.23	2.69	0
		(36.27)		(36.54)		(35.66)		(37.42)		(37.28)		(37.06)		(36.11)		
	Syntax	11.16	2.27	12.50	0.72	12.15	1.04	12.21	1.06	12.08	1.24	11.72	2.26	12.04		1.22
		(11.47)		(12.32)		(12.15)		(12.19)		(12.20)		(11.73)		(11.97)		

TABLE 11.11. *Continued*

Characteristics	Variable	Q-factor group													Test of significance[a]
		I-minus		I-plus		II-minus		II-plus		III-minus		III-plus		Residual		
		X	SD	X	SD	X	SD	X	SD	X	SD	X	SD	X	SD	
Laterality	Hand preference	1.85	0.43	1.65	0.72	1.43	0.81	1.76	0.44	1.91	0.30	1.60	0.71	1.79	0.57	0
	Hand asymmetry	8.5	11.3	11.2	9.7	12.1	10.2	5.3	8.8	7.6	6.9	9.7	10.8	10.6	14.3	0
		(8.34)		(11.28)		(12.11)		(5.34)		(7.59)		(9.72)		(10.60)		8,12
	Eye preference	1.48	0.82	1.42	0.69	1.29	0.64	1.40	0.76	1.40	0.79	1.65	0.49	1.46	0.74	0
Self-image	Self-concept	37.39	9.61	38.74	10.25	35.18	10.18	37.30	11.40	36.08	10.88	41.52	10.33	39.97	10.34	0
		(36.59)		(39.26)		(35.19)		(37.45)		(35.72)		(41.54)		(39.99)		
Social factor	Parent occupation	1.74	0.99	2.19	1.06	2.50	1.2	1.65	0.70	2.16	1.84	1.63	0.62	2.13	1.25	0
		(2.03)		(2.03)		(2.45)		(1.67)		(2.34)		(1.56)		(2.09)		
	Oral language reception	8.73	1.97	12.03	2.14	9.77	3.12	10.32	1.88	10.9	2.4	11.12	2.39	10.2	1.65	1,5,8,11
		(9.36)		(11.61)		(9.79)		(10.28)		(11.21)		(10.86)		(10.19)		
Teachers' classroom observations	Oral language expression	12.08	2.56	14.13	2.29	12.41	3.53	13.32	2.75	14.15	3.44	14.68	2.59	13.07	1.93	1,5
		(12.63)		(13.77)		(12.43)		(13.28)		(14.40)		(14.41)		(13.03)		
	Behavior	14.65	1.93	17.73	2.01	16.73	3.01	16.36	2.61	16.77	3.22	17.04	2.57	16.23	2.11	1,5
		(15.41)		(17.25)		(16.75)		(16.31)		(17.10)		(16.73)		(16.18)		
	Motor development	5.44		6.08		5.77		5.64		5.69		6.00		5.47		
		(5.61)		(5.96)		(5.78)		(5.63)		(5.77)		(5.99)		(5.45)		
Diagnosticians' observations during testing with Dia-Gjessing	Approach to reading	1.38	0.74	4.03	1.74	3.74	1.82	2.35	1.35	2.90	1.73	2.28	1.02	2.46	1.45	1–2,6,8,10–11
		(1.58)		(3.92)		(3.76)		(2.35)		(2.92)		(2.22)		(2.44)		
	Sounding out	3.33	1.49	4.47	1.16	3.58	1.35	4.04	1.15	4.18	1.47	3.36	1,18	3.35	1,23	1,10,11
		(3.32)		(4.48)		(3.58)		(4.04)		(4.17)		(3.37)		(3.35)		
	Speech: quantity	2.82	0.59	3.00	0.59	3.00	0.75	2.72	0.96	3.40	0.84	2.88	0.85	2.92	0.78	0

	1	2	3	4	5	6	7	
Speech: quality	2.61 0.50 (2.72)	3.05 0.33 (2.98)	2.77 0.44 (2.77)	2.94 0.42 (2.94)	3.18 0.75 (3.22)	2.96 0.37 (2.95)	3.00 0.49 (2.99)	1
Articulation	2.82 0.40 (2.89)	3.00 0.33 (2.95)	2.74 0.56 (2.73)	2.96 0.21 (2.96)	2.82 0.41 (2.85)	3.00 0.32 (3.01)	2.96 0.46 (2.94)	0
Personal interaction	1.64 0.58 (1.72)	2.18 0.63 (2.12)	2.27 0.96 (2.28)	1.67 0.58 (1.68)	1.88 0.84 (1.90)	2.06 0.43 (2.03)	2.00 0.62 (1.99)	1
Achievement attitude	2.05 0.69 (2.19)	2.91 0.68 (2.81)	2.73 0.70 (2.75)	2.75 0.64 (2.77)	2.36 0.51 (2.39)	2.60 0.60 (2.58)	2.27 0.63 (2.27)	1,3,11
Social contact	3.00 0.55	3.41 0.86	3.33 0.49	3.16 0.60	3.78 0.83	3.10 0.63	3.27 0.72	0
Persistence	2.60 0.75 (2.80)	3.50 0.75 (3.36)	2.88 0.70 (2.90)	3.25 0.64 (3.28)	2.50 1.00 (2.56)	3.19 0.66 (3.17)	2.91 0.81 (2.88)	1,9
Work adjustment	3.40 0.82	3.74 0.69	3.50 0.61	3.62 0.67	3.46 0.69	3.42 0.77	3.37 0.79	0
Concentration	2.73 0.65 (2.82)	3.39 0.56 (3.33)	3.06 0.80 (3.06)	3.11 0.57 (3.11)	2.83 0.72 (2.87)	3.06 0.66 (3.05)	2.92 0.78 (2.91)	1
Parents' observations reported during case history								
Age of talking	2.68 0.90 (2.74)	2.92 0.74 (2.89)	2.53 0.70 (2.52)	3.00 0.60 (3.00)	2.83 1.03 (2.86)	3.00 0.78 (3.00)	2.82 0.77 (2.81)	0
Headaches	2.60 0.75	2.79 0.57	3.00 0.00	2.59 0.62	2.80 0.42	2.95 0.23	2.84 0.47	0
Sleep disturbances	2.85 0.37	2.86 0.45	2.59 0.71	2.69 0.70	2.40 0.97	2.95 0.22	2.72 0.61	0

TABLE 11.11. *Continued*

Characteristics	Variable	Q-factor group													Test of significance[a]
		I-minus		I-plus		II-minus		II-plus		III-minus		III-plus		Residual		
		X	SD	X	SD	X	SD	X	SD	X	SD	X	SD	X	SD	
Parents' observations (*continued*)	Restless sleep	2.90	0.45	2.82	0.55	3.00	0.00	2.88	0.33	2.80	0.63	2.90	0.31	2.96	0.20	0
	Poor appetite	2.85	0.37	2.93	0.26	2.88	0.34	2.63	0.62	2.80	0.63	2.80	0.53	2.75	0.53	0
	Stomachaches	2.76	0.54	2.86	0.35	2.69	0.70	2.61	0.50	2.90	0.32	2.85	0.49	2.79	0.51	0
	Enuresis: nocturnal	3.00	0.00	2.83	0.47	2.47	0.83	2.58	0.77	2.80	0.63	2.81	0.51	2.83	0.48	0
	Enuresis: diurnal	3.00	0.00	3.00	0.00	3.00	0.00	2.88	0.50	3.00	0.00	2.76	0.44	2.96	0.20	0

[a] Numerical code for the test of significance between pairs of Q-factor groups. The numerals indicate a statistically significant difference between the following pairs:
1. QI-minus versus QI-plus.
2. QI-minus versus QII-minus.
3. QI-minus versus QII-plus.
4. QI-minus versus QIII-minus.
5. QI-minus versus QIII-plus.
6. QI-minus versus residual group.
7. QI-plus versus QII-minus.
8. QI-plus versus QII-plus.
9. QI-plus versus QIII-minus.
10. QI-plus versus QIII-plus.
11. QI-plus versus residual group.
12. QII-minus versus QII-plus.
13. QII-minus versus QIII-minus.
14. QII-minus versus QIII-plus.
15. QII-minus versus residual group.
16. QII-plus versus QIII-minus.
17. QII-plus versus QIII-plus.
18. QII-plus versus residual group.
19. QIII-minus versus QIII-plus.
20. QIII-minus versus residual group.
21. QIII-plus versus residual group.

Table 11.11 shows the summary statistics for the achievement tests, including the means corrected for differences in mean WISC-Total IQs for the various groups. Here, again, the QI-minus group does particularly poorly across a variety of achievement variables, such as spelling, oral reading, word pronunciation, and listening comprehension (oral language reception). This group also scored low in syntax and sounding out. This pattern of low scores supports the notion of generalized audiophonological problems, that is, auditory dyslexia.

The WISC and VADS profiles for the QI groups are contrasted in Figure 11.4. The WISC profiles for both are the same as those for the entire dyslexia sample. The VADS profile, however, does show that the QI-minus group deviates markedly from the general trend. This group scored much higher on Aural-Oral than on the other three subtests. In contrast to the other subtests, Aural-Oral does not require any reading or writing, which are areas in which the QI-minus group did particularly poorly. This finding suggests good correspondence between VADS and other literacy skills variables.

The data from the indirect variables appear to support the earlier conclusion that the QI-minus group is a variant of auditory dyslexia, a group with severe reading and spelling difficulties and related audiolinguistic problems as well as low scholastic aptitude. These children have particularly poorly developed literacy skills in both phonological and orthographic areas in the primary grades.

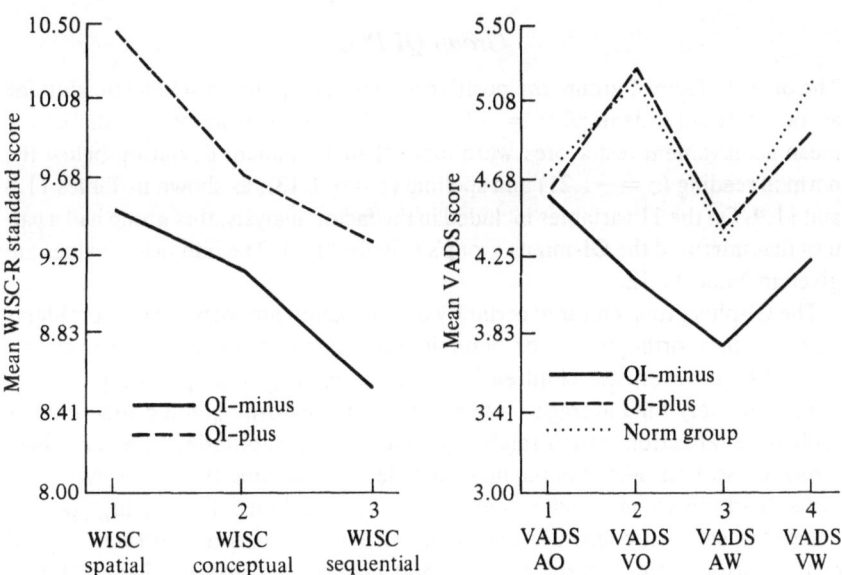

FIGURE 11.4. Mean profiles of the three-way split of the WISC (Wechsler Intelligence Scale for Children) subtests and the four VADS (Visual Aural Digit Span Test) subscores for the Q-factor groups I-minus and I-plus. AO, Aural-Oral; VO, Visual-Oral; AW, Aural-Written; VW, Visual-Written.

TABLE 11.12. Q-factor group mean scores on the 11 direct achievement variables identified in the R-factor analysis, corrected for initial mean differences in scholastic aptitude ($n = 181$)

Variables	Q-factor group						Residual
	I-minus	I-plus	II-minus	II-plus	III-minus	III-plus	
Complex phonological functions	−1.33	0.70	−0.38	0.50	−0.36	0.22	0.05
Phonological cluster functions	−1.07	0.66	−0.15	0.35	−0.22	0.27	−0.26
Phonological assimilation	0.17	−0.09	0.11	0.00	−0.29	0.10	−0.07
Orthographic error detection	−0.16	0.24	0.10	0.02	0.58	−0.58	−0.04
Severe reading problems	0.17	−0.17	0.26	0.02	0.49	0.09	−0.42
Semantic literacy functions	−0.03	0.15	−0.40	0.18	0.09	0.23	−0.26
Reversals	−0.39	0.29	−0.24	0.22	0.11	−0.10	−0.02
Attentiveness	0.01	0.16	−0.56	0.03	0.03	0.23	−0.04
Orthographic speed	−0.08	0.17	0.82	−0.82	−1.13	0.36	0.11
Phonological dependence	−0.22	0.21	0.40	0.12	0.41	−0.64	−0.12
Complex orthographic functions	−1.27	1.01	0.75	−0.59	0.15	−0.23	−0.19

Group QI-Plus

The other Q-factor I group, the positive loading group, had a scholastic aptitude average virtually identical ($\bar{z} = -0.04$) to the cohort mean of $z = 0$. But the mean achievement test scores were more than 1 standard deviation below the norm in reading ($z = -1.21$) and spelling ($z = -1.13$), as shown in Tables 11.8 and 11.9. On the 11 variables included in the factor analysis, this group had a pattern that mirrored the QI-minus group's (Figure 11.3). The numerical values are given in Table 11.12.

The QI-plus group children certainly do not exhibit any very serious problems with complex orthographic or phonological functions. Despite these relative strengths, however, the children have severe reading and spelling problems. Their relatively high average on factor 11, complex orthographic functions, is probably a reflection of their relatively high scholastic aptitude as well as of high scores on several other nonreading variables. At the time these data were collected (early in second grade), these children, with their relatively high performances in scholastic aptitude and their other desirable qualities such as good concentration, achievement attitude, and classroom behavior (Table 11.11), were able to compensate for their visuoorthographic weaknesses. As the demands for a sight vocabulary and reading speed increase with age, it is our opinion that their relative scores in variables 10, phonological dependence, and 11, complex orthographic functions, will gradually decline, making their pattern of scores consistent with a diagnosis of visual dyslexia.

Additional data relating to this group can be found in Table 11.10 and Figure 11.4. There were slightly more girls in this group than had been predicted from the sex ratio in the total dyslexia sample; this was also true of the clinical visual dyslexia group.

The data for the various language variables show the QI-plus group doing best on word pronunciation, syntax, listening comprehension, and sounding out. The children in the clinical visual dyslexia group also did particularly well on these variables, consistent with the underlying dyslexia theory.

This group's performance on WISC and VADS is shown in Figure 11.4. The WISC pattern was consistent with that of the total dyslexia sample, whereas the VADS profile coincided with that of the norm group.

In summary, the two Q-factor I groups appear to represent two different dyslexia syndromes, one visual and one auditory.

Q-Factor II

The two pupil groups selected by means of the second Q-factor also had profiles that were mirror images of each other. These profiles are shown in Figure 11.5. The profile drawn with a solid line represents the Q-factor group II-minus, while the dashed lines represent the Q-factor group II-plus. The predominant trend in these profiles is for the first group to have low scores on the left side of the profile and high scores on the right side, while the second group has the opposite pattern.

On the basis of the description of the 11 variables that make up these profiles, the immediate reaction would be that the first profile represents auditory dyslexia and that the second, group II-plus, represents visual dyslexia. The data in Table 11.8 show that these two groups were quite similar with respect to mean scholastic aptitude scores, with means of $\bar{z} = -0.44$ and $\bar{z} = -0.38$, a difference that was not statistically significant. But the results of the achievement tests in reading and spelling were quite different for the two groups (Table 11.9). These differences were consistent with our dyslexia theory, in that the pupils with auditory dyslexia had even lower scores in spelling than in reading.

Group QII-Minus

This group had its lowest scores on variables 1, 2, 6, 7, and 8, measuring complex phonological functions, phonological cluster functions, semantic literacy functions, reversals, and attentiveness. They scored highest on variables 9, 10, and 11, dealing with orthographic speed, phonological dependence, and complex orthographic functions. Of all the seven Q-factor groups, this group scored lowest on variables 6, semantic literacy functions, and 8, attentiveness, whereas it had the highest average on variable 9, orthographic speed. Group QII-minus appears, then, quite clearly to represent auditory dyslexia.

Among the indirect variables that could contribute to a better understanding of this group it would seem reasonable to focus on tests and observations relating to audiolinguistic functions. Table 11.11 shows that in comparison with the other six Q-factor groups, the II-minus group did particularly poorly in melody reproduction and articulation. In addition, they were rated relatively low in auditory

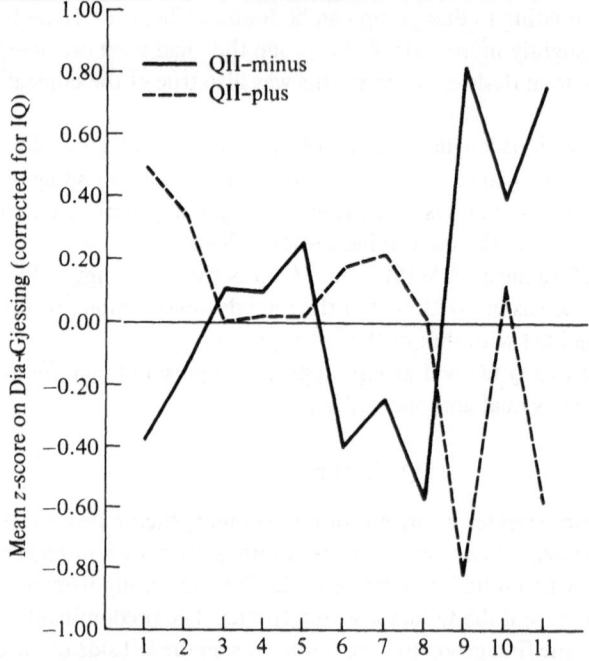

1. Complex phonological functions
2. Phonological cluster functions
3. Phonological assimilation
4. Orthographic error detection
5. Severe reading problems
6. Semantic literacy functions

7. Reversals
8. Attentiveness
9. Orthographic speed
10. Phonological dependence
11. Complex orthographic functions

FIGURE 11.5. Direct variables profiles for the Q-factor groups I-minus and II-plus.

discrimination, word pronunciation, oral language reception, oral language expression, and age of talking. These findings clearly support the notion that these pupils have problems primarily in the area of audiolinguistic functioning. This group also received very low ratings in persistence with respect to school work.

The results of WISC and VADS are shown in Figure 11.6, constructed the same as Figure 11.4. As can be seen, neither of these two instruments makes much of a contribution toward the differential diagnosis of these two groups.

Group QII-Plus

Group II-plus had a profile quite consistent with the theory relating to visual dyslexia, especially at the two ends of the profile. Its most extreme score was the low score on variable 9, orthographic speed. Extremely slow writing is quite typical of pupils with visual dyslexia, especially in the lower grades.

This group performed quite well on a variety of indirect variables relating to audiolinguistic functioning. Table 11.11 shows these factors to be word pronunci-

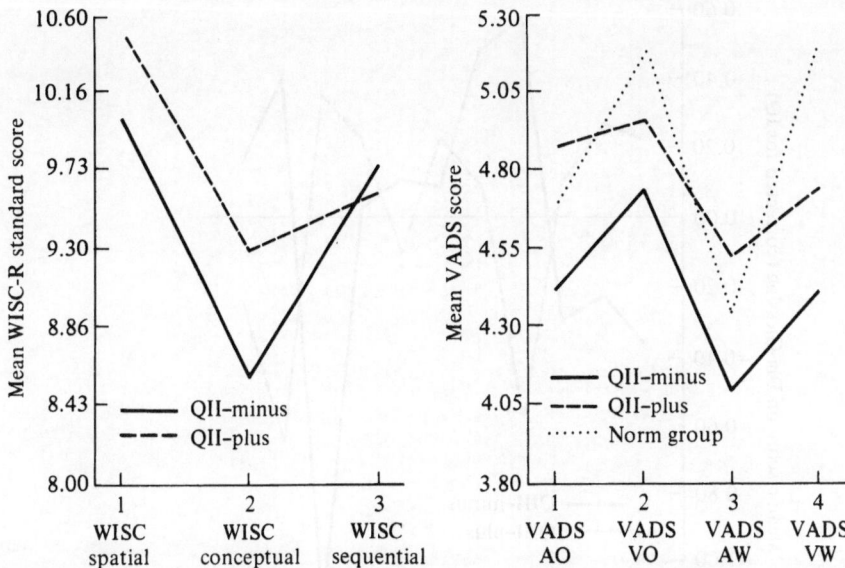

FIGURE 11.6. Mean profiles of the three-way split of the WISC (Wechsler Intelligence Scale for Children) subtests and the four VADS (Visual Aural Digit Span test) subscores for the Q-factor groups II-minus and II-plus.

ation, melody reproduction, auditory discrimination, syntax, articulation, and age of talking.

In summary, Q-factor II has identified two pupil groups of clearly different profiles across the 11 direct variables that came out of the R-factor analysis. The profiles of these two groups appear to be rather obvious examples of auditory and visual dyslexia, according to our clinical model.

Nevertheless, the group profiles did have some unique features. The II-minus group, auditory dyslexia, had relatively low means in the middle of the profile. This was particularly true of variables 6, semantic literacy functions; 7, reversals; and 8, attentiveness. On the other hand, this group had a particularly high score on 9, orthographic speed. The II-plus group, visual dyslexia, also deviated from the predicted profile by not scoring low on 7, reversals, and 10, phonological dependence.

Q-Factor III

Factor III in the Q-factor analysis also identified two groups with opposite profiles. Figure 11.7 shows the mean profiles over the 11 direct variables, the III-minus group being shown with a solid line and the III-plus group with a dashed line.

The two groups differed somewhat on mean scholastic aptitude, the III-minus group having a mean of $z = -0.69$ and the III-plus group a mean of $z = -0.43$, a difference that was not significant. The groups also differed very slightly on the reading test; both averaged lower in spelling than in reading.

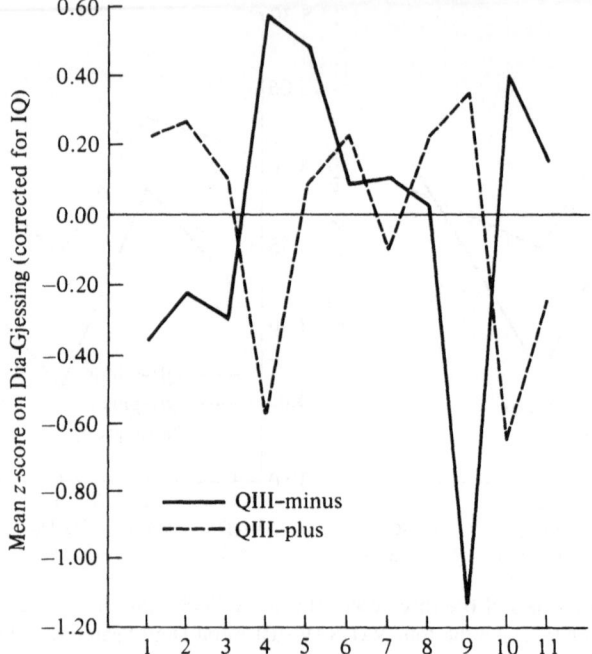

1. Complex phonological functions
2. Phonological cluster functions
3. Phonological assimilation
4. Orthographic error detection
5. Severe reading problems
6. Semantic literacy functions
7. Reversals
8. Attentiveness
9. Orthographic speed
10. Phonological dependence
11. Complex orthographic functions

FIGURE 11.7. Direct variables profiles for the Q-factor groups III-minus and III-plus.

By viewing the two variables at each end of the profile (1, 2, and 10, 11), it appears that again we have an auditory dyslexia group, the III-minus, and a visual dyslexia group, the III- plus.

Group QIII-Minus

The III-minus group had a rather pronounced profile. Three of the profile points were higher than for any other group. These high points covered orthographic error detection (variable 4), severe reading problem (5), and phonological dependence (10). This group also had two points that were the lowest of any group, orthographic speed (9) and phonological assimilation (3). The III-minus group, then, appears to have a profile that suggests some variant of auditory dyslexia, with the unique feature of extreme difficulties and slowness with writing and spelling.

The most distinctive aspect of the III-minus profile is, nevertheless, the weak phonological functions (1 and 2) and the strong visual functions (10 and 11).

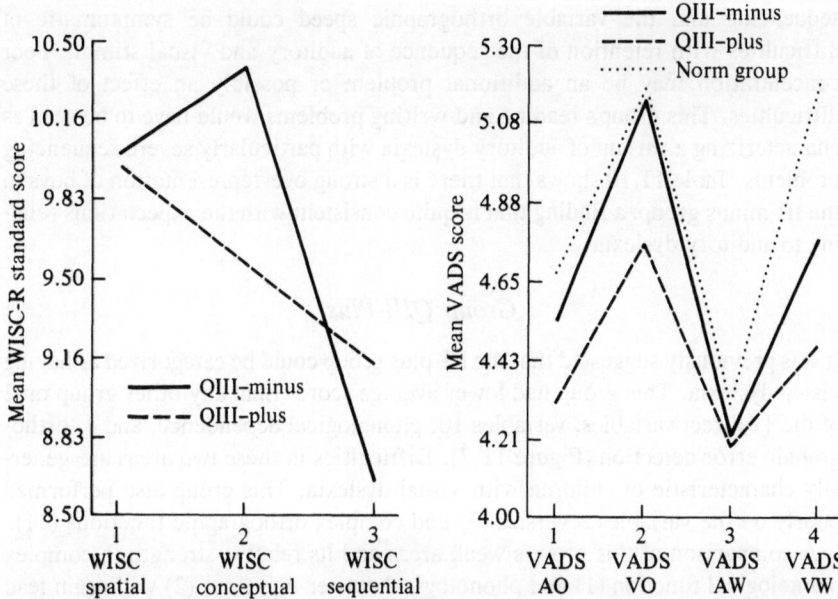

FIGURE 11.8. Mean profiles of the three-way split of the WISC (Wechsler Intelligence Scale for Children) subtests and the four VADS (Visual Aural Digit Span test) subscores for the Q-factor groups III-minus and III-plus. AO, Aural-Oral; VO, Visual-Oral; AW, Aural-Writing; VW, Visual-Writing.

With regard to the indirect variables, this group was the highest rated auditory group with respect to oral language variables (Table 11.11).

Figure 11.8 depicts the WISC and VADS profiles. Although the VADS data do not seem to provide additional insights into this group, the WISC results, viewed in conjunction with the data from the direct variables, appear to yield some interesting data. The III-minus group averaged above the norm of 10 in the conceptual area, the spatial average was at the norm, and the sequential score was markedly low. The sequential tests include the scales coding and arithmetic. These scales contain a significant speed factor, since they have time limits. In addition, the coding test requires quick spatial orientation, not too dissimilar from the letter and letter-combination identification involved in the variable orthographic speed, on which group III-minus received an especially low score. Both sets of tasks also require concentration on mental school tasks. This gets us back to the very low rating that the group received on the indirect variable concentration. The group also rated particularly low in persistence.

In the interpretation of the III-minus data there was considerable emphasis on the first three direct variables shown in Figure 11.7. These involved the assessment of phoneme-grapheme relationships, phonetic analysis and blending, consonant clusters, and the ability to read nonsense words. Difficulties in these areas reflect the problems just mentioned with regard to coding and orthographic speed. On the other hand, the problems reflected in the WISC category of sequencing and the variable orthographic speed could be symptomatic of difficulties with retention of the sequence of auditory and visual stimuli. Poor concentration may be an additional problem or possibly an effect of these difficulties. This group's reading and writing problems would have to be seen as characterizing a variant of auditory dyslexia with particularly severe sequencing problems. Table 11.10 shows that there is a strong overrepresentation of boys in the III-minus group, a finding that is quite consistent with the expectations relating to auditory dyslexia.

Group QIII-Plus

It was previously suggested that the III-plus group could be categorized as having visual dyslexia. This group had lower average scores than any other group on 2 of the 11 direct variables, variables 10, phonological dependence, and 4, orthographic error detection (Figure 11.7). Difficulties in these two areas are generally characteristic of children with visual dyslexia. This group also performed poorly on the variables reversals (7) and complex orthographic functions (11).

A comparison of this group's weak areas and its relative strength in complex phonological function (1) and phonological cluster functions (2) will again lead to the conclusion that this is a group of visual dyslexics. Although the children in this group exhibited most of the characteristics of visual dyslexia, they did surprisingly well on variable 9, orthographic speed, an area in which visual dyslexics tend to perform quite poorly.

Data from the indirect variables appear to provide little additional information of interest (Table 11.11 and Figure 11.8).

Residual Q-Group

The residual Q-group consisted of the dyslexic children who had the lowest loadings in the Q-factor analysis (no loadings above 0.20). This group's mean profile is shown in Figure 11.9. In comparison with the profiles of the previous six groups, this profile is quite flat. The biggest deviation was on variable 5, severe reading problems. This group's profile fits neither the auditory nor the visual dyslexia pattern. Our dyslexia theory suggests that this group represents the non-modality-related groups emotional dyslexia, educational dyslexia, and other rare forms of dyslexia.

As can be seen in Table 11.8, this group had the second highest mean scholastic aptitude score of all seven Q-factor groups. The fact that the group performed quite poorly on the literacy skills tests suggests rather complex and diffuse relationships, which are reflected in the somewhat diffuse literacy skills variable severe reading problem.

Summary of the Q-Factor Group Data

A Q-factor analysis of the same 74 variables on which the R-factor analyses in Chapter 9 were based identified seven different pupil groups. On the basis of the group profiles across the 11 variables identified in the R-factor analysis, six of the

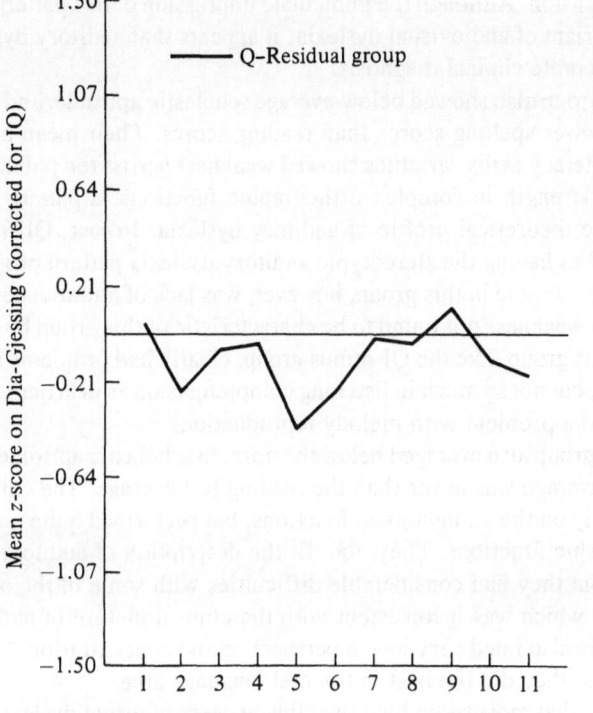

1. Complex phonological functions
2. Phonological cluster functions
3. Phonological assimilation
4. Orthographic error detection
5. Severe reading problems
6. Semantic literacy functions
7. Reversals
8. Attentiveness
9. Orthographic speed
10. Phonological dependence
11. Complex orthographic functions

FIGURE 11.9. Direct variables profile for the residual Q-factor group.

pupil groups could be characterized as having either visual or auditory dyslexia. There were three variants of each of these major types. The seventh group, the residual Q group, appeared to have a nonmodality-related dyslexia.

The three Q groups that were most similar to clinically identified cases of auditory dyslexia had the following unique features:

The QI-minus group had relatively low scholastic aptitude, along with very severe spelling problems. The children had rather extreme difficulties on the variables complex phonological functions and complex orthographic functions. But past clinical experiences suggest that at this early stage of reading development, weaknesses with visuoorthographic skills occur also among pupils who basically have auditory dyslexia. This is particularly true of pupils who pay little or no attention to phonetic analysis and who tend to guess, sometimes rather wildly, at words on the basis of the word's visual configuration. This group also had some difficulties with oral language, particularly with reception, that is, listening comprehension. Although the immediate impression of this pattern may be that this is a variant of audiovisual dyslexia, it appears that auditory dyslexia may be a more accurate clinical diagnosis.

The QII-minus group also showed below-average scholastic aptitude, and these children too had lower spelling scores than reading scores. Their mean profile across the direct literacy skills variables showed weakness across the phonological functions and strength in complex orthographic functions, a pattern quite consistent with the theoretical profile of auditory dyslexia. In fact, QII-minus could be described as having the stereotypic auditory dyslexia pattern proposed by Gjessing (1977). Of note in this group, however, was lack of attentiveness for school activities, a weakness not found to be characteristic of this group by clinical experience. This group, like the QI-minus group, clearly had problems in the oral language area, but not so much in listening comprehension as in articulation. The group also had a problem with melody reproduction.

The QIII-minus group also averaged below the norm in scholastic aptitude, and its spelling score average was lower than the reading test average. The children did relatively poorly on the phonological functions, but performed quite well on complex orthographic functions. They, too, fit the description of auditory dyslexia quite well. But they had considerable difficulties with some of the orthographic functions, which was inconsistent with the clinical picture of auditory dyslexia. They were also rated very low in persistence and concentration. Of the three minus groups, they did the best in the oral language area.

The three groups that most resembled the clinical cases of visual dyslexia had the following unique features:

QI-plus had the highest scholastic aptitude average of all seven Q-factor groups. The children did about equally poorly on the achievement test in reading and spelling, but they revealed several positive attributes. Their profile across the 11 literacy skills variables showed the highest averages for complex phonological as well as complex orthographic functions, phonological cluster functions, and reversals. At this point in their schooling these children do not appear to represent the visual dyslexia pattern unequivocally. It was assumed that they had compensatory qualities that covered up many of their difficulties. Our hypothesis was that as reading demands increased in volume and speed, these children would eventually develop a much more typical pattern of visual dyslexia, showing considerable weakness in the visuoorthographic areas. Even though they only partially fit the expected profile of visual dyslexia, our total clinical evaluation was that they would best fit the general pattern of this type.

QII-plus averaged somewhat below the norm in scholastic aptitude, with reading and spelling scores being about equally poor. This group's mean profile across the 11 literacy skills variables showed trends that were most consistent with the clinical pattern of visual dyslexia. Its main deviation from the typical pattern was that it was not overly dependent on phonics and showed little or no tendency toward reversal errors.

QIII-plus resembled QII-plus with respect to scholastic aptitude and reading, but was a bit lower in spelling. Of all the clinical groups, III-plus resembled the visual dyslexia syndrome the most. Its performance across the 11 direct literacy skills variables was particularly poor on the variables phonological dependence, orthographic error detection, complex orthographic functions, and reversals, a pattern quite common in visual dyslexia.

These first six Q-groups were all considered variants of modality-related types of dyslexia. A study was made of the 11 direct variables to determine which, if any, differentiated the groups. A discriminant analysis showed that three variables discriminated most sharply among them—variables 1, 9, and 11 (complex phonological functions, orthographic speed, and complex orthographic functions, respectively). The next three variables in order of strength of differentiation were phonological dependence (10), phonological cluster functions (2), and orthographic error detection (4).

The residual Q-group differed from the other six by not being modality related. It appeared to represent the emotional, educational, and rare forms of dyslexia groups in the dyslexia model.

The Q-factor analysis did yield additional differentiation within the clinical subgroupings. But in a practical diagnostic setting, such further differentiation would typically also take place. It was important, however, to extract the more robust nuances the Q-factor analysis provided.

Agreement Between Clinical and Statistical Grouping of Dyslexia Type

Table 11.13 provides a cross-tabulation of the children grouped in the two classification systems. It summarizes how the children in the four clinical groups were distributed across the seven Q-factor groups. It shows quite clearly that within six of the seven Q-groups there was a piling up of pupils from either the auditory or the visual dyslexia clinical subgroup. This finding is consistent with the analysis of the data pertaining to each of the Q-groups, although the fits were far from perfect.

Of the 26 children in the first Q-factor group (I-minus), 20 had been classified as auditory dyslexics in the clinical analysis, and none had been diagnosed as visual dyslexics. This affirmed our conclusion that the I-minus group represented a variant of auditory dyslexia.

A mirror situation was found in the fourth Q-group (II-plus). Of the 25 children in this group, 16 were diagnosed as visual dyslexics and none as auditory dyslexics.

For the remaining Q-groups there was also considerable agreement between the two approaches to classification. The residual Q-group did not, however, comply with this general trend, as can be seen in Table 11.13.

Since the most clear-cut differentiation appeared to be along the auditory-visual dichotomy, a further analysis was made of such a classification system. All the children in the three Q-groups with presumed auditory problems were pooled, as were all the children with presumed visual problems. By counting only

TABLE 11.13. Overlap in group membership between the four clinical groups and the seven statistical groups ($n = 181$)

| Clinical dyslexia group | Statistically selected group | | | | | | Residual group N (%) | Total N (%) |
| | Q-factor I | | Q-factor II | | Q-factor III | | | |
	Minus N (%)	Plus N (%)	Minus N (%)	Plus N (%)	Minus N (%)	Plus N (%)		
Auditory	20 (76.9)	9 (22.5)	18 (81.8)	0 (0)	8 (61.5)	6 (24.0)	12 (40.0)	73 (40.3)
Audiovisual	2 (7.7)	1 (2.5)	0 (0)	4 (16.0)	0 (0)	4 (16.0)	7 (23.3)	18 (9.94)
Visual	0 (0)	19 (47.5)	2 (9.1)	16 (64.0)	1 (7.7)	12 (48.0)	3 (10.0)	53 (29.3)
Other	4 (15.4)	11 (27.5)	2 (9.1)	5 (20.4)	4 (30.8)	3 (12.0)	9 (26.7)	37 (20.44)
Total	26 (100)	40 (100)	22 (100)	25 (100)	13 (100)	25 (100)	30 (100)	181 (100)
Chi-square test	$\chi^2 = 86.63$		df = 18		$p < .001$			

TABLE 11.14. Overlap in group membership between the clinical auditory and visual groups and two pooled statistical groups, one related to visual and one to auditory patterns $(n = 111)$

Clinical dyslexia group	Statistically selected group				Total	
	Auditory related (all minus groups)		Visual related (all plus groups)			
	N	%	N	%	N	%
Auditory	46	(75.4)	15	(24.6)	61	(100)
(%)	(93.9)		(25.2)		(55.0)	
Visual	3	(6.0)	47	(94.0)	50	(100)
%	(6.1)		(75.8)		(45.0)	
Total	49	(44.1)	62	(55.9)	111	(100)
(%)	(100)		(100)		(100)	

Chi-square test: $\chi^2 = 53.7$ $df = 1$ $p < .001$
Contingency coefficient $C = .57$, $C_{max} = .707$ $C/C_{max} = r = .81$

those children who had been diagnosed clinically as belonging to one of these groups, a 2 × 2 cross-tabulation table was worked out, encompassing 111 of the original group of 181 children (Table 11.14). The highest agreement was found between the clinical visual dyslexia group and the pooled statistical plus groups (I, II, and III), with 47 children falling in this group, or 94% of all cases diagnosed as visual dyslexia. Of the 61 pupils who were classified as auditory dyslexic, 46 or 75.4% were in the three statistical minus groups. This level of agreement is certainly quite high. Expressed as a contingency coefficient the agreement had a value of $C = .57$. Since the maximum C value for this situation is .707, the estimated correlation between these two classification approaches is $r = .81$.

This number is, of course, an overestimate of the total situation, since it involved only two clinical groups and six statistical groups. The correspondence was not nearly as great for the remaining two clinical types of dyslexia, audiovisual and other forms, versus the seven Q-factor groups, as shown in Table 11.13.

Even though there were some disagreements between the results of the clinical and the statistical groupings, the agreement is certainly high enough to warrant the conclusion that it was not accidental or coincidental. Coupled with the results of the interscorer agreement in the clinical classification, these findings clearly support the notion that the phonological-auditory versus orthographic-visual distinction is a useful and appropriate point of departure for the classification of dyslexic children.

This research supports the notion that during research on subtypes of dyslexia it is beneficial to utilize clinical subgroupings based on an underlying dyslexia theory as well as statistical subgroupings that may be independent of any theory about such subtypes. Using both types of subgroupings with the same sample of children, as was done here, can lay a good foundation for comparative studies, for finer differentiations among types, and for new hypotheses, as well as for a mutual validation of the subgroupings.

CHAPTER 12

Eye Examinations

H. Aasved

Issues and Methods

It is well-known that certain eye conditions result not only in personal discomfort but also in difficulties with reading. Impaired vision can, of course, cause reading problems, since it limits differentiation of details. However, when people of limited sight manage to read with or without visual aids, they usually read normally, although perhaps slower than those with normal vision. Eye characteristics that result in more specific disturbances of the reading processes include especially latent strabismus, that is, a tendency toward squinting, and insufficient convergence, which involves impaired ability to fixate both eyes on the same target at near point.

The most common symptoms of these two conditions are eye fatigue, with burning, itching, and discomfort around the eyes, and possibly headache. For some individuals reading also may be disturbed as a result of double vision, letters and words that appear to overlap, letters and lines that appear to be crooked, parts of words that disappear, letters that become unclear, and problems with finding the next line of print. The fact that discomfort and disturbances of the reading process are connected with problems of simultaneous vision as the result of latent strabismus and insufficient convergence can be discovered simply by covering one of the eyes—the difficulties disappear.

Ever since reading and spelling problems became the subjects of investigation, eye difficulties have been a central issue. A great deal of disagreement has concerned the importance of a variety of eye conditions in reading and writing problems. Some of the more controversial issues relate to refraction, latent strabismus, insufficient convergence, impaired fusion, visual suppression, eye dominance, brain dominance, mixed dominance, saccadic eye movements and optometric training programs (American Academy of Pediatrics, 1973; Benton, 1973; Benton, 1965; Berner & Berner, 1953; Bettman et al., 1967; Bishop et al., 1979; Bø, 1972; Brod & Hamilton, 1971; Delacato, 1966; Dunlap, 1965; Dunlop, 1979; Dunlop & Dunlop, 1974, 1976; Dunlop et al., 1973; Eames, 1955, 1959; Flax, 1973; Fowler & Stein, 1980; Goldberg, 1959, 1968; Goldberg & Arnott, 1970; Griffin et al., 1974; Hallgren, 1950; Helveston et al., 1970;

Keeney & Keeney, 1968; Keogh, 1974; Norn et al., 1969; Orton, 1925, 1928; Park, 1948; Rubino & Minden, 1973; Shearer, 1966; Skydsgaard, 1942; Stromberg, 1938; Subirana, 1958; Udnaes et al., 1977). In addition, there are a number of neurologically oriented controversial issues such as minimal brain dysfunction, anatomical and electrophysiological brain changes (Drake, 1968; Duffy et al., 1980a, 1980b; Galaburda & Kemper, 1979; Hagberg, 1975; Hier et al., 1978; Leisman & Schwartz, 1978; Preston et al., 1974; Yeni-Komshian, 1975).

A review of the literature thus provides little security with regard to the importance of a variety of visual characteristics in reading and writing problems. Some earlier research is not comparable with current research. Furthermore, the criteria for what constitutes dyslexia are unclear and varied, as pointed out earlier in this book. Different professions will, of course, approach the problem from different viewpoints; the fact that treatment is being attempted may in individual cases have a considerable psychological effect.

In view of this background, it was of great interest to carry out a series of eye examinations in conjunction with the very large Bergen Project. The first such examinations were done while these pupils were in the first grade, by orthoptists and people specializing in ophthalmology. A sample such as this should make possible objective studies of eye characteristics in relation to educational and psychological analyses and analysis of the relationships, if any, between these eye characteristics and the diagnosis of dyslexia and dyslexia types.

Data from the initial eye screening examinations of the entire cohort were subjected to extensive statistical analyses and correlated with data from the educational and psychological tests. These analyses showed no particular relationship between eye characteristics and achievement in reading and spelling from dictation. Table 12.1 summarizes some of the eye characteristics found in children at different levels of reading ability, reading level 1 representing the poorest readers and level 5 the best readers. As the table shows, there were no statistically significant differences in any of these characteristics among the different groups. These

TABLE 12.1. Relationship between reading level and certain visual characteristics at the time of the initial eye examination ($n = 2,590$)

Reading level (1 = low)	Stereopsis negative (%)	Straabismus: ⅓ meter			Convergence >20 cm (%)	Central suppression (%)
		Manifest (%)	Intermittent (%)	Latent (%)		
1	5.6	3.3	1.3	83.8	1.3	10.3
2	7.3	3.2	2.3	83.2	0.3	10.1
3	8.4	3.2	1.4	79.5	0.2	8.2
4	4.9	2.1	1.6	79.8	0.3	7.4
5	5.3	2.7	1.3	79.4	0.3	7.9
N	153	72	39	2,097	11	218
P (chi-square test)	.13	.74	.80	.33	.58	.45

results do represent groups, however, and the possibility exists that there may be a connection between eye difficulties and reading and writing difficulties for individual pupils.

In this chapter we present data from extensive follow-up eye examinations of pupils who were identified by the educational and psychological tests as having specific and general learning disabilities. These examinations were undertaken at the Department of Ophthalmology, Haukeland Sykehus (the Bergen University Hospital) and included thorough orthoptic examinations along with eye examinations by one of the supervising physicians in ophthalmology. The children were in the second and third grades (i.e., 1 to 2 years after the initial screening examination done at the end of the first school year).

Finally, 5 years after the extensive eye examinations of the learning disability cases we performed another follow-up of those pupils for whom previous results had indicated the need for further evaluation and possible treatment.

Eye Functions Examined

The following eye examinations were given:

1. Visual acuity. This characteristic was examined with a Snellen chart for each eye separately and for both eyes simultaneously at a far point of 6 meters (20 feet) and a near point of ⅓ meter (1 foot). The child used glasses if this gave better vision.

2. Eye refraction. This was measured objectively by means of special equipment (retinoscope or skiascope). Eye drops were placed in the eyes prior to the examination to immobilize the ciliary muscles. This procedure allows refraction characteristics to be measure without any interference from the accommodation muscles.

3. Eye position. The child viewed an object with both eyes at distances of ⅓ meter and 6 meters while the eyes were alternately covered, to reveal possible squint (strabismus).

4. Simultaneous vision. Simultaneous vision and eye position were examined in a special orthoptic apparatus called synoptophore. This apparatus has two movable arms on which one can place pictures. Small openings allow one eye to see the picture on one arm and the other eye to see the picture on the other arm. If there is a deviation in the position of the eyes, the two arms can be moved so that the angle between them corresponds to the squinting angle of the eyes. This apparatus therefore can be used to evaluate conditions such as primary position and latent and manifest strabismus, and squinting angle can be given in degrees. By means of a variety of pictures one can determine the extent of simultaneous vision. The weakest degree is called simultaneous perception, which implies that the two eyes are perceiving separate pictures simultaneously. Our examination determined if there was simultaneous perception in both eyes' macula lutea, if there was simultaneous perception outside this area in one eye, or if there was no simultaneous perception.

The next step in the examination related to fusion, where two pictures that differ in only one detail are merged and perceived as one picture. By varying the angle between the arms of the synoptophore one can determine the degree of fusion. The eyes follow until the deviation in the angle in relation to the primary position exceeds the child's degree of fusion, so that the pictures perceived by the two eyes will separate. Fusion can then be determined in degrees corresponding to the angle between the arms of the synoptophore. If the child can handle an angle of 20 degrees or more, fusion is considered normal.

The most advanced degree of simultaneous vision gives stereoscopic vision, or depth perception. This can also be determined by the synoptophore by means of special pictures, with which one can also measure the degree of stereopsis. In this examination the results of the stereopsis examination were reported in five gradations: normal, acceptable with one error, acceptable with stimulation, slow with some errors, and poor or no measurable stereopsis.

5. Convergence. An object was brought in toward the base of the nose. The extent of conversion was given as distance in centimeters from the base of the nose. In addition, the pupil's ability to carry out voluntary convergence of the eyes was recorded as possible, impossible, or no voluntary convergence. The last is, of course, a characteristic of manifest strabismus.

6. Eye motility. An object was moved from side to side and up and down while the child watched the object. Eye movements were registered as normal or abnormal. Abnormal movements could be poor pursuit (paralysis), jerkiness (saccadic), or flickering (nystagmus).

7. Accommodation. In accommodation, the eye's refraction is automatically altered so that vision is sharp at all distances. Accommodation was measured by determining how close a pupil could hold reading material and read rather fine print. The closest distance was recorded in centimeters. Children normally should be able to accommodate to within 10 centimeters of the reading material.

8. Dominant eye. In a one-eyed situation, eye preference was determined by having the child look at an object some distance away through a long, thin cylinder. In addition it was noted if the child had good or poor ability to perform this task with the nondominant eye.

Considerable interest has been shown recently in the concept *reference eye test* (Bishop et al., 1979; Fowler & Stein, 1980; Dunlop, 1979; Dunlop & Dunlop, 1974, 1976; Dunlop et al., 1973; Udnaes et al., 1977). By means of this examination one tries to determine the dominant eye during simultaneous vision. For this examination one also uses the synoptophore. Pictures are used in which the details stimulate the middle 2 degrees of the retina, which are of most significance. An evaluation of this characteristic is not particularly simple. In this project it was part of the general follow-up eye examination. To get more reliable information, however, the students were brought in again and the test was carried out 10 times for each. During this time the examination was also carried out on a comparable control group of children. This control group was as similar to the dyslexia group as possible except for the fact that the control group had no perceptible reading or spelling disabilities. The label *normal reference eye* was used when the dominant eye was on the same side as the dominant hand. *Crossed correspondence* refers to the reference eye and dominant hand on opposite sides. *Alternating correspondence* means that the reference eye shifts from one side to the other during the showing of the pictures. *Shifting correspondence* means that in the course of the 10 trials, the same result was obtained less than seven times. One possible outcome of this examination is that a reference eye is not developed or that the examination may not be possible because of the suppression of central vision in one eye as in, for example, manifest strabismus.

9. Prism reflex test. The eyes' position was examined by the use of prismatic correction while vision was fixated on objects at ⅓ meter distance and 6 meters distance. The results were measured in prismatic strength in diopter units.

10. Simultaneous vision during prismatic fusion. Degree of simultaneous vision was measured in prismatic diopters by varying the strength of the prism during testing.

11. Bifoveal fixation. This was tested with prismatic glasses of strength 4 diopter with base to the outside. One could thereby determine if the child could fixate with both eyes simultaneously or if there was central visual suppression in one eye.

Subgrouping of the Pupils

The Sample and Its Subtypes

The learning disability cases discussed in this chapter and the next consisted of the total group of 259, as described in the Appendix, Table A.1. All these children were classified on the basis of educational and psychological tests according to the Gjessing dyslexia model (see Chapter 8). This classification involved four dyslexia types: auditory, audiovisual, visual, and "others." The sizes of these four groups will differ from those described in previous chapters, since the retarded children were included here, although most of them were classified in the category "others." The first three types are, from a medical point of view, generally thought of as genetic, specific dyslexia, whereas "others" is often considered to be secondary reading and writing disabilities.

The educational-psychological evaluations were also the bases for grouping the students by scholastic aptitude (IQ) and by degree of educational progress in reading and spelling.

Educational Progress Groups

On the basis of achievement tests administered during the first four grades, the pupils were divided into three groups according to their educational development:

Group 1 consisted of learning disability cases with poor educational progress, about 25% of the total group. Group 2 included the middle 50% of the children, who had average development. The remaining 25% made up group 3, which showed good educational progress.

Aptitude Level

On the basis of evaluation with a scholastic aptitude (IQ) test in the first and second grades, the pupils were divided into four ability groups. The dividing lines were respectively +1 standard deviation, −1 standard deviation, and −2 standard deviations from the mean of the total cohort of pupils in the project. According to common international practice, the tabulations in this chapter relate to those students in the higher ability group, that is, those who scored higher than −1 standard deviation below the mean. (This corresponds to about the 16th percentile rank, and would generally translate on an aptitude test to an IQ of about 85.) The same analyses were done for the pupils in the lower ability group, that is, those who scored below −1 standard deviation. The results for the latter group will be detailed later in this chapter.

Grouping of Eye Data

We found it helpful to analyze the visual data by the four-way dyslexia subgrouping of the pupils. Findings include the relationship of eye characteristics to dyslexia types and educational progress. Additional eye examinations were performed on individual pupils, specifically to determine if certain eye conditions were important for reading and writing. Part of this section involves an evaluation of 16 children with poor educational progress who went through an experiment of use of an eye patch over one eye for 3 weeks. With such a patch, symptoms connected with latent strabismus and insufficient convergence eventually disappear, because the problem associated with lack of simultaneous vision is canceled.

The Follow-Up Sample

The total learning disabled group (dyslexics plus retarded) involved 259 pupils (approximately 8% of the cohort), 162 boys (62.5%) and 97 girls (37.5%). Of these 259, 253 participated in the initial eye examination and 204 went through the extensive follow-up examinations. There were 131 pupils in the higher ability group (above −1 standard deviation from the cohort mean), and 73 pupils in the lower ability group.

For a variety of reasons, 49 dyslexia cases were not followed. They were analyzed separately on the basis of the educational-psychological data and eye data from the screening test. As a group they made excellent progress in reading and writing, which may have led their parents to conclude that there was no need for any additional eye examinations.

TABLE 12.2. Distribution of pupils by type of dyslexia and educational progress ($n = 259$)

Educational progress	Dyslexia type				Total	
	Auditory*	Audiovisual	Visual	Other	N	(%)
Poor	25	9	16	13	63	(24.3)
Moderate	45	10	38	33	126	(48.7)
Good	28	3	15	17	63	(24.3)
Unknown	1	0	2	4	7	(2.7)
(%) N	(38.2) 99	(8.5) 22	(27.4) 71	(25.9) 67	259	(100.0)

Eye Conditions Related to Dyslexia Types and Educational Progress

The distribution of the 259 pupils in the follow-up study by dyslexia type and by education progress is given in Table 12.2. The category "auditory dyslexia," comprised 38.2% of the total dyslexia group.

The eye conditions of the 131 children who scored above -1 standard deviation on the WISC-R (above 85 IQ) were analyzed as a group. The results of the examinations of these 131 children are discussed below.

Visual Acuity

Table 12.3 shows the distribution of the various combinations of visual acuity of the two eyes within our sample according to the four dyslexia groups. Of the total sample, 92.4% had normal vision in both eyes. No child had weaker acuity than 20/30 in the best eye or 20/60 in the weaker eye. Surprisingly, the best acuity occurred among the 30 pupils whose educational progress was lowest—only two of these children had the combination 20/20, 20/30 and none had poorer acuity than that, whereas 5 of the 10 pupils who had some visual impairment were among the 31 pupils with the best educational progress.

TABLE 12.3. Comparison of visual acuity of children in the various dyslexia groups ($n = 131$)[a]

Acuity, each eye meters (feet)	Dyslexia type				Total	
	Auditory	Audiovisual	Visual	Other	N	(%)
6/6–6/6 (20/20–20/20)	51	10	37	23	121	(92.4)
6/6–6/9 (20/20–20/30)	3	0	1	1	5	(3.8)
6/6–6/12 (20/20–20/40)	0	1	1	0	2	(1.5)
6/6–6/18 (20/20–20/60)	0	0	1	0	1	(0.8)
6/9–6/9 (20/30–20/30)	0	0	0	1	1	(0.8)
6/9–6/12 (20/30–20/40)	0	1	0	0	1	(0.8)

[a] Only those children are included for whom complete records were available.

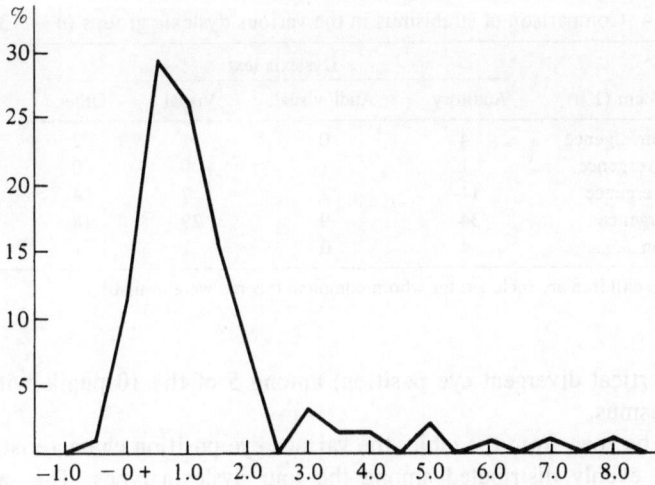

FIGURE 12.1. Spherical refraction of 131 dyslexics.

Eye Refraction

The refraction characteristics of the two eyes for all students were found to be very similar. Figure 12.1 shows the distribution of spherical refraction in the right eye for all 131 pupils for whom complete records were available, and whose IQs were above 85. Most of the children were slightly hypermetropic, +0.5 and +1. Only one pupil was on the myopic side, skiascopically −0.5 in both eyes; this child belonged to the audiovisual dyslexia category. Only eight children had hypermetropia of more than +4, with a maximum in one child of +8 in both eyes. Of these eight, three were of the dyslexia type "other", while the remaining five were distributed among the three other dyslexia categories.

Among these 131 pupils, astigmatism occurred in at least one eye in 31 (23.7%), of whom 5 had astigmatism of 2 diopters or more. The children with astigmatism were quite evenly distributed among the various dyslexia groups as well as educational progress groups.

For the total evaluation of refraction characteristics there was, then, an even distribution for the different dyslexia groups as well as educational progress groups.

Eye Position

Table 12.4 shows the incidence of eye position characteristics in the various dyslexia groups. The testing was done at a distance of 33 centimeters. Examinations at 6 meters revealed about the same incidences for manifest strabismus but a somewhat lower incidence for latent strabismus, the same situation found during the screening examination of the entire cohort. In addition to some cases of significant convergent and divergent strabismus, there was also some hyper-

TABLE 12.4. Comparison of strabismus in the various dyslexia groups ($n = 131$)[a]

Distance 33 cm (1 ft)	Dyslexia text				Total (%)	
	Auditory	Audiovisual	Visual	Other		
Manifest convergence	4	0	2	2	8	6.1
Manifest divergence	1	1	0	0	2	1.5
Latent convergence	11	2	7	4	24	18.3
Latent divergence	34	9	29	18	90	68.7
No deviation	4	0	2	1	7	5.3

[a] Only those children are included for whom complete records were available.

tropia (vertical divergent eye position) among 5 of the 10 pupils with manifest strabismus.

As can be seen from the table, the various eye position characteristics were relatively evenly distributed among the four dyslexia types. The same was also true when the patterns were compared across the three educational progress groups.

Squinting Angle

At all three educational progress levels combined, there were, according to the examination with the synoptophore, only four children who had a squinting angle of 10 degrees or more. Of these, two had manifest convergent strabismus, one each from the auditory and visual dyslexia groups, and the other two with auditory dyslexia, had exophoria (latent divergent strabismus) or exotropia (manifest divergent strabismus). With the use of prismatic correction at an examination distance of 33 centimeters, another child had manifest strabismus with a squinting angle of 12.5 degrees. He was in the auditory dyslexia group and in the high educational progress group.

Eye Motility

Abnormal eye motility was noted in 13 children. Of these, seven had manifest strabismus, five latent strabismus, and one was in the primary position (no strabismus). These 13 pupils were evenly distributed according to dyslexia type, but most of them (nine) were in the "moderate" educational progress group.

Convergence

The vast majority, 90.8% of all pupils examined, had normal convergence, with a near-point convergence of 8 centimeters or less. Only three children had near-point convergence of 12 to 26 centimeters. Of these three, one was in each educational progress group and one had audiovisual and two had visual dyslexia.

The frequency of voluntary convergence of the eyes was found to be relatively evenly distributed among the various subgroups. Among 43 pupils without manifest strabismus, voluntary convergence was noted to be impossible. This group was also quite evenly distributed among the various dyslexia groups as well as educational progress groups.

Accommodation

All 131 students were able to accommodate at 10 centimeters or less.

Simultaneous Vision Evaluated With Synoptophore and With Prismatic Correction

Simultaneous Vision

Among the first three dyslexia types, only five of the 131 pupils had abnormal or no simultaneous vision. All had manifest strabismus and were distributed among the poor and moderate educational progress groups.

Fusion

The examinations with the synoptophore revealed that only five pupils had either peripheral or no fusion. Additional examinations with the use of prismatic glasses indicated two additional pupils who did not show normal fusion. All seven children had manifest strabismus and were distributed across all dyslexia types and educational progress groups. The two examination methods revealed approximately the same information.

Stereoscopic Vision

Altogether eight of the 131 pupils had poor or no demonstrable stereoscopic vision. Of these, six had manifest strabismus and two had exophoria (latent divergent strabismus). These children were distributed across the first three dyslexia types and all three educational progress levels.

Dominant Eye

When given a choice of eye for looking at an object through a tube; 82 of the 131 pupils (62.6%) indicated right-eye dominance. There was no statistically significant difference among dyslexia types or educational progress groups. The same situation held true with regard to the ability to switch dominant eye.

Reference Eye Test

Figures 12.2 and 12.3 show the results of the reference eye test. Figure 12.2 indicates the condition for the 110 pupils in the higher ability group who were brought in for additional evaluation with the reference eye test. The results were compared with those from a comparable control of 89 children.

Only one child registered alternating reference eye; in Figure 12.2 the categories "alternating" and "shifting" reference eye are combined. As can be seen

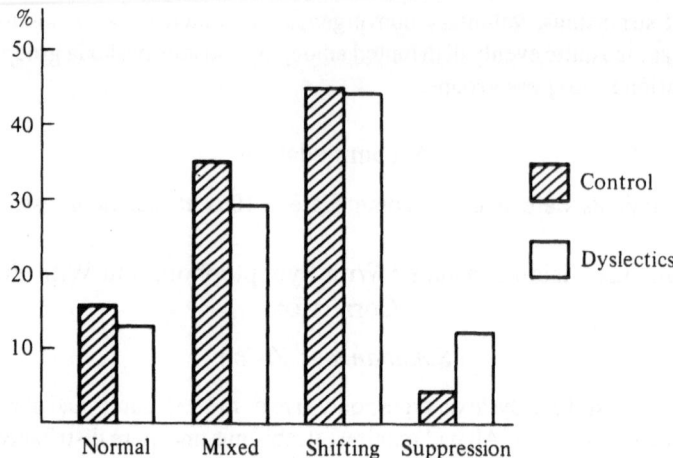

FIGURE 12.2. Reference eye test for 110 learning disability pupils and 89 controls.

from the figures, the reference eye test data are pretty much the same for the dyslexia group as for the control group. Figure 12.3 reveals the same data by dyslexia group. For all groups, shifting reference eye had the highest frequency, but there were no significant differences among the various dyslexia groups. Nor were there significant differences among the three educational progress groups with regard to the reference eye test.

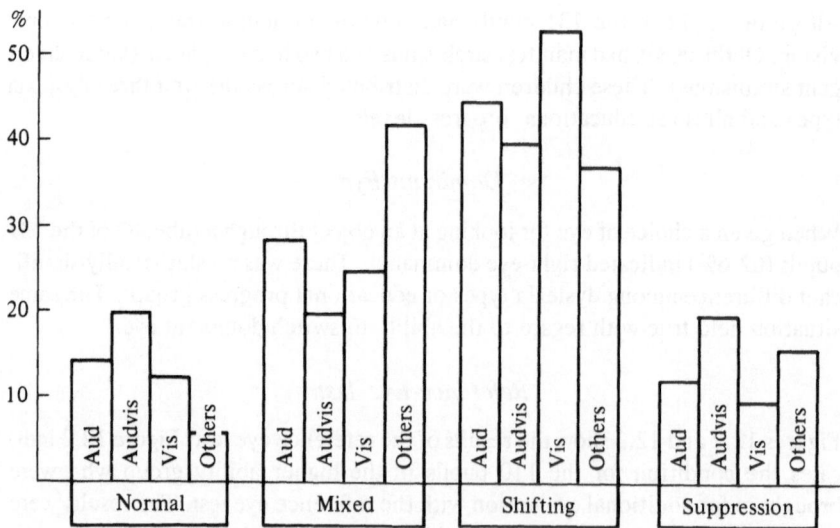

FIGURE 12.3. Reference eye test for 110 dyslexic pupils by type of dyslexia.

Central Visual Suppression

Tests with prismatic glasses 4D with base out indicated central visual suppression among 11 children (8.4%) out of 131, the cases being evenly distributed among the various dyslexia types. Of these, there were five in each of the two lowest educational progress groups and only one in the "good" group. Eight of the 11 children had manifest strabismus, two with exophoria and one with esophoria.

Dyslexia Pupils With Low School Ability

The follow-up studies included, as mentioned earlier, 73 learning disability cases whose school ability test scores were more than 1 standard deviation below the cohort mean, or IQ 85 or lower. The same analyses and evaluations were performed for this group as for the 131 pupils in the higher ability group. There were no significant differences between the two groups with regard to the various eye characteristics tested, nor any tendency for overrepresentation in any of the dyslexia groups with regard to any visual characteristics.

Data for 49 Learning Disability Cases Who Did Not Participate in the Follow-Up Examination

The group of 49 pupils who did not participate in the follow-up examination showed generally somewhat better educational progress than the remaining pupils. Only 15% were in the "poor progress group," in contrast to 27.5% of the 204 pupils who were in the follow-up examination. The eye data for these 49 pupils from the screening testing were analyzed as they related to the four dyslexia types and the three educational progress groups. Only one pupil had manifest strabismus; he was in the dyslexia group "other" and in the "middle" educational progress group. Otherwise there was relatively even distribution of the various eye conditions across the four dyslexia types. Most of the pupils with latent strabismus were in the "moderate" educational progress group.

Summary of Eye Conditions by Dyslexia Type Compared to the Total Cohort

Table 12.5 compares the frequencies of some eye conditions as they occurred in the various dyslexia groups with the screening data for the entire cohort. To facilitate comparisons, the frequencies are given only in percentages. The table indicates a tendency toward somewhat higher frequencies of some eye problems in some of the dyslexia types than in the total cohort (limited acuity in one or both eyes, manifest strabismus, and latent convergent strabismus). Differences are not statistically significant, however, for any of the groups.

TABLE 12.5. Percent incidence of eye conditions in the 253 learning disability cases by dyslexia type compared with the total cohort of 2,740

Characteristic	Total cohort	Dyslexia type			
		Auditory	Audiovisual	Visual	Other
Acuity ≤ 6/9 (20/30) in one or both eyes	4.2	5.1	9.1	2.9	4.8
Manifest strabismus	3.9	7.1	9.1	4.3	7.9
Latent strabismus					
Convergent	11.1	20.2	18.2	13.0	19.0
Divergent	69.8	64.6	68.2	78.3	61.9
Convergence ability					
≥ cm	3.6	3.0	4.5	4.3	1.6
Simultaneous perception prism ≥ 20 diopters	2.3	4.0	4.5	1.4	4.8
Prismatic fusion ≤ 20 diopters	6.1	6.1	9.1	2.9	6.3
Poor stereopsis	5.9	7.1	9.1	1.4	7.9
Central suppression	8.3	10.1	13.6	7.2	9.5
Number	2,740	99	22	69	63

Limited acuity and manifest strabismus were among the characteristics that occurred with somewhat higher frequency among the 73 pupils in the lower ability group compared with those in the higher ability group.

Follow-Up of Children With Convergence Problems

At the time of the screening examinations in first grade, the 11 children with a near-point convergence of more than 20 centimeters from the eye showed remarkably poor reading ability. Four of these children were in the lowest reading level group. These four pupils were among the dyslexia cases followed up. It was found at follow-up that two of the four pupils had near-point convergence of 6 centimeters, that is, excellent convergence ability. One had visual dyslexia and was placed in the "good" educational progress group; the other was in the dys-

TABLE 12.6. Distribution of visual problems among various dyslexia types in 55 children found at follow-up examination to have eye conditions requiring examination and possible treatment

Visual problem	Dyslexia type				Total
	Auditory	Audiovisual	Visual	Other	
Refraction (acuity)	14[a]	0	4	8	26
Manifest strabismus	7	2	2	4	15
Latent strabismus	8[a]	3	2	4	17[a]
Total	26	5	8	16	55

[a] Three pupils with latent strabismus also had acuity problems.

lexia group "other" with "moderate" educational progress. The other two had convergence near-point of 16 and 18 centimeters, respectively. One of these children had visual dyslexia and the other auditory. They both showed "moderate" educational progress. These follow-up examinations, therefore, gave no support to the notion that there is a high relationship between convergence and dyslexia. This finding is consistent with data found in other places in this chapter relating to convergence.

Follow-Up of Eye Conditions Requiring Additional Examinations

At follow-up of the 204 learning disability cases, 55 children had eye conditions requiring further examination, evaluation, and possibly treatment. Among these were 26 children with refraction problems, 15 with manifest strabismus (esotropia), and 16 with latent strabismus (esophoria). Two of the pupils in the last group also had problems with refraction. For the rest of the 204 children the follow-up examination revealed normal eye characteristics. One case of latent strabismus (esophoria) was of such low degree and without symptoms of fatigue that treatment was contraindicated.

Table 12.6 shows the distribution of these 55 pupils according to the four dyslexia groups [three pupils are counted twice because they had both refraction problems and latent strabismus (esophoria)]. The largest number are in the auditory group (47.3%). (In comparison with the total group there are relatively more pupils in the dyslexia group "other.") The distribution according to dyslexia type was approximately the same for the 34 children in the higher ability group as for the 21 children in the lower ability group, the dividing line being, again, −1 standard deviation below the cohort mean on a school ability test (IQ 85).

These 55 children were followed up again approximately 5 years after the first follow-up. The main issues at this second follow-up pertained to the extent to which the pupils had eye problems, whether they used the prescribed glasses, and what the parents thought about their child's reading ability. The children were in grade 8 at the time.

Some of the points in conjunction with this second follow-up are summarized in Table 12.7. Of the 26 pupils who required the second follow-up with regard to refraction problems, corrective glasses had been prescribed earlier for 24. Of the two who did not have glasses prescribed, one had unilateral astigmatism without discomfort, the other had anisometropia. Both of these children reported at this 5-year follow-up good reading ability and no visual discomfort. Of the 24 for whom glasses were prescribed, only 8 were wearing glasses 5 years later; four were using them only occasionally and the remaining four wore them regularly. Three of the four with glasses had hypermetropia of over +4.0 diopters, and one had pronounced astigmatism. Among the 16 who at the time of follow-up reported that they never used glasses, six had hypermetropia from +0.75 to +2.5 diopters and the remaining 10 had astigmatism ranging from 0.5 to 3 diopters. The circumstances regarding the need for and use of glasses were very simi-

TABLE 12.7. Visual problems of 55 dyslexic children 7 years after screening

Aptitude level (IQ)	Number	Surgery	Glasses 1980	Glasses 1985	Prismatic glasses 1980	Prismatic glasses 1985	Reading ability 1985 Good	Reading ability 1985 Average	Reading ability 1985 Poor
Refraction acuity problems									
> −1 SD	15		13	4			12	3	0
< −1 SD	11		11	4			4	3	4
Manifest strabismus									
> −1 SD	10	3	5	5			8	2	0
< −1 SD	5	1	3	1			2	1	2
Latent strabismus									
> −1 SD	11		2[a]	1	2	1	7	4	0
< −1 SD	6		1[a]	0	5	1	0	2	4

[a] One pupil had surgery who previously wore prismatic glasses.

lar for the two ability groups. Reporting of reading ability, however, showed rather marked differences. Of the 15 pupils in the upper ability group, 12 reported good reading ability and none reported being a poor reader. In the lower ability group there was an even distribution across the three groups according to the educational progress levels poor, moderate, and good.

Of the 15 pupils with manifest strabismus, surgical correction had been performed on four. Eight children had received glasses for the correction of hypermetropia; of these eight, three also were operated on. At the last follow-up, six of these eight continued to wear glasses. Here, too, the report regarding reading ability varied by aptitude group, with good reading ability among 8 of the 10 pupils in the higher aptitude group and poor reading ability among two of the five in the lowest group.

Two of the 16 pupils with latent strabismus had received glasses 5 years before, and one of them continued to use the glasses at the last follow-up. Altogether six pupils had received prismatic glasses, and one pupil had been operated on before receiving the prismatic correction. As was found earlier, the higher aptitude children had good reading ability whereas the children in the low aptitude group had significantly lower reading ability.

Eye Patch Experiment

As mentioned previously, the covering of one eye aides in the discovery of the extent to which problems of simultaneous vision play a role in reading difficulties.

An experiment was carried out in which an eye patch was placed over one eye for 3 weeks in each of 16 children with dyslexia while they were in the fifth grade. Their reading ability was then compared with that of a control group of 14 pupils without dyslexia. Three of the 16 dyslexia pupils showed across-the-board improvement in reading ability and fewer errors with eye patch than without. All three belonged to the higher school aptitude group, and all three had auditory dyslexia. In one case the decrease in pronunciation errors during reading aloud could probably be ascribed to a considerably reduced reading speed. This child had at the time of the last follow-up a noncorrected astigmatism with acuity of 20/40 in the right eye and 20/30 on the left. With correction the pupil had 20/15 acuity in both eyes. Later the pupil put the glasses away and reading ability was reported by the parent to be "moderate." The other two children had somewhat faster reading speed and fewer pronunciation errors when one eye was covered than without. One of these had slight latent convergent strabismus (esophoria), not treated, and moderately good reading ability was reported at the follow-up. The other had latent divergent strabismus (exophoria) in addition to slight astigmatism that was corrected with glasses. She reported some help from glasses for a while, but at the time of the final follow-up she never used glasses and reported good reading ability.

Comments and Evaluation

Several of the tests used in the follow-up examination were also part of the screening testing done in the schools. A comparison of the data showed that for most of these examinations the results for the total learning disability sample were nearly the same as the screening data for the entire cohort. This was true of visual acuity, eye dominance in one-eyed situations, stereoscopic vision, prismatic correction, prismatic fusion, convergence, and central visual suppression. Only with regard to strabismus was there some difference between the groups, in that it occurred slightly more frequently in the disability group in the form of manifest convergent and divergent strabismus and divergent strabismus (exotropia), as well as latent convergent strabismus. For all of these strabismus conditions, as well as for results of additional eye tests, there was an even distribution by dyslexia type. There was therefore no particular tendency for special eye difficulties to occur in any one dyslexia group. This was true of the total of 204 pupils who went through the follow-up examination and the 49 pupils who were not followed personally but whose visual characteristics from the grade 1-2 screening test were analyzed. Nor did a division of the dyslexia pupils by school aptitude level show any main difference in eye data. On the basis of the reading and spelling test from grade 1-2 to grade 3-4, there was an even distribution among the three educational progress groups.

Educational progress was somewhat slower in the lower aptitude group than in the higher, but no influence of eye problems could be discerned.

Most of the pupils with eye difficulties found in the screening examination were not part of the total disability group. For example, 123 pupils had manifest or intermittent strabismus at the time of screening, but only 16 were among the disability cases.

In recent years there has been a great deal of interest in the reference eye test. The first reports were very positive, and it appeared that we had found an eye condition which was associated particularly with visual dyslexia. The initial research seemed to indicate that crossed reference eye occurred with particularly high frequency in this type of dyslexia (Dunlop & Dunlop, 1974). Later observations seemed to indicate that unstable reference eye also occurred in visual dyslexia (Fowler & Stein, 1980). Later investigations raised doubt about the validity of these observations (Bishop et al., 1979; Udnaes et al., 1977). This was why we brought in as many cases as possible for repeated examinations with respect to the reference eye test and put them all through 10 consecutive examinations with the special pictures in the synoptophore. As the analysis shows, we were not able to demonstrate that different forms of reference eye behavior had any kind of relationship to any particular type of dyslexia. It would appear, therefore, that we still have not established a definitive positive relationship between eye characteristics and dyslexia in general, nor any particular relationship to specific dyslexia types.

Analysis of individual cases in a follow-up examination in grade 3-4 and a second follow-up 5 years later yielded meaningful information in addition to the more general analysis of group data. Of the 204 pupils who were followed up, 55 had visual characteristics that required further examination. They either had received some treatment earlier or treatment had been initiated in conjunction with the first follow-up or some time thereafter. The remaining pupils had such normal visual characteristics at the visual screening that there was no need for a second follow-up. The visual problems of the 55 pupils were distributed in three areas: refraction and manifest and latent strabismus. These problems were distributed fairly evenly according to dyslexia type as well as across the educational progress level of the children. The final follow-up showed that most of the pupils who had had glasses prescribed for them did not use these 5 years later, and most of them had used glasses only a short time. This was true of pupils with minor refraction problems, as well as pupils with latent strabismus who had had prismatic glasses prescribed. Those who continued to wear glasses had extreme refraction problems and felt dependent on glasses, or had manifest strabismus.

A division on the basis of scholastic aptitude showed that the visual characteristics of the high and low groups were quite similar. They differed appreciably, however, with regard to reading ability as reported at the time of the final follow-up. This information was for the most part given by the parents, partly also by the students. Otherwise information was obtained from the teacher. Reading ability at the final follow-up was clearly poorer in the lower school aptitude group than in the higher. In the latter group no one reported poor reading ability at the time of follow-up and most indicated reading ability was "good." This tendency was quite similar for the three categories of visual problems.

For those pupils who had worn glasses temporarily and later put them away, only one reported that glasses had been of help. It was more common to hear that other events had been more important and had contributed more to the improvement in reading ability, for example, change of school and environment and illness, which precipitated reading for recreation.

It is difficult to evaluate objectively how many pupils' reading benefited from prescribed glasses or other prescribed treatment regarding the eyes. It would seem reasonable to assume that the 15 students who at the final follow-up continued to wear glasses, had felt the need for this aid for reading. But one cannot therefore conclude that this has been a main treatment for reading and writing difficulties. These students were distributed in the various dyslexia groups about the same as the total group. For the 22 students who wore glasses only a short time and later discarded them, it would seem reasonable to assume that the glasses were of no significance with regard to reading difficulties. It is of course possible that treatment for eye problems generally, including temporary use of glasses, can give a stimulus to a greater effort in learning to read and in that way contribute to some improvement in reading ability. Parental reporting of appreciable improvement in reading ability in conjunction with the use of glasses, including prismatic glasses, may be colored by wishful thinking that the eye characteristics were a main cause of reading difficulties, without there being much foundation for such an assumption.

On the basis of the extensive statistical analysis and individual evaluation one can conclude the following:

Dyslexic children did not differ from other children with regard to eye characteristics.

Most children with eye problems do not have dyslexia.

In general, there appears to be no particular causal relationship between eye characteristics and reading and spelling difficulties as revealed by the educational-psychological examinations in this project. It is entirely possible that in certain individual cases the eye difficulties may have been an additional burden. In such cases optimal treatment of eye problems should be rendered, so that the students are as best equipped as possible to receive other, more relevant treatment for their reading and spelling difficulties. For this reason all learning disability cases should be given thorough visual examination with an evaluation of possible need for special treatment.

The results of this investigation are consistent with most of the earlier medical studies regarding the relationship between eye characteristics and dyslexia.

The reading and spelling difficulties in children must continue to be viewed as mainly an educational problem, and educators must take the main responsibility for the treatment of these children.

The population that was the subject of these analyses in the Bergen Project would be an interesting group to follow later in life from the view point of educational level attained, psychological makeup, and medical history, including eye characteristics. This is especially true, of course, for the students with dyslexia in the first years of school. The data that have been gathered from the first school years should form a good basis for follow-up during the entire growth period of the child and into adulthood.

Acknowledgments. Collaborators in the clinical eye-examinations at the Department of Ophthalmology, Haukeland Hospital, Bergen: Wendy Evans Lothe (orthoptist), Magnus Odland, Torstein Bertelsen, Johan H. Seland.

CHAPTER 13

Neurological Examinations

P.E. Waaler, K. Helland-Hansen, H. Miljeteig, O. Opshaug,
J.L. Larsen, H. Bruland, and L. Irgens

Purpose of the Investigation

In 1896 the concept of word blindness was introduced by British physicians
(Morgan, 1896). Since then there has been a great deal of interest among pediatric neurologists in the medical correlates of children's reading and writing
problems (herein referred to as dyslexia). Several investigators have found that
among selected groups of these children there is a higher than normal incidence
of signs of minimal brain dysfunction (MBD) (Ingram, Mason & Blackburn,
1970; for general overview see e.g., Duffy & Geschwind, 1985). Localized brain
damage has been found in a few individuals with reading and writing problems
(Galaburda, Sherman, Rosen, Aboitiz, & Geschwind, 1985).

In the past the majority of neurological studies have been carried out on dyslexics who have been referred for neurological examination because of their
learning problems. The Bergen Project provided a unique opportunity to study *all*
learning disability cases within an entire cohort of a population. We were
interested in the prevalence of neurological symptoms in the children with learning disabilities. Of particular interest was a clarification of possible connections
between MBD and learning disabilities. The following is a brief summary of the
most important findings from our pediatric neurological examinations. Our
results may be compared with parts of the most important previous epidemiologi-
cal study that involved children with reading and writing problems, the Isle of
Wight study of children's health from 1964 to 1974 (Rutter et al., 1970; Rutter &
Yule, 1975).

Methods

Sample Selection Criteria and Plan of the Investigation

The neurological investigations were carried out during the spring of 1982, when
the children in the Bergen Project were in the fifth grade. At this time 24 of the
259 learning disabled originally in the project were no longer under study for various reasons. The 149 boys and 86 girls (235 children) still in the project were

invited by letter to appear for an examination. This letter summarized the aims of the investigation and contained the essential practical information.

A total of 164 children were examined (69.8% of the disability group)—107 (65.2%) boys and 57 (34.8%) girls. In the case of children who did not appear, some parents stated that they did not wish to be involved in any more examinations and some indicated that their child was fully recovered or so much improved in reading and writing that the parents considered further examinations unnecessary. In many cases no particular reason was given.

A control group of 19 boys and 22 girls was selected randomly by statistical methods. These children attended the same classes and went through the same examination schedule as the learning disabled. In our investigation system it was not possible to conceal from the examining physician whether a given child belonged to the disability or to the control group.

The children were examined at school during school hours, each examination lasting about 1 hour. In most cases one or both parents accompanied their child to the interview. A few interviews were given as home visits. The practical work with interviews and neurological examinations was divided among three of us (K.H.-H., O.O., and H.M.)

Interview and Neurological Examination

The parents answered 126 questions regarding disorders in the family, pregnancies, birth and perinatal period, growth and development (motor, language, toilet training, etc.), behavior and emotional characteristics, diseases, and injuries of the child.

We employed an examination schedule that is usual in practical child neurology. In addition, some ideas and tests were taken from various sources, especially from Touwen (1979) and Rasmussen and Gillberg (Rasmussen, 1982). Some tests were also taken from a neuropsychological test battery (Reitan & Davison, 1974). Every child went through 128 separate examinations. These examinations can be grouped as follows: (a) height, weight, and head circumference; (b) general medical examination (heart, lungs, etc.); (c) various external anomalies; for example, simian crease, epicanthus, hypertelorism; (d) reflexes; (ed) cranial nerves (mostly motoric functions of eyes and face); (f) gross motor functions, balance, and gait; (g) tests relating to coordination, fine motor, and cerebellar functions; (h) tests of laterality (hand, foot, eye); (i) tests of fine sensation [gnosia, graphesthesia, form perception (stereognosis)]; (j) right–left discrimination; (k) observations of general behavior, language, articulation, writing, drawing, concentration, and motor activity.

The entire battery of 128 examinations will not be described in detail here. The following are brief descriptions of some of the tests that showed significant differences between the learning disabled and controls or between subgroupings by dyslexia type:

1. Pegboard. Small pegs are placed in small holes with a special pattern in the shortest possible time.

2. Finger tapping. The child hits a mechanical counter with the index finger as many times as possible in a given amount of time.

3. Prechtl's test. The child stretches the arms forward, spreads the fingers, and holds the arms and fingers still.

4. Diadochokinesis. The child twists the hand and forearm alternately back and forth as quickly as possible.

5. Figure copying. The child copies 11 figures from developmental drawings, University of Wisconsin.

6. Follow-the-finger test. The child mimics the movement of the examiner's index finger in a certain pattern.

7. Cut a circle. The general ability of the child with scissors and the tendency to notches are registered.

8. Finger agnosia. One of the child's fingers is touched without the child looking. Which finger?

9. Graphesthesia. A numeral is written on the tip of the finger without the child looking. Which numeral?

10. Stereognosis. An object is placed in the child's hand without the child looking. Which object?

11. In-between test. Two fingers, for example, thumb and fourth finger, are touched without the child looking. How many fingers are there in between? (Kinsbourne & Warrington, 1963).

12. Right–left discrimination. The child points to right and left parts on his or her own body and on a drawing with the eyes open and thereafter with the eyes closed.

Ratings of Observations

A suitable and reliable grouping of the results from the various questions and tests was achieved by use of a *qualitative* classification: (a) normal, (b) slight/possible problem (slightly/possibly abnormal), (c) definitive problem (definitely abnormal), (d) unknown (this alternative was used only in the interview part). The qualitative classification was used for the majority of the variables.

Some tests were scored in time or by points. We called these tests *quantitative* and classified responses as good or poor. Performance was classified as poor when the time used for a given task exceeded the 75th percentile or the number of points obtained was less than the 25th percentile for the control group norm.

Additional Examinations

A selected group of the children also went through computerized tomography (CT) of the brain and/or electroencephalography (EEG). The criteria for participation in these examinations were definite signs of neurological dysfunction during the clinical examination and/or unsatisfactory results of the remedial instruction that had been instituted to deal with the children's reading and spelling difficulties.

The results of CT and EEG examinations were compared with corresponding data from special control groups. For ethical reasons it was not possible to examine children from the same school classes as the dyslexics. As a comparison group for the CT material we used the results of CT examinations of 52 children aged 8 to 12 years. Most of these children had been examined because they suffered from headache or epilepsy. As a comparison group for the EEG material we used the EEG curves from 8 to 12-year-old children ($n = 104$). Most of these children had been examined because they suffered from headache. There were no dyslexics among the children in the CT and EEG comparison groups.

Statistical Methods

When learning disabled children were compared with controls we used simple Chi-square tests or Chi-square tests in a simple logistic model. When subgroups according to dyslexia types were compared (and the controls excluded), we employed chi-square tests in log-linear models using three-way contingency tables with the following classification variables: (a) sex, (b) results of various neurological examinations, and (c) subgroups of dyslexia types.

Results

It should be pointed out again that the children studied here were the 259 learning disability cases (less the 24 cases lost through attrition). The dyslexics and the retarded were not analyzed as separate groups. Every one of the 235 remaining cases was classified by type of dyslexia, a process which differed from the separate analyses reported previously for the educational and psychological data. (The retarded students were, for the most part, classified as dyslexia type "others."). The main thrust of the neurological study was the comparison between the learning disabled and the controls. Because of the large quantity of data, only the results that showed significant differences between these two main groups are tabulated.

Reading and Writing Problems in the Family

Part of the interview related to the presence of reading and writing difficulties among close relatives of the children. Ninety (56%) of the learning disabled and 6 (15%) of the control children had one or more first-degree relatives (parents, siblings) with such problems. In the Isle of Wight study (Rutter et al., 1970), 33% of the children with reading and writing difficulties had parents and/or siblings with similar problems.

Motor Impairments

Several studies of children with reading and writing problems have shown that some of these children have impaired motor functions (for a general overview see, e.g., Duffy & Geschwind, 1985). This was confirmed in our study. The

TABLE 13.1. Comparison of 164[a] children with learning disabilities and 41 control children in terms of their parents' information about their fine and gross motor functions

Ability	Group	Normal N (%)	Unknown[b] N (%)	Slight/ possible problem N (%)	Definite problem N (%)	P (Chi-square test)
Handwriting	Disabled	102 (63)	10 (6)	44 (27)	5 (3)	< .005
	Control	39 (95)	0	2	0	
Use of puzzles, building blocks, etc.	Disabled	140 (86)	7 (4)	16 (10)	0	< .05
	Control	38 (93)	3 (7)	0	0	
Walking, running	Disabled	150 (91)	5 (3)	6 (4)	3 (2)	< .05
	Control	41 (100)	0	0	0	
Physical education skills	Disabled	144 (88)	1 (1)	16 (10)	3 (2)	< .01
	Control	41 (100)	0	0	0	

[a] For handwriting test, total was 161; for puzzles and so on, total was 163.
[b] Results not included in chi-square tests.

TABLE 13.2. Comparison of 164 children with learning disabilities and 41 control children on qualitative tests for fine motor coordination and cerebellar functions

Ability	Group	Normal N (%)	Slightly/ possibly abnormal N (%)	Definitely abnormal N (%)	P (Chi-square test)
Follow-the-finger test, dominant hand	Disabled	145 (88)	19 (12)	0	< .05
	Control	41 (100)	0	0	
Follow-the-finger test, non-dominant hand	Disabled	139 (85)	23 (14)	2 (1)	< .001
	Control	41 (100)	0	0	
Diadochokinesis, dominant hand	Disabled	116 (71)	46 (28)	2 (1)	< .01
	Control	37 (90)	4 (10)	0	
Diadochokinesis, nondominant hand	Disabled	81 (49)	71 (43)	12 (7)	< .001
	Control	31 (76)	10 (24)	0	
Diadochokinesis, mirror movements, dominant hand	Disabled	86 (52)	71 (43)	7 (4)	< - .05
	Control	29 (71)	12 (29)	0	
Handwriting	Disabled	101 (62)	55 (34)	8 (5)	< .001
	Control	37 (90)	3 (7)	1 (2)	
Cutting a circle	Disabled	101 (62)	55 (34)	8 (5)	< .0001
	Control	39 (95)	2 (5)	0	
Notches in circle	Disabled	74 (45)	71 (43)	19 (12)	< .01
	Control	28 (68)	12 (29)	1 (2)	

problems were particularly pronounced with regard to fine motor coordination, but gross motor coordination was also involved. It should be pointed out, however, that many dyslexics had perfectly normal coordination; in fact, some of them were particularly competent in this area.

Table 13.1 gives the parents' information about certain fine motor skills in their child. Some of the children had difficulties with handwriting, doing puzzles, and using building blocks. There were no significant differences between learning disabled and controls in the following tasks: tying shoelaces, buttoning, eating, drawing, doing crafts, and showing general judgment regarding manual skills.

Tables 13.2 and 13.3 show the results of some qualitative and quantitative tests for fine motor coordination. The disabled had the most problems with figure copying, handwriting, cutting a circle, and, for the nondominant hand, diadochokinesis and following the finger. Several tests did not show significant differences between the two main groups: finger-nose test, finger opposition, grip of a pencil, follow a line, gest imitation, losing pegs (in the pegboard test), mirror movement in diadochokinesis test (nondominant hand), and finger tapping (dominant hand).

Tables 13.3 and 13.4 show the results of some qualitative and quantitative gross motor tests. Few learning disabled had definite problems in these areas. Sixteen other tests for gross motor functions did not show significant differences between learning disabled and controls.

With regard to motor activities of the face and eyes, there were significant differences between learning disabled and controls with regard to the ability to move the tongue and the ability to differentiate tongue movements from head movements (Table 13.4). Fifteen other tests showed no significant differences.

TABLE 13.3. Comparison of 164[a] children with learning disabilities and 41 control children on quantitative tests for fine and gross motor coordination

Ability	Group	Good N (%)	Poor N (%)	P (Chi-square test)
Figure copying	Disabled*	60 (37)	103 (63)	< .001
	Control	29 (71)	12 (29)	
Pegboard, dominant hand	Disabled	90 (55)	74 (45)	< .05
	Control	30 (73)	11 (27)	
Pegboard, nondominant hand	Disabled	77 (47)	87 (53)	< .05
	Control	27 (66)	14 (34)	
Finger tapping, non-dominant hand	Disabled	95 (58)	69 (42)	< .05
	Control	31 (76)	10 (24)	
Catching a ball, dominant hand	Disabled	143 (87)	21 (13)	< .01
	Control	41 (100)	0	

[a] For figure copying, total was 163 children.

TABLE 13.4. Comparison of 164 children with learning disabilities and 41 control children on qualitative tests for gross motor coordination and motor functions of the face

Ability	Group	Normal N (%)	Slightly/ possibly abnormal N (%)	Definitely abnormal N (%)	P (Chi-square test)
Balance, right	Disabled	138 (84)	24 (15)	2 (1)	
foot	Control	39 (95)	2 (5)	0	< .05
Balance, left	Disabled	124 (76)	37 (23)	3 (2)	
foot	Control	39 (95)	2 (5)	0	< .01
Walking a line	Disabled	150 (91)	13 (8)	1 (1)	
	Control	41 (100)	0	0	< .01
Prechtl's test,	Disabled	141 (86)	23 (14)	0	
arm deviation	Control	40 (98)	1 (2)	0	< .05
Prechtl's test,	Disabled	124 (76)	36 (22)	4 (2)	
choreiform movements	Control	37 (90)	4 (10)	0	< .05
Tongue move-	Disabled	136 (83)	25 (15)	3 (2)	
ments	Control	41 (100)	0	0	< .001
Dissociation	Disabled	94 (57)	61 (37)	9 (5)	
between head and tongue movements	Control	35 (85)	6 (15)	0	< .001

Fine Sensation and Right-Left Discrimination

The tests for agnosia, graphesthesia, stereognosis, and the in-between test demand a high degree of interplay between the finger/hand sensitivity, processing in the brain, and language functions. As shown in Table 13.5, there were marked differences between learning disabled and controls with regard to agnosia and graphesthesia. The table also shows that some dyslexics had problems with right-left discrimination. Stereognosis turned out to be a less sensitive test for these children. The following examinations did not show significant differences between the two groups: stereognosis and in-between test (both hands); stereognosis, number of errors (nondominant hand).

Speech

The frequencies of certain speech problems among learning disabled and controls are given in Tables 13.6 and 13.7. The parents reported definite delay of speech development in 16% of the disabled and none of the controls. In the Isle of Wight study (Rutter et al., 1970), 33% of the children with reading and writing problems had delayed speech development. As can be seen from Table 13.6, some of the disabled had a variety of articulation problems and some had limited vocabulary. Practically none of these problems were present in the control group.

TABLE 13.5. Comparison of 164 children with learning disabilities and 41 control children on sensation and for right–left discrimination

Ability	Group	Good N (%)	Poor N (%)	P (Chi-square test)
Agnosia, dominant hand	Disabled	50 (30.5)	114 (69.5)	< .0001
	Control	26 (63)	15 (37)	
Agnosia, nondominant hand	Disabled	37 (23)	127 (77)	< .0001
	Control	22 (54)	19 (46)	
Graphesthesia, dominant hand	Disabled	63 (38)	101 (62)	< .001
	Control	28 (68)	13 (32)	
Graphesthesia, non-dominant hand	Disabled	37 (23)	127 (77)	< .0001
	Control	26 (63)	15 (37)	
Stereognosis, number of errors, dominant hand	Disabled	130 (79)	34 (21)	< .05
	Control	38 (93)	3 (7)	
Right–left discrimination	Disabled	100 (61)	64 (39)	< .01
	Control	35 (85)	6 (15)	

TABLE 13.6. Parents' information about speech problems for 164[a] children with learning disabilities and 41 control children

Variable	Group	Normal N (%)	Unknown[b] N (%)	Slight/ possible problem N (%)	Definite problem N (%)	P (Chi-square test)
Age of fluent speech[c]	Disabled	98 (61)	4 (2)	37 (23)	25 (16)	< .01
	Control	30 (75)	1 (2)	10 (25)	0	
Vocabulary	Disabled	119 (76)	10 (6)	23 (15)	5 (3)	< .0001
	Control	39 (95)	2 (5)	0	0	
Stammering	Disabled	151 (92)	2 (1)	10 (6)	1 (1)	< .05
	Control	41 (100)	0	0	0	
Lisping	Disabled	146 (89)	2 (1)	13 (8)	3 (2)	< .01
	Control	41 (100)	0	0	0	
Indistinct speech	Disabled	120 (74)	6 (4)	34 (21)	3 (2)	< .0001
	Control	40 (98)	1 (2)	0	0	
Other speech problems	Disabled	138 (85)	6 (4)	15 (9)	4 (2)	< .05
	Control	39 (95)	1 (2)	1 (2)	0	

[a] For vocabulary category, total was 157; for indistinct speech and other speech problems, total was 163.
[b] Results not included in chi-square test.
[c] Rating of age of fluent speech: < 4 years = normal; 4 years = possibly abnormal; > 4 = abnormal.

TABLE 13.7. Parents' observations about speech functions, concentration, and behavior for 164 children with learning disabilities and 41 control children

Variable	Group	Normal N (%)	Slightly/ possibly abnormal N (%)	Definitely abnormal N (%)	P (Chi-square test)
Pronunciation	Disabled	145 (88)	18 (11)	1 (1)	
	Control	41 (100)	0	0	< .01
Maturity of language	Disabled	145 (88)	15 (9)	4 (2)	
function	Control	41 (100)	0	0	< .01
Concentration	Disabled	132 (80)	30 (18)	2 (1)	
	Control	40 (98)	1 (2)	0	< .01
Duration of attention	Disabled	127 (77)	28 (17)	9 (5)	
	Control	41 (100)	0	0	< .0001
Motor activity	Disabled	132 (80)	22 (13)	10 (6)	
	Control	39 (95)	1 (2)	1 (2)	< .05
General behavior	Disabled	132 (80)	22 (13)	10 (6)	
	Control	40 (98)	1 (2)	0	< .01
Contact	Disabled	146 (89)	17 (10)	1 (1)	< .01
	Control	41 (100)	0	0	< .01

Concentration, School Achievements, Behavior, and Emotional Problems

These areas are covered in other parts of this book. However, our investigations uncovered some additional data of interest.

As shown in Tables 13.7 and 13.8, many of the learning disabled had problems with concentration and school achievements. According to their parents, the concentration problems were mostly present when the children were engaged in school work and to a much lesser extent when they were involved in other activities. Some of the disabled showed increased motor activity during the examination.

TABLE 13.8. Parents' information about school achievements and concentration for 164 children with learning disabilities and 41 control children

Variable	Group	Normal N (%)	Unknown N (%)	Slight/ possible problems N (%)	Definite problems N (%)	P (Chi-square test)
School achievements,	Disabled	33 (20)	18 (11)	91 (55)	22 (13)	
language	Control	38 (93)	1 (2)	2 (5)	0	< .0001
School achievements,	Disabled	103 (63)	14 (9)	34 (21)	13 (8)	
mathematics	Control	39 (95)	0	2 (5)	0	< .0001
Concentration, home	Disabled	54 (33)	10 (6)	83 (51)	17 (10)	
lessons	Control	32 (78)	0	9 (22)	0	< .0001

[a] Results not included in chi-square test.

TABLE 13.9. Parents' information about behavior and emotional problem areas for 164 children with learning disabilities and 41 control children[a]

Variable	Group	Normal N (%)	Unknown[b] N (%)	Slight/ possible problems N (%)	Definite problems N (%)	P (Chi-square test)
Age of bladder control[c]	Disabled	130 (79)	0	16 (10)	18 (11)	< .01
	Control	36 (88)	0	3 (7)	2 (5)	
Age of bowel control[d]	Disabled	146 (90)	0	10 (6)	7 (4)	< .05
	Control	39 (95)	0	2 (5)	0	
Loneliness	Disabled	139 (85)	4 (2)	–	21 (13)	< .05
	Control	39 (95)	1 (2)	–	1 (2)	
Aggressiveness	Disabled	137 (84)	2 (1)	22 (13)	3 (2)	< .05
	Control	40 (98)	0	0	1 (2)	
Other behavioral problems	Disabled	150 (92)	2 (1)	8 (5)	3 (2)	< .05
	Control	39 (98)	1 (2)	0	0	
Frequent headaches	Disabled	139 (85)	1 (1)	13 (8)	11 (7)	< .05
	Control	38 (93)	1 (2)	2 (5)	0	

[a] For bowel control and other behavioral problems, total for disabled children was 163. For other behavioral problems, total for controls was 40.
[b] Not included in chi-square test .
[c] Rating of bladder control: < 4 years = normal; 4–6 years = possibly abnormal; > 6 years = definitely abnormal.
[d] Rating of bowel control: < 4 years = normal; 4 years = possibly abnormal; > 4 years = definitely abnormal.

The parents generally viewed their child's learning disabilities with optimism. The children were in the fifth grade at the time of our examination. The parents reported improvement in reading and writing problems in 92% of the children, no change in 6%, and worsening in only 2%.

Tables 13.7 and 13.9 show that several learning disability children had behavioral and emotional problems. The following variables within these areas did not show significant differences between the two groups: (a) (information from parents) well-being, bullying, ability to contact, dependency, pain in the stomach or in other locations, anxiety, inhibitions, divorced parents; (b) (during the examination) ability to cooperate.

Laterality

There has been much debate about the possible connections between laterality and learning disabilities. Table 13.10 suggests a slightly higher tendency among the learning disabled to prefer the left hand and foot. Using the .05 level of significance, the Chi-square test showed no statistically significant differences between the two groups with respect to choice of hand for writing and for ball throwing.

TABLE 13.10. Hand or foot preferred by 164 children with learning disabilities and 41 control children

Activity	Group	Right[a] N (%)	Left[b] N (%)	Ambidextrous[c] N (%)	Various combinations[d] N (%)
Writing	Disabled	141 (86)	23 (14)	0	–
	Control	39 (95)	2 (5)	0	–
Catching a ball	Disabled	143 (87)	18 (11)	3 (2)	–
	Control	39 (95)	2 (5)	0	–
Throw/cut/hammer	Disabled	142 (87)	11 (7)	0	11 (7)[e]
	Control	39 (95)	1 (2)	0	1 (2)
Hop on one foot/	Disabled	107 (65)	15 (9)	1 (1)	41 (25)[f]
trample/kick	Control	32 (78)	2 (15)	1 (2)	6 (15)[e]

[a] *Right:* right hand or foot was consistently chosen.
[b] *Left:* left hand or foot was consistently chosen.
[c] *Ambidextrous:* either right or left hand or foot might be chosen.
[d] *Various combinations:* right hand or foot was used in some activities and left hand or foot in others.
[e] One child was ambidextrous for one of the three functions.
[f] Six children were ambidextrous for one function, and one child was ambidextrous for two of the three functions.

Previous Illnesses and Injuries

Among the children with learning disabilities there were isolated examples of abnormal pregnancies, deliveries, and neonatal problems. A few children had experienced serious illnesses or injuries. It is difficult to judge whether these problems contributed to or resulted in reading and writing problems in specific cases, since group data showed no significant differences between this group and the controls.

EEG and CT Findings

EEG records showed definite abnormalities in 18.4% and possible abnormalities in 26.2% of the 103 disabled children examined. These figures were higher than those in our special control group of 104 patients, in which 7.7% had definite and 19.2% had possible abnormalities. The most frequent location of clearly abnormal changes among the disabled was in the temporal region, observed in 16 boys and 5 girls. The most common finding was slow activity, whereas spikes were infrequent. The abnormalities occurred with equal frequency on the right and left side.

With regard to CT examinations, 30.5% of the 105 disabled examined had definite (19%) or possible (11.4%) abnormalities. This was a much higher frequency than in the comparison group of 52 children (1.9% definite and 5.8% possible abnormalities). The most frequent finding in the learning disabled related to the ventricular system; particularly common were small enlargements in the frontal areas. These enlargements were often unilateral but could occur on either side. In some cases the enlargements were bilateral. Three of the children had abnormal findings in the brain itself (two minor and one large older infarction). In summary, the changes identified by the CT examinations were localized in different areas of the brain, sometimes on the right side, sometimes on the left, and occasionally bilateral.

As far as we know, similar series of CT studies in children with learning disabilities have not appeared in the literature. A detailed report of our EEG and CT studies in learning disabilities will appear elsewhere. It should be mentioned that autopsy studies of a few dyslexic persons who died in accidents have revealed structural changes in localized areas of the brain (Galaburda et al., 1985). It is also of interest to mention that CT studies of children with minor neurodevelopmental disorders (Bergstrøm, Bille, & Rasmussen, 1984) showed results similar to those in our series of CT examinations.

Neuropediatric Findings Within Subgroups of Dyslexics

So far in this chapter, *all* the disabled children examined have been evaluated as a group and compared with the controls. It is also of considerable interest to study neurological findings within subcategories of dyslexia. The following is a brief summary of our findings. Again, it must be remembered that the entire learning disability group, including the retarded, was classified as to dyslexia type.

Subclassification According to Dyslexia Types

The size of the study group allowed the study of the four-way dyslexia classification: auditory, visual, audiovisual, and others, the last being a grouping of several types including educational and emotional dyslexia.

It proved very difficult to find any clear patterns when comparing the various dyslexia types. However, in some areas the *visual* group stood out as better than the auditory group: (a) (according to parental reports) incidence of articulation problems and delayed speech; (b) (results of examinations) certain motor tests and some tests of finer sensation. It is quite possible that these differences might be the result of the fact that the visual group functioned at a higher average intellectual level than the auditory group.

Subclassification According to Intelligence

The learning disabled were divided into subgroups by means of their individual results on the Wechsler Intelligence Scale for Children, Revised, total score (WISC-Total). In a number of areas the performance of the disabled with WISC-Total score over 85 (which is −1 SD) was significantly better than for the dyslexics who scored 85 or lower. As shown in Tables 13.11, 13.12, and 13.13, this related to tests and examinations in the areas of fine motor functions, fine sensation, right-left discrimination, and a few other abilities. In addition to the variables shown in these tables, similar differences were found for the variables

TABLE 13.11. Qualitative tests in 158 children with learning disabilities divided into subgroups according to performance on the Wechsler Intelligence Scale for Children (WISC-R)

Ability	WISC– Total score, N of children	Normal N (%)		Slight/ possible problems N (%)		Definite problems		P (Chi-square test)
Dissociation between	> 85, 110	103	(94)	6	(5)	1	(1)	
head and eye	≤ 85, 48	39	(81)	8	(17)	1	(2)	< .05
movements								
General evaluation	> 85, 110	104	(95)	4	(4)	2	(2)	
of language	≤ 85, 48	38	(79)	9	(19)	1	(2)	< .05
General behavior	> 85, 110	97	(88)	8	(7)	5	(5)	
	≤ 85, 48	33	(69)	10	(21)	5	(10)	< .05
Concentration	> 85, 110	96	(87)	13	(12)	1	(1)	
	≤ 85, 48	34	(71)	13	(27)	1	(2)	< .05
Duration of attention	> 85, 110	95	(86)	12	(11)	3	(3)	
	≤ 85, 48	30	(62.5)	12	(25)	6	(12.5)	< .01

"cutting a circle" and "follow a line while writing." However, the analysis showed that for these two variables there was a significant difference between boys and girls, the boys having the most problems.

In one area the children with the lowest WISC-Total score were better than the ones scoring above 85 IQ: Only 2 (4%) of those in the lowest intelligence group had problems with enuresis after 4 years of age. Such problems were found in 15 (14%) of the children with WISC-Total score above 85. These observations are difficult to explain. However, in addition to maturational delay, it is usual to regard emotional problems as causes of enuresis in many children. (It should be noted, however, that all the retarded pupils were in the below 85 IQ group, while

TABLE 13.12. Quantitative motoric tests in 158 children with learning disabilities divided into subgroups according to performance on the Wechsler Intelligence Scale for Children (WISC-R)

Ability	Total WISC-score, N of children	Good N (%)	Poor N (%)	P (Chi-square test)
Manipulation of a ball	< 85, 110	102 (93)	8 (7)	
	≤ 85, 48	39 (81)	9 (19)	< .05
Figure copying	< 85, 109	61 (56)	48 (44)	
	≤ 85, 48	10 (21)	38 (79)	< .01
Pegboard, dominant	< 85, 110	59 (54)	51 (46)	
hand	≤ 85, 48	16 (33)	32 (67)	< .05
Finger tapping	> 85, 109	80 (73)	29 (27)	
dominant hand	≤ 85, 48	25 (52)	23 (48)	< .05

TABLE 13.13. Quantitative tests for fine sensation, right–left discrimination, and in-between test investigated in 158 children with learning disabilities divided into subgroups according to performance on the Wechsler Intelligence Scale for Children (WISC-R)

Ability	WISC–Total score, N of children	Good N (%)	Poor N (%)	P (Chi-square test)
Agnosia, dominant hand	> 85, 110	39 (34.5)	71 (65.5)	< .05
	≤ 85, 48	9 (19)	39 (81)	
Agnosia, non-dominant hand	> 85, 110	30 (27)	80 (73)	< .05
	≧ 85, 48	6 (12.5)	42 (87.5)	
Graphesthesia, dominant hand	> 85, 110	53 (48)	57 (52)	< .001
	≦ 85, 48	10 (21)	38 (79)	
Graphesthesia, non-dominant hand	> 85, 110	31 (28)	79 (72)	< .01
	≦ 85, 48	4 (8)	44 (92)	
Stereognosis, dominant hand	> 85, 110	76 (69)	34 (31)	< .05
	≦ 85, 48	25 (52)	23 (48)	
Stereogenesis, non-dominant hand	> 85, 110	81 (74)	29 (26)	< .05
	≦ 85, 48	27 (56)	21 (44)	
Stereogenesis, no. of errors, non-dominant hand	> 85, 110	100 (91)	10 (9)	< .01
	≦ 85, 48	36 (75)	12 (25)	
Right–left discrimination	> 85, 110	74 (67)	36 (33)	< .05
	≦ 85, 48	22 (49)	26 (51)	
In-between test	> 85, 109	63 (58)	46 (42)	< .05
	≦ 85, 47	17 (36)	30 (64)	

all the children above 85 IQ were dyslexic, making it statistically possible for all enuretics to be dyslexic.)

Subclassification According to Presence (Hereditary) or Absence (Not Hereditary) of Parents and/or Siblings With Reading and Writing Problems

No clear patterns differentiated these two subgroups, but those in the "hereditary" group had significantly more problems than the "not hereditary" group with respect to the following variables: (a) various complications at the neonatal stage, (b) being bullied, (c) loneliness, (d) school achievement in mathematics, (e) age at bowel control, (f) writing ability, and (g) balance, dominant foot.

Subclassification According to Assessed Development in Reading and Spelling Up to Grade 3-4

To measure the development of reading and spelling abilities among the children with learning disabilities, the results of achievement test scores in these two areas in grade 1-2 were compared with the grade 3-4 results by means of a "developmental score" (described in Chapter 6). The disabled children were ranked and divided into three groups according to their developmental scores (fast, medium, slow). No pattern identified any of these groups as being unique with regard to their results in the neurological examinations. The "fast" group scored higher than the other two groups only on one test (handwriting).

Subclassification According to Sex

Chi-square tests showed that learning disabled boys scored significantly lower than learning disabled girls on the following variables: (a) Age at bowel control; (b) presence of various types of seizures; (c) aggressiveness; (d) finger opposition, both hands; (e) finger/nose test, nondominant hand; (f) writing test; (g) staying on the line while writing; (h) motor activity; and (i) finger tapping, nondominant hand.

The disabled girls, on the other hand, scored significantly lower than the disabled boys on the following variables: (a) Abnormal birth presentation; (b) being reserved; (c) pencil pressure while writing; (d) pegboard, both hands combined; and (e) in-between test, dominant hand.

It is of interest that the boys showed more aggressiveness, whereas the girls were more reserved. Otherwise, no clear patterns of sex differences emerged from the data.

Discussion

There are several methodological problems involved in our investigations:

1. We investigated neurological problems in learning disabled children as a group. It was therefore natural to choose statistical methods for the workup. Such methods provide the possibility of discovering neurological disturbances that may be present in only one or a few cases. On the other hand, we were able to demonstrate the neurological problems that were of practical significance for several of these children. To a certain degree we were also able to demonstrate the extent of neurological signs in these children.
2. Parents' information concerning pregnancy, birth, and the child's first years might be inaccurate, and slight problems might be forgotten. However, this caveat applies to both the disabled and the controls.
3. A qualitative classification of results (normal, slightly abnormal, definitely abnormal) cannot give exact results. Again, this caveat applies to both groups.
4. Bias problems: Both parents and doctors will have a tendency to expect normal results from the controls and abnormal results from the disabled. Furthermore, it is probable that in the families of learning disabled children more attention is paid to the existence of reading and writing difficulties than in the families of the control children. Definitions of reading and writing problems also are variable, but this will be the case in the families of both groups.

Our study gives information about nearly 70% of the 235 learning disability cases who were invited for investigation. We found children with neurological dysfunctions in one or several of the following areas: fine motor coordination, gross motor coordination, fine sensation, right-left discrimination, speech, concentration, school achievements, behavior, and emotional characteristics. In addition, abnormal observations were made in EEG and CT studies of several of the children selected for these examinations. Our observations confirm the results reported in the literature (for general summary, see, e.g., Duffy & Geschwind, 1985) and give a picture of the extent of additional problems that affect many children with learning disabilities in a cohort of the population. It is important to take such additional problems into account when an individual plan of treatment is worked out.

Our study gives no secure information about possible neurological problems in the 71 children with learning disabilities who did not appear for investigation. We know that the sex distribution in these 71 was similar to that in the 164 children who were included in the investigation. The parents of some of the 71 thought that the reading and writing difficulties of their children had improved or disappeared. However, similar conclusions were also drawn by a large majority of parents of the 164 learning disabled who were investigated by us.

The clearest differences between the children with learning disabilities and controls were found when all disabled children were kept together as one group. When the children were divided into subgroups, it was as a rule difficult to discover significant differences between the individual groups. An exception was subdivision according to intelligence (see Tables 13.11, 13.12, and 13.13). The children with the lowest WISC-Total scores clearly had more problems than children with normal WISC-Total scores in areas such as fine motor coordination, right–left discrimination, and fine sensation. All these functions demand integration of several different parts of the brain and collaboration with the peripheral nervous system. The combination of these functional problems and subnormal intelligence might indicate more extensive cerebral dysfunction in these children; lesions do not seem to be limited to any special parts of the brain. It should be mentioned that, in the Isle of Wight study (Rutter & Yule, 1975), quite similar observations were reported. In that study manual skills, for example, showed the poorest results in the group with the lowest intelligence (this group was called "backward readers" by Rutter and Yule). In our study poor manual skills were also found in some learning disability cases WISC-Total score within the normal range (above 85).

It is well accepted that reading and writing problems in children can have several different causes. The learning disability cases in the Bergen Project were selected from a cohort of children by means of a procedure that stressed a reading and writing performance. As expected, the results of our investigations did not indicate a functional disturbance or anatomical lesion localized to one or a few areas of the brain.

Summary and Conclusions

This neuropediatric study comprised 164 11-year-old children with reading and writing disabilities and 41 control children from the same school classes. The study included 69.8% of all learning disability cases in an annual cohort of school children.

The following lists the variables that differentiated best between dyslexics and controls:

1. Reading and writing difficulties among first-degree relatives (parents, siblings).
2. Fine motor coordination (copying designs, handwriting, cutting a circle with scissors, follow-the-finger test, diadochokinesis, tongue movements, head–tongue dissociation).
3. Gross motor coordination (physical education skills, balance).
4. Fine sensation (agnosia, graphesthesia).
5. Right–left discrimination.
6. Speech functions (age of clear speech, vocabulary, articulation).
7. Information regarding school achievements (language and mathematics) and ability to concentrate.
8. Behavior and emotional problems (age at bladder control, general behavior, and ability to sustain social contact during the examination).
9. Sex (higher frequency of dyslexia in boys than in girls).

On the basis of our results the following conclusions may be drawn:

1. In severe cases of learning disabilities a neuropediatric examination is indicated to diagnose and deal with possible signs of minimal brain dysfunction.
2. Reading and writing problems are a group of disorders that may involve different causative factors.
3. A brain lesion may be associated with learning disabilities. It can occur in different parts of both hemispheres.
4. Learning disability cases of normal intellectual ability score higher than those of low intellectual ability in fine motor functions, fine sensation, and several other functions.

Acknowledgments. This investigation has received financial support from "Åndssvakesakens forskningsfond" and "Cerebral pareseforeningen i Bergen." It has received consultant services from Section of Medical Informatics and Statistics, University of Bergen.

CHAPTER 14

Growth and Efficacy Data: Results of the Total Experimental Program

H.-J. Gjessing and H.D. Nygaard

As in the case of many other studies of children with specific learning disabilities in the literacy skills, there was also in the Bergen Project a great deal of interest in how these children developed over time. Follow-up was certainly appropriate in this longitudinal study — it was possible to follow the children from grade 1 to grade 9. Special methodological problems associated with studies of this kind are discussed here. Also presented in this chapter is a brief review of the follow-up literature, and our follow-up data.

Follow-Up Studies of Children With Dyslexia

There have been quite a few follow-up studies of children with dyslexia. Fairly recent detailed reviews of the literature can be found in Spreen (1982) and in Schonhaut and Satz (1983). Follow-up studies vary widely in quality with respect to design and research methodology. Some studies focus primarily on the effects of various remedial programs, instructional plans, and treatments (e.g., Balow & Blomquist, 1965; Kline & Kline, 1975; Koppitz, 1971; Monroe, 1932).

Most follow-up studies are, however, primarily prognostic and descriptive; the question of growth is not necessarily tied to any particular treatment effect. This is especially true when follow-up is long (e.g., Howden, 1967; Rawson, 1968; Spreen, 1978). In addition to being interested in the development of reading skills, investigators have looked at such issues as school dropout rates, advanced education, adult socioeconomic status, personal adjustment, and antisocial (criminal) behavior. The variability in quality of research methodology relates to conceptualization and definition of the issues, instrumentation (tests, question-naires, interviews), and research techniques (sampling, control, statistical sophistication). One also finds considerable variation in sample size, which can range from about 30 to 3,400, including controls. Most samples are clinical refer-ral samples, which introduces biases of relatively unknown type and magnitude.

The ages of the children studied also vary considerably, starting from the primary grades (e.g., Rawson, 1968) to early secondary school age (e.g., Trites & Fiedorowicz, 1976). Quite a few studies have had small samples with a wide age range, which would lead to rather tenuous conclusions. Much evidence points to the fact that the problems of dyslexics vary greatly with age and achievement level, which would, of course, influence prognosis and development.

The time spans of follow-up studies also vary considerably, ranging from a few months to many years. Obviously, a longer time span is desirable in most situations. A long span makes possible study of the long-range growth of the children and of concurrent problems along the way (e.g., antisocial behavior, adjustment, dropout).

A long period between the initial study and follow-up has the disadvantage that the results of specific interventions become blurred over time. The most desirable thing would be periodic reevaluations, but this has rarely been done. If a project involves a particular treatment program over a specified time interval, some immediate postintervention is particularly desirable. This is also true of diagnostic methods. The long-range effects of such a program also need to be studied.

Discussion of Three Follow-Up Studies

Instead of providing another survey of the follow-up research, we have chosen to review three studies. These studies are particularly relevant to the Bergen Project.

Monroe followed up (1932) on her initial study of a large group of dyslexics in the Chicago area. Her diagnostic approach and remedial program were worked out in collaboration with Orton (1925). She used individually prescribed instruction based on the particular problems exhibited by each child.

Monroe's sample of 189 pupils was divided into three groups. The 89 pupils in group 1 were treated at a clinic by specially trained tutors. Group 2 consisted of 50 children who received special help from their regular classroom teachers. These teachers had received some special training, and they kept in touch with the clinic. These two groups, then, received similar treatment, the differences being the setting and the degree of specialization of the teachers. The 50 children in group 3 served as controls, receiving whatever instructional program was available at their regular school. All 189 children underwent the same diagnostic workup and all complied with the selection criteria for inclusion in the study. The three groups were equated after the pretesting so as to make them comparable.

The results of follow-up were not particularly surprising. Group 1 showed the most progress, 1.39 years in grade equivalents over a 7-month period of special help. During the same time span group 2 had an average gain of 0.79 year, whereas group 3 gained an average of only 0.14 year.

Monroe provided a rather detailed description of the remedial programs used with the two treatment groups, but no information as to what happened to the control group.

Kline and Kline (1975) have also been associated with what is now called The Orton Dyslexia Society. They did a follow-up study of 216 dyslexics of varying ages selected from a clinical referral sample of 750 who had been referred to their clinic by family physicians because of severe learning disabilities. The study sample had all been diagnosed as having "developmental dyslexia" (Critchley, 1970), and they were provided with help from specially trained clinicians who used the Orton Gillingham approach, a remedial program with a very strong phonics emphasis.

The program was carried out with the 92 persons who agreed to participate; they were referred to as the "clinic group." There were 29 persons in the "school group" who did not participate in the clinic program. The latter group did, for the most part, receive some form of special help at school.

The posttests were administered by people who did not know if the students belonged to the clinic group or the school group. The growth in reading achievement at the time of the posttest was categorized as "some," "marked," or "dramatic." The percentages of pupils who actually showed growth from pretest to posttest were 95.7 and 44.8 for the clinic and school groups, respectively. The category "dramatic" was used for 17.5% of the clinic group and 3.4% of the school group. Using another dyslexia sample of 95 as a comparison group it was found that only 4.3% of the clinic sample showed no progress, whereas this was the case for 49% of the dyslexics who did not participate in the clinic program.

Schonhaut & Satz (1983) studied the entire cohort of kindergarten-age boys in Alachua County, Florida. They were pretested in the second grade with a standardized reading test. Four groups were formed on the basis of the test results:

Group 1 Severely retarded in reading $N = 49$
Group 2 Mildly retarded in reading $N = 62$
Group 3 Average reading ability $N = 252$
Group 4 Superior reading ability $N = 63$

Follow-up testing was done 3 years later. On the basis of the test results in grade 5, the pupils were again classified into four categories, as they had been 3 years earlier. Of the 49 children who were originally in the severely retarded in reading group, only 6% scored average or higher, while 18% of those mildly retarded in reading had reached the average or higher level. The investigators interpreted their finding as discouraging, concluding that there is a "grim prognosis" for children with reading difficulties in the second grade.

The results of this third study are much at variance with the first two reviewed here. Some factors obviously played a major role.

First, the first two studies entailed extensive, systematic individualized diagnosis and remedial treatment. This was not the case in the Schonhaut & Satz study. Second, the time interval between the pretest and posttest was much shorter in the first two studies, although this varied a bit in the Kline and Kline study. The favorable results may be temporary, a conclusion supported by the follow-up study by Balow and Blomquist (1965). The short-term changes could simply be a novelty effect or perhaps a Hawthorne effect, which would, of course, diminish over time. There could also be some methodological problems that explain the lack of long-term effects; these are discussed below.

TABLE 14.1. Scale of criteria for rating follow-up studies developed by Schonhaut and Satz, 1983

Criteria	Score
I. Length of follow-up period	
A. Follow-up from before age 8 to after age 20	3
B. Follow-up period at least 10 years	2
C. Follow-up period at least 5 years	1
D. Follow-up period less than 5 years	0
II. Size of sample	
A. At least 100 subjects	2
B. At least 50 subjects	1
C. Less than 50 subjects	0
III. Adequacy of sampling procedure	
A. Population consisting of entire school class(es)	2
B. Sample drawn from an entire school class	1
C. Clinic sample	0
IV. Adequacy of control	
A. Matched control group of average readers	2
B. Some control group or means of comparison	1
C. No control group	0
V. Adequacy of criteria for defining learning disabilities	
A. Objective well-defined criteria	2
B. Some attempt at systematic definitional criteria	1
C. No attempt at systematic definitional criteria (e.g., vague criteria, diagnosis according to referral problem, etc.)	0

Criteria for Methodology in Follow-Up Research

The basis for this discussion of criteria for good follow-up research is the analysis by Schonhaut and Satz (1983). They listed five prerequisites for a good follow-up study:

1. An adequate follow-up period.
2. A sufficiently large sample size.
3. A satisfactory method of sample selection.
4. An adequate comparison group.
5. A valid and objective measure of reading/learning ability.

It should be pointed out here that these criteria were designed for use only in prognostic follow-up studies, and not in efficacy studies that would entail the use of specific remedial and treatment programs.

On the basis of these five criteria, Schonhaut and Satz devised a scale that rates prognostic follow-up studies on a scale from 0 to 11 (Table 14.1).

They used this scale to evaluate 18 different follow-up studies published between 1962 and 1978. They rated four studies 1, two studies 2, two 3, two 4, three 5, one 6, none 7, and two 8. Two received the highest ratings of all 18 studies, 9 out of 11 points.

The results from most of these 18 studies confirm that the prognosis for children who are poor readers in the early grades is, for the most part, quite discouraging. The prognosis in five studies was "good," two studies reported "mixed" prognosis, and in 11 studies the prognosis was "poor."

Among the eight studies rated highest there was only one in which the prognosis was "good." In other words, prognosis tended to vary inversely with the quality of the study. This tendency was particularly pronounced with respect to size of sample, adequacy of sampling procedure, and adequacy of control.

The Bergen Project can now be viewed against the background of these studies, although it was not primarily an efficacy study nor basically a prognostic study: It had components of both designs, including a short-term and a long-term follow-up.

The project involved extensive diagnostic evaluations (pretests) of the entire dyslexic sample, on the basis of which an individual prescriptive remedial program was laid out for each child. Part of the program involved advisory conferences with the parents and the teachers, all worked out by specially trained teachers and school psychologists.

All the dyslexic children were treated within the framework of the Norwegian public schools, although done differently in the various schools. Some schools set up reading clinics; others provided individual and/or group instruction from special teachers in a pull-out program. Some students received help in their own classrooms where there was a two-teacher team, one of them typically a specially trained reading teacher. The special instruction lasted anywhere from a few months to several years, depending on the need.

This entire project was rated by us, using the criteria set forth by Schonhaut and Satz. The results are shown in Table 14.2. We rated the Bergen Project 9 on the 11-point scale, which placed it among the top-rated studies reviewed by

TABLE 14.2. Methodological merit of the Bergen Project as evaluated by the Schonhaut and Satz rating scale (see Table 14.1)

Criteria	Score
I. Length of follow-up period	
C – Follow-up period at least 5 years	1
II. Size of sample	
A – At least 100 subjects	2
III. Adequacy of sampling procedure	
A – Population consisting of entire school classes	2
IV. Adequacy of control	
A – Matched control group of average readers	2
V. Adequacy of criteria for defining learning disabilities	
A – Objective, well-defined criteria	2
Total	9

Schonhaut and Satz. The project also had some important qualities that are not taken into consideration in this rating scale.

First, follow-up evaluation was done twice, at grade 3-4 and again at grade 9. Second, both the pretest at grade 1-2 and the first follow-up entailed double testing to ascertain reliable assessment and to reduce the regression effect. This selection process was used with all the pupil groups involved in the project. Furthermore, the final selection of the dyslexia sample was validated against the opinions of teachers and parents, which resulted in a somewhat smaller sample.

Despite the high rating of this project, as an efficacy study it was encumbered by the problems characteristic of such studies. Two difficulties were particularly bothersome.

First, there was no systematic control of the extent to which the remedial programs were executed. The school system provided the necessary financial support so that every child with a learning disability could receive the kind of help prescribed in the initial diagnosis. The remedial programs were kept track of by the special educators and school psychologists, but the quality of this effort probably varied considerably.

The other difficulty entailed the lack of a dyslexic control group for which no special treatment was provided. From a purely experimental viewpoint this is, of course, a major weakness, but one that was accepted from the very beginning as unavoidable. A group of children with a problem as serious and consequential as dyslexia could not remain untreated over a span of several years; it would have been considered unethical and, in the real world, impractical.

Much of the follow-up evaluation of this project was based on interviews with the parents, teachers, school psychologists, and special educators, as well as follow-up assessments. These are all discussed in the subsequent sections of this chapter, along with an interpretation of how they all fit into a practical, clinical context.

Evaluation by the School and the Parents of the Development of the Dyslexics and the Practical Value of the Project

The Bergen Project was a very extensive and demanding long-term research project which affected the daily school routines over an extensive period. Its practical execution was completely dependent upon close and systematic cooperation by a variety of people, particularly the teachers, school psychologists, and parents. It was natural, therefore, as well as necessary to get the opinion of these groups regarding their experiences with and evaluations of the project. They were seen as the *consumers* of our findings.

These evaluations were gathered under two major headings. First there was the question of the *value* of this approach to alleviate or reduce learning disabilities and their social and emotional concomitants. The other major question related to the practical *implementation* of the project, dealing with such issues as the value of the guidelines provided, time utilization, use of diagnostic and remedial aids, and so on.

Resources for Gathering Systematic Information
From the Consumer Groups

To collect the opinions and impressions of the main consumer groups—parents, teachers, and educational specialists—a series of questionnaires, interviews, and report forms were developed, as described in the following.

1. School psychologists and other specialists gave the teachers feedback about the test results obtained on their pupils at the end of grade 1 and the beginning of grade 2. This feedback dealt with individual pupil data as well as classroom averages. The big emphasis was, of course, on the learning disabled, although no such classification was made without consulting the teacher and the respective parents.

2. Questionnaires were sent to all teachers during April and May of second grade regarding the implementation of the project up to that time. The issues covered at that time related to the adequacy of the feedback they had received, to the scope of the classroom investigations, and to certain census-type information such as class size, teachers' backgrounds, and so on. Opinions were also gathered relating to the instructional program associated with the project.

3. Questionnaires were sent to the educational specialists involved in June of second grade. Information gathered at this time related to their experiences with the feedback process, cooperation with the schools and the teachers, and implementation of the individual assessments which they had been responsible for during the fall of second grade. They were also asked for their opinions about the group and individual tests used so far.

4. Each classroom teacher filled out another questionnaire during February-March of third grade. This dealt with the development of each class as a whole and of the dyslexic children in particular. The questions regarding the dyslexic children related to their educational progress, how the special instructional program was worked out in each classroom, the type and degree of cooperation with the homes, the usefulness of the special instructional materials provided, and their value for each pupil's achievement and school adjustment.

5. A questionnaire was sent to the parents of every dyslexic child in September of the fourth grade. The parents were asked fairly detailed questions regarding their child's development from before the special educational program was initiated at the beginning of second grade to the present. They were asked to evaluate the severity of their child's learning disabilities in second and fourth grade, the child's development during this time span, what factors they felt were involved in the child's development, their views of the guidance they had received from the school and how they felt the child was adjusting to the school situation, intellectually and emotionally.

6. Another questionnaire was sent to the parents of each dyslexic student in April-May of ninth grade. This questionnaire was similar to the one they received in fourth grade, but was limited to school achievement and adjustment.

7. A questionnaire was sent to the teachers in April-May of ninth grade. As mentioned elsewhere, the children in Norwegian schools generally had the same teacher several years in a row, but by ninth grade their teachers had not known

the children during the elementary school years, so this questionnaire was limited to a status report relating to the dyslexic children's achievement in the literacy skills.

The results of these questionnaires were analyzed, summarized, and interpreted, forming the basis for the discussion here. As in any longitudinal study spanning many years, one would, of course, expect a certain amount of attrition. Further, many parents avoided some of the more detailed questions but answered the major ones. The response return for the main questions over the entire follow-up time span was about 85%, although the rates for some of the detailed questions were considerably lower. The response rates for the 147 teachers of the 181 dyslexic pupils was 91% for the questions answered most often, less than that for other questions. It should be remembered that this project dealt with a very stable population, and that the attrition rate in all aspects of this research was basically an insignificant factor.

The Consumer Groups' Views on the Dyslexic Pupils' Development

Parents

The questionnaires to the parents in the fourth and the ninth grades asked about the children's literacy skills problems in the second grade. The children were reported to have had "severe" or "very severe" learning disabilities by 64% and 57% of the parents at the time of the two questionnaires, respectively. This difference in judgment would certainly be considered slight, considering the fact that there was a 5-year time interval between the two opinions. These figures also suggest that the parents were generally aware of the problem at an early time in the child's schooling. There is, of course, also more emphasis on these basic skills in the early grades. The slight decline in these percentages may also be a reflection of what the parents saw as very positive growth in their children's acquisition of literacy skills. The percentage of parents who reported severe or very severe learning disabilities by the fourth grade dropped to 18%; by the ninth grade the incidence was 9%.

The other options for answers to the questions regarding the severity of the children's learning problems were "minor," "insignificant," and "none." For the last two ratings combined, 6% of the parents checked these in the second grade, 37% in the fourth grade, and 58% in the ninth grade. The replies from the parents suggested very positive growth for about half the children who were labeled learning disabled in the second grade.

Teachers

The teachers were not asked about the degree of difficulty with literacy skills, as were the parents. They were simply asked whether the dyslexic pupils had shown improvement in these skills. Affirmative answers to this question were given by 83% of the teachers, supporting the parents' impressions of positive growth, although the respective percentages are not comparable because of the way the question was asked. But the ninth-grade data were comparable, since the teachers were now asked to rate the severity of the pupils' problems. The combined incidence of "severe" and "very severe" problems in reading was judged by the teachers to be 20%, while the same rating of spelling difficulties was 37%. The parents were not asked to differentiate between reading and spelling; their 9% incidence figure represented a combination of the two subjects.

Comparison of Parents' and Teachers' Responses

The evaluations of the teachers and the parents of the children in the ninth grade differed considerably. The teachers still rated 37% of the dyslexic sample as having spelling difficulties. Reading is undoubtedly the more important skill at this time for the acquisition of educational, vocational, and social skills and information. About 20% of the children were still considered to have severe or very severe reading difficulties, while a total of 39% of them had reading difficulties rated as insignificant or none.

The parents viewed their children's development more positively than did the teachers, but which rating is more accurate? The ninth-grade teachers had known these students for only the better part of a year; they were also teaching in a departmentalized school in which classes were fairly large. The teachers obviously did not know the children as well as did the parents; on the other hand, the teachers had the benefit of a more or less normative frame of reference through the other students. The teachers were probably better judges of how these children performed in school in comparison with their peers and in relation to what is ordinarily expected of students in the ninth grade. But the children's overall adjustment to the entire school and social situation was probably perceived more accurately by the parents.

Parents are further in the position to observe how their child functions in everyday life, with respect to not only school performance but also the daily application of literacy skills. The Bergen Project entailed considerable parent contacts, and the parents were strongly urged to discuss the learning difficulties with their children. It would seem reasonable to assume that the opinions expressed by the parents also reflect to a large extent how the children themselves viewed their achievement. The parents were no doubt more subjective than the teachers, but their highly positive impressions may be valuable to their children's self-concepts.

The parents gave very positive statements not only about their children's school achievement, but about the children's school attitudes as well. Before the special program was initiated in the second grade, the parents who reported that their child did not enjoy school (ratings of "not well" and "poor") were 18%. By the fourth grade this percentage had dropped to 4%. But it was up to 13% in the ninth grade. The ninth-grade figure could, of course, indicate simply that by this stage of development an increasing number of students do not enjoy school. It is also important to notice that by this time the special remedial help offered these students at an earlier age had gradually disappeared. The teachers' judgment regarding the extent to which the students did not enjoy school was about the same as that reported by the parents.

Since there was no parent control group, it is difficult to evaluate the ninth-grade data. It may be of interest, however, to compare these data with the results of a school attitude study done in Norway in the 1960s (Sandven, 1968). Ninth-grade students were asked directly to what degree they liked or did not like school. For the entire ninth-grade sample ($n = 3,364$), the percentage of students who did not enjoy school ("rarely like school" and "like school only occasionally") was 29%. For pupils who were taking the lower track, which typically included the low achievers, the percentage was 37%.

One cannot draw any hard and fast conclusions about these data since the two studies differed in so many respects—time of data collection, the rating scales themselves, and respondents (students vs. parents). But it would appear that the 13% figure for the dyslexic children for ninth grade was quite low, especially for a group of learning disabled students.

In Norway, children start first grade at age 7; the ninth grade is the end of obligatory schooling. By the end of ninth grade there was still a significant number of students in the Bergen dyslexia sample who had serious reading difficulties—9% according to the parents, 20% according to the teachers. The teachers were also asked to judge this incidence for all ninth graders. This turned out to be 1%, which is probably an underestimate—some pupils undoubtedly developed literacy skills problems later on in their schooling. It seems reasonable to assume that this study identified most potential learning disability cases in the initial testing in grades 1 and 2. Our best judgment as to the incidence of what one might call hard-core dyslexia in this particular cohort of children is probably not over 2% by the end of compulsory schooling.

Before we initiated the Bergen Project we estimated that 5% of the ninth-grade pupil population had severe learning disabilities. This means that even using the most pessimistic judgments—those of the ninth-grade teachers—three of five children with potential learning disability would no longer qualify as having "severe or very severe reading problems." From a research point of view it would have been advantageous to have had a nontreated dyslexic control group. Nevertheless, it appears safe to conclude that on the average the cohort involved in this project was considerably better off than what had been the case. It also seems reasonable to ascribe the positive changes to the intervention associated with this project.

The Consumer Groups' Evaluation of the Project's Practical Outcome

Parents

The fourth-grade parental questionnaire asked for opinions with respect to a variety of reasons for the children's progress or lack of progress. The parents were presented with many alternatives, such as the special instruction provided, home–school cooperation, parental support, the quality and appropriateness of the regular education, the child's attitudes and reactions to the special help provided, and the child's general development. The parents were asked to check one or more options on the questionnaire.

Of the 148 parents who responded, 115 (78%) replied that their child had made good school progress, 24 (16%) replied that their child had not shown particularly good progress, and 9 (6%) were uncertain. Among the 115 who checked good progress, the "special instruction provided" was emphasized by 62%. In fact, 25% checked only that particular alternative. On the other hand, 38% did not indicate that the special instruction had been a significant factor for their child's development. The alternatives checked by these parents were about evenly distributed between three factors: home–school cooperation, the quality of the regular classroom instruction, and the child's own unique growth pattern. But only 3% checked the developmental pattern, "the child simply grew out of it," to the exclusion of all other options. An additional 13% checked additional factors, for a total of 16%. In other words, 84% of the parents had the opinion that the school's contribution was the primary deciding factor in their child's positive development, with special instruction as the single dominant factor.

Twenty-four parents (16%) felt that their child had made little or no progress. Among these, nine ascribed the lack of school progress to the child's anxiety and lack of self-confidence. About half of the 24 indicated that the main reason for the child's lack of success in school was simply a lack of interest in reading and writing. Seven parents checked lack of support from the school as a major factor, eight checked lack of home–school cooperation, and one checked lack of effort by the home.

This summary of the parents' opinions about possible reasons for their child's progress or lack of such indicates that progress was mainly attributed to the school's effort, particularly the special instruction, while few parents attributed lack of progress to a lack of effort by the school. Most parents felt that lack of progress was related to characteristics of the child, such as lack of interest, anxiety, and lack of self-confidence.

The parents' evaluation is clear testimony that the school had done a good job for the members of the cohort with dyslexia. On the other hand, some children's lack of interest, anxiety, and lack of self-confidence are often the result of the school's inability to help and support these pupils. These problems were not studied in sufficient depth to determine whether they were the cause or the result of the learning problems, or simply occurred concurrently with them.

Teachers

According to the teachers' replies to the questionnaire at the end of third grade, 100 pupils had made more progress than they otherwise would have made without the special program and 21 pupils showed no effect of the special program. The teachers did not respond in the case of 60 children. It should be pointed out that most of the teachers had taught these same children since the beginning of first grade, which gave them a better basis for comparison than if they had taught them in third grade only.

It was the opinion of the teachers, then, that the program had been beneficial for 83% of the dyslexic children. In reply to the question of whether the special instructional program was necessary, 89% of the teachers answered affirmatively. With respect to the advice the teachers had been given by the research team, 98% of them considered it relevant. The teachers expressed the opinion that the special help that had been provided met the needs of the vast majority of the children. Some teachers did not answer these questions, usually justifying their lack of response by stating that they had taken over the class at a later stage and had insufficient experience with the children to answer the questions.

The teachers were also asked if the dyslexic pupils had problems other than those studied in this project. A "no" answer was given by 74%. Among the problems mentioned by the remaining 26% were social and emotional problems, poor concentration, and difficulties in learning mathematics.

The teachers were asked how they thought the dyslexic pupils had reacted to the special instructional program provided for them. The teachers thought that 76% had reacted positively and had shown increased motivation to learn; they had no clear feeling about 22% of the children. In only 2% of cases did the teachers report negative reactions among these pupils. The teachers also expressed the opinion that about 40% of the dyslexic pupils had improved their school attitudes and their self-confidence as a result of the special program. In the case of about 1% of the pupils the teachers felt that the special program contributed to lower self-confidence and less enjoyment in school.

The teachers had been informed about the project in a variety of ways—at faculty meetings by members of the research team, in information bulletins, from the minutes of the board of education, and from the principals, who had attended special meetings related to the project. Seventy-nine percent of the teachers felt that the communication was good or excellent; the remaining 21% considered it inadequate or poor. Criticism of poor or inadequate communication from the administration appeared to be fairly common, so the 21% should probably be interpreted as acceptable.

At the transition from first to second grade a fairly extensive program of testing and observations was implemented in every classroom. The purpose was to obtain normative data on school achievement and school and social adjustment; the main focus, of course, was the identification of children in need of special help with literacy skills. When asked about this phase of the project, 25% of the teachers said that the study had yielded more information about their pupils than they would have obtained otherwise. About 50% said that they had not gotten any new information, while the remaining 25% were unsure about this point.

With respect to teachers gaining insight about specific pupils, about 50% of them replied affirmatively to this, about 30% replied negatively, and 20% were not sure. When asked about the effectiveness with which the project was able to identify pupils in need of special instruction, 43% of the teachers felt that the project had not been effective. Since 43% is a large number, we analyzed the comments of these teachers in some detail. Some teachers stated that they had already identified the learning disabled children independently of the project. Others thought that some children identified were not those who needed help the most, that they had other pupils who should have been included but were not.

Much of this additional information came to light when the teachers were asked if they had other pupils who should have been referred to the school psychologists because of learning difficulties. Thirty-one teachers replied affirmatively to this inquiry; altogether they had 51 pupils with a variety of problems. More than half the children were reported to have reading and writing difficulties, while others had behavior problems or difficulties with mathematics. In some classes the teachers identified as many as three pupils who they thought should have been identified by the project; several of these pupils had more than one specific school-related problem.

It should be pointed out, however, that it was not the purpose of this research project to attempt to identify, diagnose, and treat all children in the cohort who needed help. The project attempted only to identify, on the basis of specific criteria, all children with specific learning problems with literacy skills (underachievers in reading and spelling), plus those who had general learning disabilities (retarded) on the basis of low scores on scholastic aptitude (IQ) tests. The project had no responsibilities for pupils with other, special needs, but teachers were encouraged to refer these pupils to the school psychologists according to the procedures already in effect, independent of the Bergen Project.

The teachers' opinions reviewed so far pertain to relatively global aspects of the project. They were also asked very specific questions regarding the various instruments used in the screening testing. These instruments consisted of the following:

1. Two rating scales. Scale I was modeled after an American rating scale by H.R. Myklebust, covering understanding and use of oral language, motor coordination, and school behavior. Each area was rated on a 5-point scale, from "much above average" to "much below average." Scale II rated pupil achievement in mathematics, spelling, and reading on a 3-point scale (above average, average, below average) and also rated the degree to which achievement was consistent with expectations based on the pupils' judged aptitude for schoolwork.
2. Two sociometric tests, in which pupils were to identify the three classmates they would prefer to study or play with. Both tests entailed pictorial stimuli.
3. A school-attitude survey dealing with school in general as well as specific school subjects.
4. A self-concept test.
5. A group intelligence test (a somewhat abbreviated version of the Sandven test, a Norwegian test).
6. Achievement test in mathematics, silent reading, and spelling from dictation.

The teachers' opinions about the two rating scales were very favorable – "very good" (53%) and "very useful" (69%). They particularly liked scale II.

The sociometric tests were given favorable ratings by only 30% of the teachers. The remaining 70% expressed little or no use for this kind of information. There were unfavorable comments relating to these tests scattered throughout the various questionnaires and interviews. Many of these appeared to be related to other sociometric tests that utilize negative choices ("Who would you *not* want to . . ."). Even though the sociometric instruments we used entailed only positive choices, the main objection seemed to be against the focus on specific individuals in the classroom. The teachers were more oriented toward cooperative activities and equality among the children. Seen in this context, any focusing on individuals could be viewed unfavorably, and this attitude carried over to their judgments regarding the sociometric instruments.

With regard to the school-attitude survey and the self-concept test, between 40 and 50% of the teachers expressed the opinion that these had been "quite useful" or "very useful." They were much more positive about these instruments than about sociometry.

The intelligence test was judged "quite useful" or "very useful" by 68% of the teachers.

The achievement tests in silent reading and spelling were judged "quite useful" or "very useful" by a good 80% of the teachers; 60% assigned these ratings also to the mathematics test. When asked if such tests were useful in identifying pupils with learning disabilities, 76% gave an unqualified "yes" answer, while 3% gave an unqualified "no" answer.

The reactions from the teachers indicated that, first, most teachers (76%) considered these group assessments helpful in identifying pupils with learning disabilities. They reacted particularly positively to achievement and ability tests, whereas their reactions to social and emotional instruments were more guarded. There was general agreement, however, that this whole evaluation process was too extensive. The research team agreed that for a normal instructional program there was too much testing within a relatively short period of time. But the purpose of the Bergen Project went way beyond the normal classroom procedures, since much of the information was gathered for research purposes. There was great concern for the accuracy and reliability of data and decisions, which invariably led to extensive data gathering and testing.

Education Specialists

The education specialists in this project consisted of the staff of the school district's office of school psychology plus several special educators employed by the project, altogether 15 psychologists, 12 special educators, and 4 school social workers.

The school social workers were not queried about the special instructional program. Of the 29 psychologists and special educators, 19 expressed positive reactions to the continued use of the group tests, although not to the extent they were employed in this research project. Most were in favor of achievement and ability testing, but there was much less agreement with respect to the sociometric assessment. The opinions of these specialists coincided with those of the teachers to a very large extent.

As a whole this group of educational specialists considered the instruments used well suited to identify the pupils who were in need of special instruction. Most of them pointed out, as did the teachers, that more pupils should have been identified and helped, considering it deplorable that limited financial resources limited the number of pupils who could be provided with special instruction.

The education specialists were also asked to voice their opinions regarding the program, a process in which they themselves played a central role. They all agreed that the school psychologist should participate in reporting. The majority also thought that the special education teacher should participate, whereas about half felt a need for the school social worker as well. These data showed that these specialists considered reporting back very important, seeing it also as a good way to strengthen the cooperation between their office and the school faculty. The amount of time allocated to this process was inadequate and should have been increased.

The individual assessment of pupils selected for further study entailed the use of a variety of tests. Most of these were used exclusively by the psychologists. The instruments used to evaluate literacy and oral language skills were in most cases used by the special educators. The specialists were asked to evaluate these tests.

The psychologists all agreed that the Wechsler Intelligence Scale for Children (WISC-R) was a highly suitable instrument. They also spoke quite highly of the Bender Gestalt test, but did not consider it necessary in all cases. The special education teachers had all had experience with Gjessing's diagnostic reading and spelling test (Dia-Gjessing), and they all considered this test well suited for this task. Additional tests used included a laterality assessment and Koppitz's Visual Aural Digit Span test (VADS). A personal information questionnaire on each pupil was considered a useful adjunct to the assessment process. An interview form and a self-reporting form could have been used during the teacher interviews, but only half of the specialists chose to use these tools.

There was broad agreement among the specialists that group tests are valuable instruments, not only for the screening of pupils who may need special help, but also to gather group data on a class. Most specialists favored the continued use of such tests. (It should be pointed out here that standardized achievement and ability group tests are rarely used; as of this writing there are no achievement test batteries published in Norway.)

With respect to individual tests, the WISC-R, the Bender Gestalt test, and the Dia-Gjessing stood out as being the most desirable; their routine use was recommended. The remaining tests were judged to be most appropriate for further testing in individual cases.

There was a great deal of emphasis in this project on cooperation among the school, the parents, and the office of school psychology. The specialists found the expanded, systematic program of cooperation that this project established to be very valuable, and felt that it had led to better consultations with the teachers and the parents. The pattern of cooperation established was up to most specialists' expectations, and it had resulted in a more comprehensive picture of the pupils. It was the experience of the education specialists that the parents as well as the school intended to follow the advice provided them. But the possibilities for giving all the assistance indicated were hampered somewhat by insufficient resources. The education specialists all agreed that school psychologists as well as special educators were necessary when giving advice with respect to learning disabilities. There was also agreement that recommendations regarding special education programs should be handled by each school's special education teacher in cooperation with the office of school psychology.

The education specialists bemoaned the insufficient resources, particularly with an eye toward heavier involvement after the diagnostic phase. Working on the Bergen Project, with its very tight time schedule, was an additional burden on persons who were already very busy. Follow-up work such as done in this project will be difficult to carry out in the future with the level of financing currently available to the specialists, despite the obvious value of such effort.

Statistical Analyses of Advancement Based on Test Results

The children's growth in achievement was measured in "developmental scores," which indicate the degree to which the achievement test scores differed from the scores predicted from the pretest results. The scale used was described earlier in Chapters 1 and 6. The pretests were given in grade 1-2, and the data reported here pertain to the achievement test results obtained in grade 3-4. The main purpose was to determine if the remedial program had resulted in *positive advancement*, that is, test scores on the posttest that exceeded those predicted from the pretest.

Norms for the Developmental Scores

The developmental scores have, so far, been reported in the form of z scores based on raw score distributions. Since the posttest yielded negatively skewed distributions, the distributions were normalized by conversion to stanine scores. This was done by assigning the scores from a low of 1 to a high of 9 to these respective percentages of students: 4, 7, 12, 17, 20, 17, 12, 7, 4.

The stanine scales were developed on the basis of the entire cohort in reading, spelling, and mathematics, as shown in Figure 14.1. The pupils who had a stanine score of 1 represented the 4% of the cohort that showed the least progress (most negative development) in comparison with progress predicted from the pretest at grade 1-2 to the posttest at grade 3-4. A developmental score of 5 showed the predicted amount of growth; scores below 5 indicated negative development, that is, growth at a less than predicted rate; whereas scores above 5 indicated positive development.

Developmental Scores for the Combined Learning Disability Group (Retarded Plus Dyslexic)

The developmental score distributions for the combined learning disability group differed quite remarkably from the norm, as shown in Figure 14.2. One would

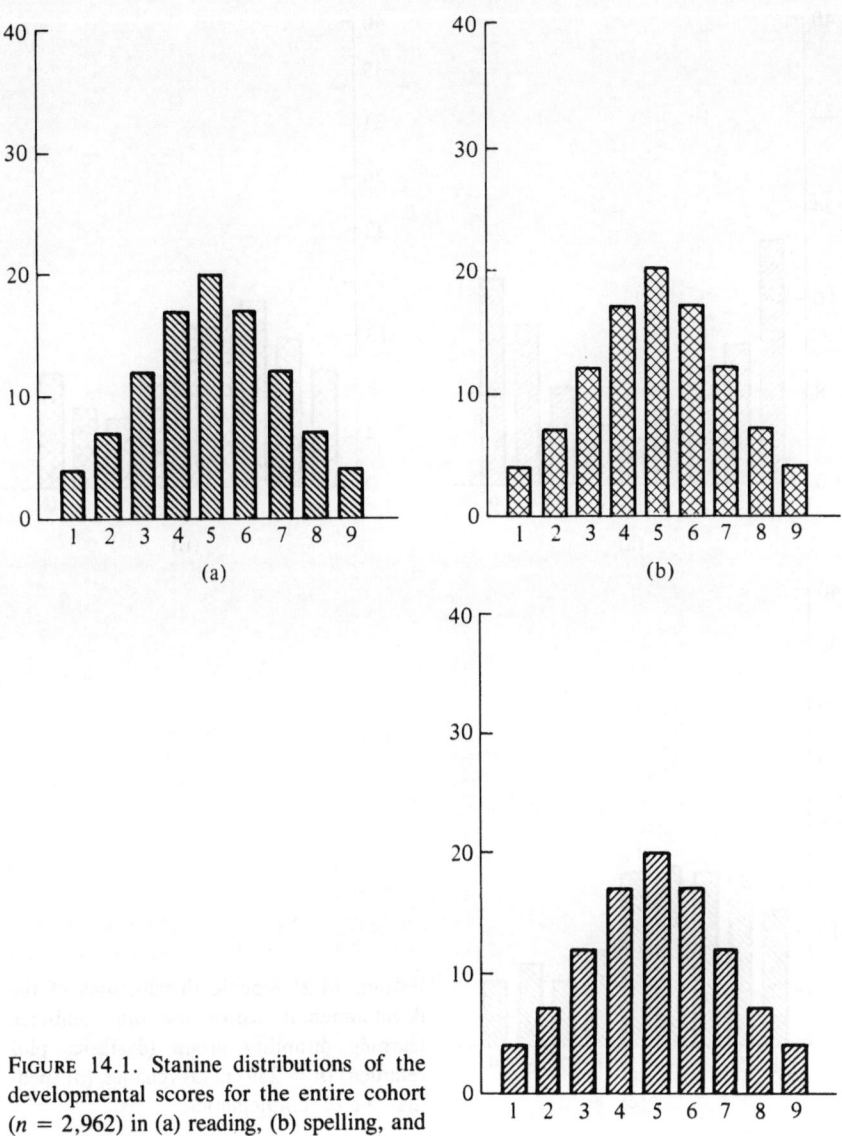

FIGURE 14.1. Stanine distributions of the developmental scores for the entire cohort ($n = 2,962$) in (a) reading, (b) spelling, and (c) mathematics.

normatively expect to find 23% in the three lowest stanines. In reading, 43.9% of the students fell in this score range, while another 40.4% scored in the top three stanines. With only 15.7% in the middle three stanines which normatively yield 54%, we have a distinctly U-shaped curve in reading.

In spelling and mathematics the situation was quite different, since in a three-way split the highest percentage was for stanines 1 through 3 and the lowest for stanines 7 through 9.

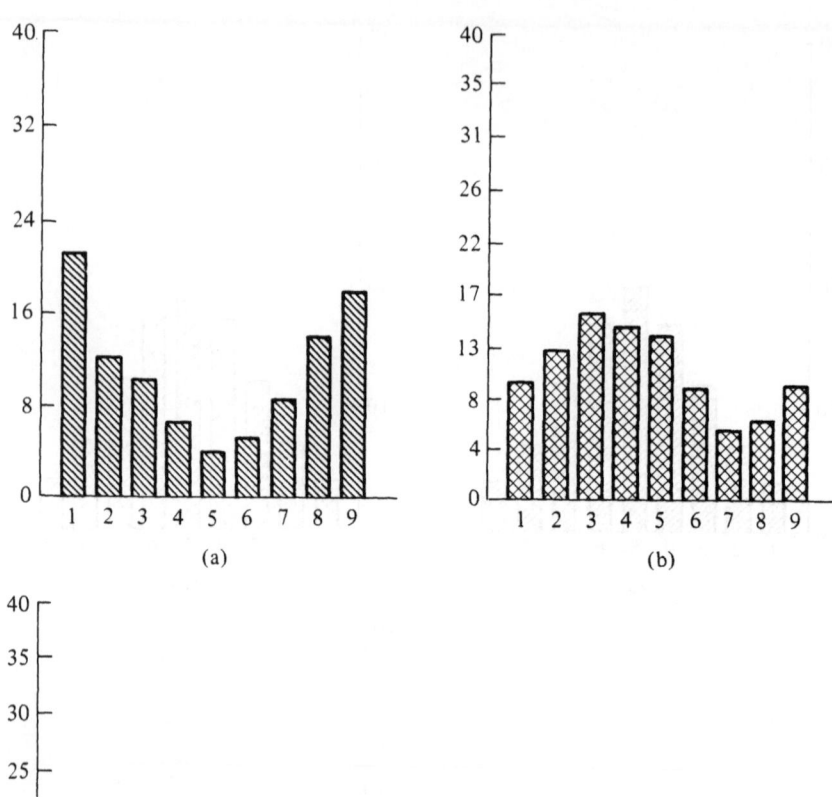

FIGURE 14.2. Stanine distributions of the developmental scores for the combined learning disability group (dyslexics plus retarded) (*n* = 259) in (a) reading, (b) spelling, and (c) mathematics.

The result for the entire cohort was, of course, normally distributed; 23% in the lowest three stanines (1–3); 23% in the top three (7–9), and 54% in the middle three. In the combined learning disability group, 38.8% fell in the bottom three stanines in spelling and 22.7% in the top three stanines. For mathematics, these percentages were 41.9% and 19%.

Growth of the Dyslexia Group Versus the Retarded Group

Children with dyslexia and those with general learning disabilities (retarded) represent two extreme groups selected on the basis of different criteria. The dys-

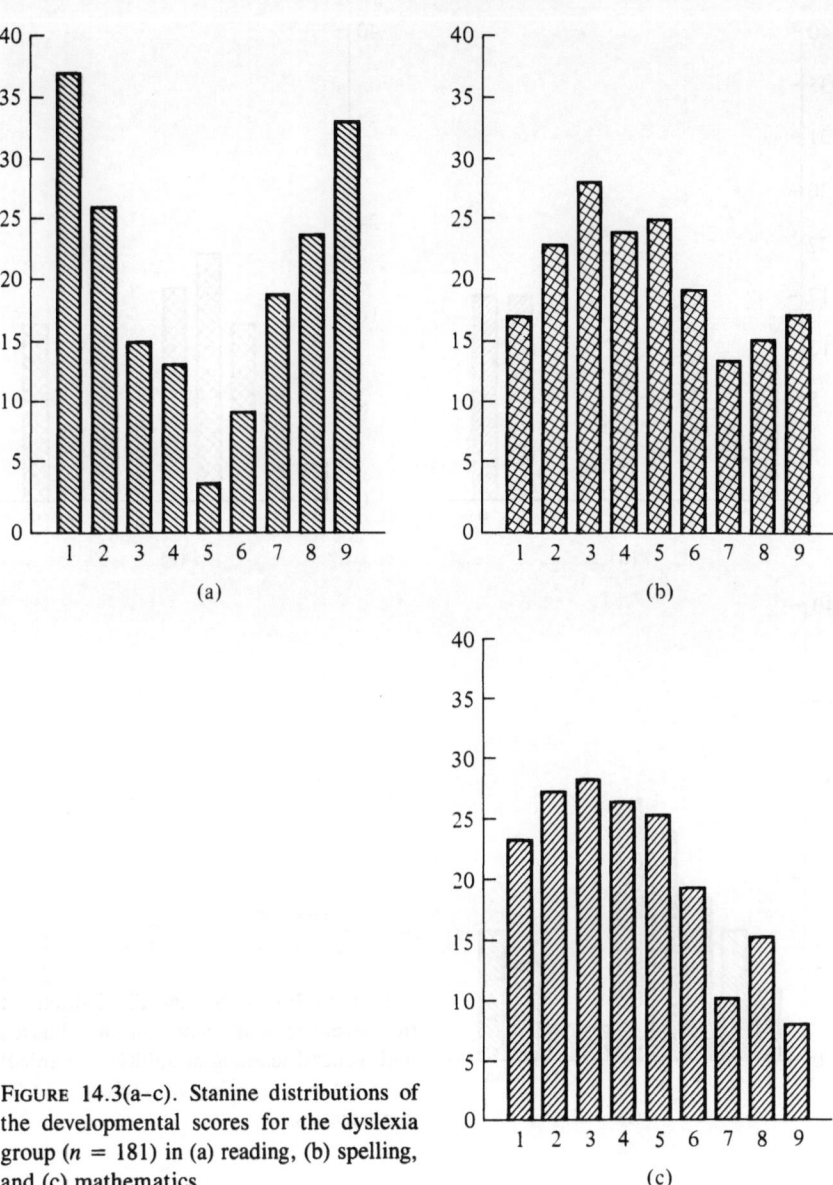

FIGURE 14.3(a–c). Stanine distributions of the developmental scores for the dyslexia group ($n = 181$) in (a) reading, (b) spelling, and (c) mathematics.

lexics had low scores in the literacy skills compared with their scholastic aptitude (IQ); the retarded had both low scholastic aptitude and school achievement. The retarded group was included in this research project for comparison purposes.

The data for the dyslexics were compared not only with those of the retarded group and the entire cohort, but also with those of a control group selected from classrooms that contained dyslexic pupils. Children in the control group had no learning problems with literacy skills; each was selected to match one dyslexic

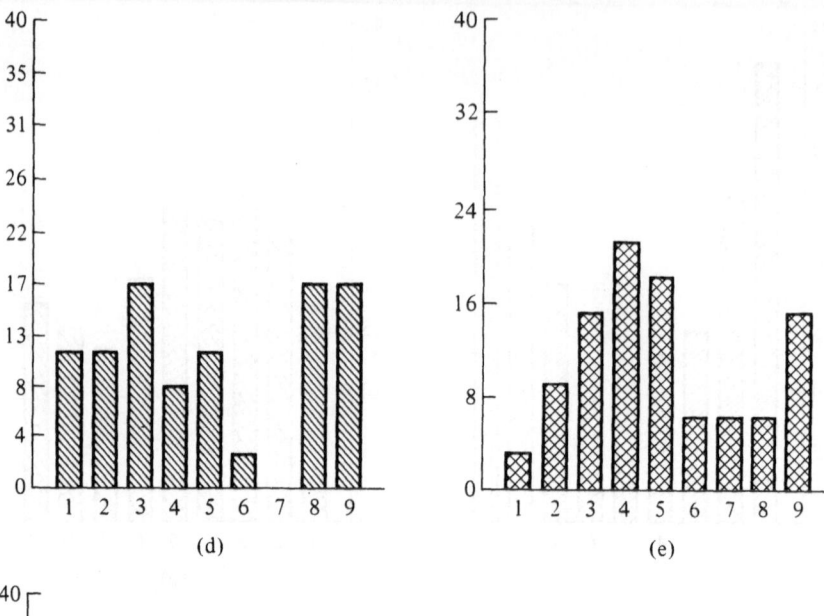

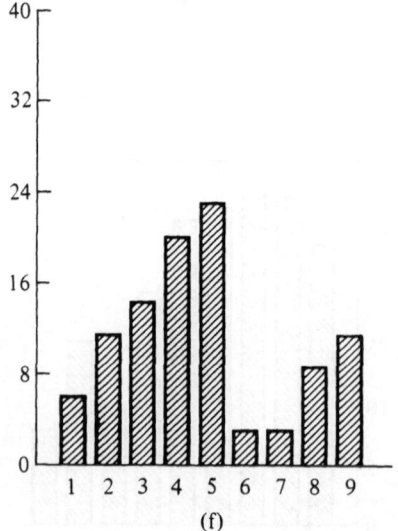

FIGURE 14.3(d–f). Stanine distributions of the developmental scores for the children with general learning disabilities (retarded) (n = 35) in (d) reading, (e) spelling, and (f) mathematics.

child on the basis of IQ and sex. It was assumed that the control group would exhibit normal growth patterns. Figure 14.3 (g–i) shows this to be the case. This figure shows the distributions of the developmental scores for the dyslexics, the retarded, and the control group across the three subject areas of reading, spelling, and mathematics. These data were analyzed by determining the percentages of children in the below-average, average, and above-average categories, which normally contain 23, 54, and 23%, respectively.

For the dyslexia group, the distribution across the three categories in reading was 43.6, 14.0, and 42.4%. The corresponding percentages for the retarded were

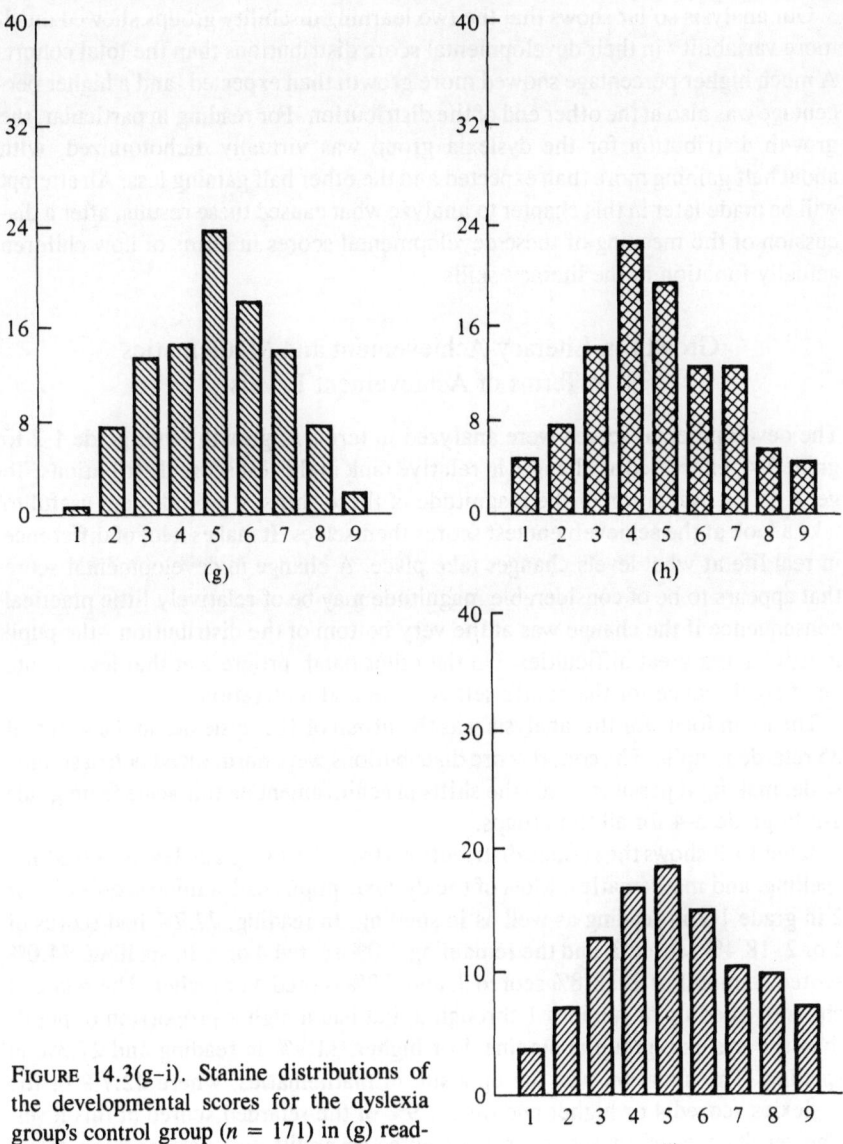

FIGURE 14.3(g–i). Stanine distributions of the developmental scores for the dyslexia group's control group ($n = 171$) in (g) reading, (h) spelling, and (i) mathematics.

41.2, 23.5, and 35.3%, whereas the control group had a distribution very close to the normal expectancy. A chi-square test of significance between the dyslexic and retarded data showed a significance level of .05.

The data from spelling and mathematics differed considerably from those from reading, close to half the scores being in the average category. The two learning disability groups did not differ significantly, although they did differ from the control group.

Our analysis so far shows that the two learning disability groups showed much more variability in their developmental score distributions than the total cohort. A much higher percentage showed more growth than expected, and a higher percentage was also at the other end of the distribution. For reading in particular, the growth distribution for the dyslexia group was virtually dichotomized, with about half gaining more than expected and the other half gaining less. An attempt will be made later in this chapter to analyze what caused these results, after a discussion of the meaning of these developmental scores in terms of how children actually function in the literacy skills.

Growth in Literacy Achievement and Mathematics in Terms of Achievement Levels

The developmental scores were analyzed in terms of growth from grade 1-2 to grade 3-4, expressed as changes in relative rank in the test score distributions. To get a better evaluation of the magnitude of these shifts, it would seem useful to take a look at the achievement test scores themselves. It makes a lot of difference in real life at what levels changes take place. A change in developmental score that appears to be of considerable magnitude may be of relatively little practical consequence if the change was at the very bottom of the distribution—the pupil is still having great difficulties. On the other hand, progress at that level could be of significance for the pupil's self-concept and motivation.

The main focus for this analysis was the group of 181 dyslexics and a group of 35 retarded pupils. The cohort score distributions were normalized onto a stanine scale, making it possible to see the shifts in achievement on this scale from grade 1-2 to grade 3-4 for all the groups.

Table 14.3 shows the stanine distributions from the two grade levels in reading, spelling, and mathematics. Most of the dyslexia pupils had stanine scores of 1 or 2 in grade 1-2 in reading as well as in spelling. In reading, 77.7% had scores of 1 or 2, 18.4% scored 3, and the remaining 4.0% scored 4 or 5. In spelling, 74.0% scored stanine 1 or 2, 18.8% scored 3, and 7.2% scored 4 or higher. The retarded children piled up at stanines 1 through 3, but had a higher proportion of pupils than the dyslexic group at stanine 4 or higher, 11.7% in reading and 27.3% in spelling. The situation was the opposite in mathematics, where 42.7% of the dyslexics scored 4 or higher and only 2.9% of the retarded scored at this level. The results are, of course, consistent with the ability test data and the selection criteria.

A shift in stanine score of 3 or lower to 4 was considered particularly critical, since this point is often used as a criterion for selecting children who need special help (Noss, 1977). Movement across the dividing line between 3 and 4 in either direction was used in this analysis. It would seem useful to also look at the transitions between 2 and 3, since about 75% of the dyslexia pupils scored 1 or 2 in grade 1-2, scores normally attained by 11% of the population. Changes at this point indicate real progress in achievement and often in pupil attitudes. Since Table 14.3 also contains the grade 3-4 data, the achievement shifts just mentioned can easily be read directly off the tables.

TABLE 14.3. Stanine distributions in reading, spelling, and mathematics in grades 1-2 and 3-4 for the dyslexic, the retarded, and the control group

Subject, group	Grade	Stanine scores [n of pupils (%)]									N
		1	2	3	4	5	6	7	8	9	
Reading											
Dyslexia	1-2	64 (35.8)	75 (41.9)	33 (18.4)	6 (3.4)	1 (0.6)					179
	3-4	57 (31.8)	43 (24.0)	38 (21.2)	21 (11.7)	13 (7.3)	3 (1.7)	2 (1.1)	2 (1.1)		179
Retarded	1-2	11 (32.4)	10 (29.4)	9 (26.5)	2 (5.9)	1 (2.9)	1 (2.9)				34
	3-4	10 (29.4)	8 (23.5)	5 (14.7)	10 (29.4)	1 (2.9)					34
Control group	1-2	1 (0.6)	10 (5.7)	23 (13.1)	38 (21.7)	41 (23.4)	34 (19.4)	21 (12.0)	5 (2.9)	2 (1.1)	175
	3-4	1 (0.6)	7 (4.0)	32 (18.3)	33 (18.9)	37 (21.1)	35 (20.0)	11 (6.3)	18 (10.3)	1 (0.6)	175
Spelling											
Dyslexia	1-2	71 (39.2)	63 (34.8)	34 (18.8)	10 (5.5)	2 (1.1)	1 (0.6)				181
	3-4	51 (28.2)	53 (29.3)	45 (24.9)	20 (11.05)	10 (5.5)	2 (1.1)				181
Retarded	1-2	7 (21.2)	11 (33.3)	6 (18.2)	7 (21.2)	2 (6.1)					33
	3-4	5 (14.3)	8 (22.9)	9 (25.7)	7 (20.0)	3 (8.6)	3 (8.6)				35
Control group	1-2	1 (0.6)	9 (5.1)	28 (15.9)	39 (22.2)	40 (22.7)	29 (16.5)	17 (9.7)	9 (5.1)	4 (2.3)	176
	3-4	4 (2.3)	12 (6.9)	26 (14.9)	36 (20.6)	41 (23.4)	26 (14.9)	19 (10.9)	3 (1.7)	4 (4.6)	175

TABLE 14.3. *Continued*

Subject, group	Grade	Stanine scores [n of pupils (%)]									N
		1	2	3	4	5	6	7	8	9	
Mathematics											
Dyslexia	1-2	30 (16.6)	38 (21.0)	36 (19.9)	38 (21.0)	24 (13.3)	13 (7.2)	2 (0.6)	0 (0.0)	1 (0.6)	181
	3-4	25 (13.8)	43 (23.8)	46 (25.4)	36 (19.9)	18 (9.9)	8 (4.4)	3 (1.7)	1 (0.6)	1 (0.6)	181
Retarded	1-2	17 (48.6)	12 (34.3)	5 (14.3)	1 (2.9)						35
	3-4	16 (45.7)	9 (25.7)	5 (14.3)	2 (5.7)	1 (2.9)	2 (5.7)				35
Control group	1-2	3 (1.7)	20 (11.4)	27 (15.3)	39 (22.2)	31 (17.6)	26 (14.8)	19 (10.8)	7 (4.0)	4 (2.3)	176
	3+4	5 (2.9)	14 (8.1)	19 (10.9)	39 (22.4)	41 (23.7)	30 (17.2)	14 (8.1)	9 (5.2)	3 (1.7)	174

The dyslexia group showed appreciable shifts upward in reading and spelling; this was also reflected in higher means. There were no such shifts in mathematics. It would seem reasonable to conclude that the shifts in reading and spelling were the results of the special instruction provided, in contrast to mathematics, where no special help was provided. Such a conclusion must be accompanied by certain reservations.

The dyslexia group was, by definition, a statistically extreme group in reading and spelling at the time of the pretest. The posttest results, therefore, would be susceptible to regression effects. As mentioned earlier, considerable efforts were made to keep the regression effect at a minimum. The initial pupil selection was based on dual testing to avoid the immediate regression effects; the selection was then validated against the judgments of teachers and parents, while at the same time the reliability of the diagnosis was evaluated. This validation process resulted in a 40% reduction in the size of the dyslexia group. Although some regression effect may still be present in our data, it must certainly be considerably less than what would have been the case if the children had simply been tested once. No other research project in this area has done as much to control for regression effect, to the best of our knowledge.

Exactly how much of the positive change that took place is real and how much is the result of regression effects is still not clear. This issue will be discussed again after additional analyses in which the shifts in achievement are corrected for regression effects.

Table 14.3 summarizes the shifts in scores from the pretest at grade 1-2 to the posttest at grade 3-4. A couple of facts are hidden in these tables. The regression effect has already been discussed. In addition, although the trend was toward a positive shift, some pupils regressed, trading places in the tables with some lower achieving pupils. Table 14.4 was worked out, therefore, to show how many of the pupils who scored below the cohort average (4–6) on the pretest had shifted into the average range and how many were still below average. Data for the retarded group are included for comparison purposes.

The dyslexia group did particularly poorly in reading and spelling, since 79.1 and 84.5% remained in stanines 1 through 3 for these two subjects. But in reading, 36 children (20.9%) had moved over into the level considered functional reading ability, represented by a stanine score of 4 or higher; the corresponding percentage for spelling was 15.5%; the corresponding numbers for the retarded were 23.3% in reading and 25.0% in spelling. The situation was reversed for mathematics, where 19.2% of the dyslexics advanced to stanine 4 or higher and only 11.8% of the retarded advanced.

A similar analysis was made to determine how many pupils had advanced from stanines 1 or 2 to 3 or higher. The percentages in reading and spelling for the dyslexic group were 35.3 and 33.6%, while the corresponding percentages for the retarded were 55.6 and 52.7%.

The problem of regression in scores was also studied for those who had stanine scores of 1 through 3 on the pretest, although only those scoring 2 or 3 could be shown to regress. About 20% of the pupils whose pretest stanine score was 2 or

TABLE 14.4. Stanine scores in grade 3-4 of the members of the two learning disability groups who scored at stanines 1-3 in grade 1-2

Subject, group	Stanine score 1-3 in grade 1-2	Stanine scores in grade 3-4 [n of pupils (%)]					Shift from 1-3 to 4+ [n (%)]
		1–3	4	5	6	7–9	
Reading							
Dyslexia	172	136	20	11	3	2	36
		(79.1)	(11.6)	(6.4)	(1.7)	(1.2)	(20.9)
Retarded	30	23	7				7
		(76.7)	(23.3)				(23.3)
Spelling							
Dyslexia	168	142	16	8	2		26
		(84.5)	(9.5)	(4.8)	(1.2)		(15.5)
Retarded	24	18	3	2	1		6
		(75.0)	(12.5)	(8.3)	(4.2)		(25.0)
Mathematics							
Dyslexia	104	84	14	3	2	1	20
		(80.8)	(10.0)	(2.9)	(1.9)	(1.0)	(19.2)
Retarded	34	30	2	1	1		4
		(88.2)	(5.9)	(2.9)	(2.9)		(11.8)

3 had a lower stanine score on the posttest in reading. The corresponding percentage for spelling was 14.3%.

The analysis of advancement and regression in rank as expressed in stanines gives some insight into the changes that took place from pretest to posttest. The *mean* stanine scores for the dyslexia group did go up. A number of children with dyslexia were documented to have advanced to the point of being considered as functioning adequately in reading and spelling. We are talking now of about 20 to 35% in reading and 15 to 34% in spelling, depending on whether we use as our criterion crossing over to stanine 4 or to stanine 3.

[The results of growth in school achievement are, in the American research literature, often reported in grade equivalent (GE) units. But the GE scale is particularly inappropriate for the study of achievement test scores at the extreme ends of the distribution. Another reason why the GE scale was not used in the Bergen Project was that no Norwegian tests provide GE norms, and none were developed specifically for this project.]

The score changes were also analyzed in light of the developmental scores, which expressed changes from those that had been predicted statistically. The developmental scores were also corrected for regression effects. This analysis showed that the majority of the pupils who shifted across the stanine thresholds in either direction also had somewhat extreme developmental scores. It was also confirmed that those dyslexia pupils who had shifted from stanine 1 or 2 to 3 or higher or from 3 to 4 or higher were pretty much in the top 23% on developmental scores. Similarly, those who made the corresponding negative shifts were, with few exceptions, in the bottom 23% on the developmental scores. These findings support the notion that the regression effect played a minor role in changing the achievement test scores.

The analysis that follows focuses on those pupils who showed the most and the least progress from the pretests to the posttests. The developmental scores were found to be the most appropriate for this analysis. The main focus in this section is the dyslexia group.

The Dyslexic Pupils' Patterns of Growth

Some dyslexics made much more progress than predicted from grade 1-2 to grade 3-4, whereas others made much less progress. This section will attempt to identify the characteristics of those pupils who obtained very high and those who received very low developmental scores. These scores were corrected for regression effect, which means that they were corrected for interpupil variation on the pretest. Since these achievement scores at grade 1-2 correlated quite highly with the scholastic aptitude test scores, this correction for regression implies that the developmental scores have also to some extent been corrected for differences in IQ.

Even though the pretest data as predictors were corrected for differences in ability, this does not remove the effect of ability differences on the developmental scores; the same variable may also contribute to changes in rank from pretest to posttest, and thus to the developmental scores. It turned out that school ability had a relatively minor positive effect on the developmental scores. In other words, if two pupils had the same pretest score but different IQ scores, the pupil with the higher ability score tended to get higher achievement test scores on the posttest. This fact was established for the cohort as a whole. How this worked for the dyslexia pupils will be discussed below.

The main impression of the connection between interpupil differences in developmental scores and the various indirect variables was that the various correlations were relatively low. Very few were significant, which means that few indirect variables appear to be good predictors of gains in achievement. The correlations between the developmental scores and the various scholastic ability, perception, and memory variables were close to zero. (A listing of these variables can be found in Table 10.1.) Among the oral language variables, the highest correlations with the developmental scores were for syntax and melody reproduction. These correlations were positive but not significant. Other factors that yielded extremely low correlations included the laterality variables, self-image, the social factor of parent occupation, and the various teacher classroom observations. There were two factors from the diagnosticians' observations during the administration of Dia-Gjessing that had particularly high correlations with growth in achievement, "approach to reading" and "speech:quantity." These correlations were both significantly different from zero. None of the factors brought out from the parents' observations reported during the case history showed any appreciable correlation with the achievement gains. Within the various groups of variables mentioned there was a scattering of individual variables, which invited further analysis.

In the analyses that follow, the dyslexia group of 181 has been divided into three stanine groups: below average, stanines 1 through 3; average, stanines 4 through 6; and above average, stanines 7 through 9. The division was done on the basis of the development of the dyslexics in reading, spelling, and mathematics. The stanine scale was again the normalized developmental score scale. The three groups consisted of 54% (97 pupils) in the average bracket and 23% (42 pupils) in each of the above- and below-average categories.

The results from these correlational analyses gave some insight into the linear relationships between gains in achievement and the indirect nonreading variables. On the basis of these correlational data one could certainly not expect many of the indirect variables to differentiate between pupil groups with different growth patterns, not even between the two extreme groups, the upper 23% and the lower 23% with respect to educational gains.

For a variable to be of interest and to be considered as a possible predictor of growth in reading or spelling, one would at least demand that the means for the two extreme groups differ appreciably. Second, one would expect enough linearity of the relationship so that the middle 54% would have a mean that would fall somewhere between the means for the extreme groups or perhaps be equal to one of them. The following analysis explores the degree to which individual variables differentiate among the three stanine groups on the basis of developmental scores. In addition, groups of variables have been analyzed to determine which individual variables had the greatest differentiating power.

The correlations and the differences among the means for the three stanine groups were analyzed for all the variables listed in Table 10.1. Similar analyses were carried out for some of the variables included in the questionnaires that the parents and teachers filled out at the time the pupils were in grades 3, 4, and 9. These included questions regarding the degree to which the pupils had reading and spelling difficulties in grades 2, 4, and 9; the types of assistance given; the duration of the special instructional program; the pupils' school attitude; and the teachers' perceptions of their own pacing of the instruction. Third, a similar analysis was made of some of the direct reading and spelling variables that were part of the individual diagnostic test, Dia-Gjessing. The results of all these analyses are summarized in the following sections.

Gains in Achievement and the Indirect Variables

This section deals with the variables listed previously under the rubrics of scholastic aptitude variables, perception and memory variables, oral language variables, laterality variables, self-image, and social factor.

Scholastic Aptitude, Perception and Memory Variables, and Gains in Reading and Spelling Achievement

In addition to the variables listed under these two main headings in Table 10.1, a variety of subscores and subscore combinations was analyzed. The WISC analysis involved all 10 subtests, the verbal versus performance discrepancy, and the three-way division of the subtests into spatial, conceptual, and sequential types. (See Chapter 11 for a discussion of this three-way split.) In addition to the seven VADS scores listed in Table 10.1, four additional scores were analyzed: "oral expression," "written expression," "intraintegration," and "interintegration." The analyses in this section involved a total of 29 variables, 17 based on the WISC, 11 on VADS, and 1 relating to the Bender Gestalt test.

Only one of these variables, the VADS "Visual-Written," had a significant correlation with the developmental scores in reading and spelling — 18 with spelling. This test requires short-term memory for a sequence of numerals. Since 29 variables were correlated with spelling and reading scores, a finding of one correlation coefficient significant at the .05 level could probably best be ascribed to chance (i.e., 1 correlation in 20 should be significant at this level by pure chance).

The WISC and Gains in Achievement

None of the WISC variables studied showed a significant correlation with growth in spelling or reading for the dyslexia sample. However, since some interesting data relating to sex differences on the WISC as well as the verbal versus performance IQ discrepancy were reported in Chapters 10 and 11, these two factors were subjected to more detailed study.

The discrepancy between the Verbal IQ (VIQ) and the Performance IQ (PIQ) on WISC has been given extensive attention in the research literature. This was discussed in Chapter 10, where we reported a mean Verbal minus Performance IQ of −4.5 IQ points; that is, the PIQ tended to be higher. It was also found that the difference was larger for girls than for boys, the mean differences being −5.45 and −3.96 IQ points, respectively.

The VIQ minus PIQ discrepancy was larger for the below-average gainers (lowest 23%) in reading than for the above-average gainers, the mean differences being −5.5 and −2.2 IQ points, respectively. The corresponding discrepancies for spelling were −5.9 and −5.0. There was, then, a tendency for the above-average gainers to have a smaller IQ discrepancy in reading than the below-average gainers. This did not appear to be the case in spelling.

The data presented in Chapter 11 show that about two thirds of the dyslexia sample had a lower VIQ, whereas about one third had a lower PIQ. Table 14.5 presents data for these two groups, divided by growth level and sex. Most of the mean IQ differences for the group with higher PIQ are in the −12 to −14 IQ points range, independent of sex, school subject, or growth level. The one exception is the difference for the above-average gaining girls, with a difference of only −7.4 IQ points. The right side of the table shows the groups with a higher VIQ. The mean differences here are in the +9 to +11 IQ points range, although the high-gaining girls showed only a +7.3 points difference.

There was a trend, mentioned earlier, that suggested that the children who were the best gainers in achievement had the smallest WISC IQ discrepancy. This

TABLE 14.5. WISC Verbal IQ (VIQ) minus Performance IQ (PIQ), sex, and stanine group achievement level

Stanine achievement level	Sex	VIQ < PIQ				VIQ > PIQ			
		N	Mean VIQ	Mean PIQ	Difference	N	Mean VIQ	Mean PIQ	Difference
Reading									
1–3	B	19	97.4	109.6	−12.2	7	103.9	92.3	+11.6
	G	10	89.0	101.5	−12.5	3	93.3	79.3	+14.0
4–6	B	36	90.1	103.1	−13.0	23	104.0	94.0	+10.0
	G	25	87.8	102.5	−14.7	11	95.2	86.1	+9.1
7–9	B	16	95.3	107.0	−11.8	10	102.7	92.4	+13.3
	G	9	85.1	92.6	−7.4	6	103.0	95.8	+7.3
Total	B	71	93.2	105.7	−12.5	40	103.6	93.3	+10.3
	G	44	87.5	100.2	−12.7	20	97.3	88.0	+9.3
Spelling									
1–3	B	15	89.1	100.3	−11.2	9	101.6	91.1	+10.4
	G	13	86.8	102.0	−15.3	2	88.0	80.5	+7.5
4–6	B	41	93.1	105.5	−12.5	24	105.0	94.3	+10.6
	G	21	86.4	97.7	−11.4	11	98.8	89.0	+9.8
7–9	B	16	95.9	110.0	−14.2	8	101.0	92.1	+8.9
	G	10	90.7	102.7	−12.0	7	97.4	88.6	+8.9
Total	B	72	93.0	105.5	−12.6	41	103.4	93.2	+10.2
	G	44	87.5	100.2	−12.7	20	97.3	88.0	+9.3

generalization appears to be true to some extent only for the girls. Otherwise, WISC IQ discrepancies appear to have no predictive value. This finding is contrary to the assertion by Lytton that a higher VIQ is predictive of success in reading (Lytton, 1972). Lytton's study involved boys only, for whom we could find no such predictability.

Chapter 11 discussed the three-way split of the WISC subtests suggested by Bannatyne (1971), reporting that the dyslexia group as a whole had a profile across the three scores that coincided with Bannatyne's data for children with learning disabilities. The highest average was in the "spatial" area, the lowest "sequential," while the "conceptual" average was in the middle.

The present analysis revealed that all three achievement growth groups had the same mean pattern as described above. This was true for reading as well as spelling. The three-way split of the WISC subtests did not contribute to differential diagnosis nor to differential prognosis.

Bender Gestalt Test and Gains in Achievement

It was reported earlier that results of the Bender Gestalt test correlated rather highly with achievement in reading and spelling for the dyslexia group as a whole (Chapter 10). The correlations with the developmental scores were, however, quite small, $-.11$ for reading and $-.08$ for spelling. Although these correlations are not significant, they are in the predicted direction in that good Bender performance (low scores) had a slight tendency to go with higher developmental scores. The means for the above-average and below-average stanine groups did not differ significantly, the above-average group having mean Bender scores of 3.0 and 3.1 in reading and spelling, while the means for the below-average groups were both 3.6. The variance in both groups was particularly large. It appears, then, that results of the Bender Gestalt test alone will not contribute significantly to a differential prognosis in dyslexia.

WISC, VADS, and Bender Scores Combined and Gains in Achievement

The analyses of the WISC, VADS, and Bender Gestalt test gave little support to the notion that these tests were of value in predicting growth in literacy achievement for a group of dyslexic children. To study the combined predictive power of these tests, a discriminant analysis was carried out among the three stanine groups. All ten WISC subtests, the four VADS subscores, and the Bender Gestalt score were included in the analysis. Again, there were no clear-cut trends in reading, although the Bender test showed up again as having some slight discriminating power. In spelling, the visual-written part of VADS had some discriminating power, along with the two WISC subtests "reasoning" and "picture completion," all scores being in the positive direction.

Oral Language Variables and Gains in Achievement

There were four oral language variables studied, word pronunciation, melody reproduction, auditory discrimination, and syntax. None of these variables correlated appreciably with growth in reading or spelling.

The analysis described in Chapter 10 revealed that all of these variables except for word pronunciation correlated rather highly with scholastic aptitude and sex. It was decided, therefore, to do a two-way analysis of variance, which in addition to dividing the sample into the three stanine groups also divided it according to sex. In addition, differences in scholastic aptitude were corrected for by using WISC-Total IQ as a covariate. Only in the case of melody reproduction did this type of analysis yield significant additional information, particularly with respect to sex. The boys did more poorly than the girls. In the case of both sexes, the higher stanine group also had higher melody reproduction scores, although the differences did not prove to be statistically significant.

Laterality Variables, Self-Image, and Social Factor and Gains in Achievement

In the area of laterality, four variables were studied: hand preference, hand asymmetry, foot preference, and eye preference. Only hand asymmetry had a positive but not significant correlation with gains in reading and spelling. All these factors had large variances within each of the stanine groups, but there were no significant differences between the above- and below-average stanine groups. The same finding was also true for self-image.

Data for the one social factor studied—parent occupation—had also been gathered on the entire cohort, making comparisons between the dyslexics and the general population possible. Parent occupation was classified on a 5-point scale that placed much emphasis on parental educational level, with 5 being the highest level. In the case of the dyslexia group, there was no significant correlation between parent occupation and the developmental scores. The different occupational groups were about equally divided across the various stanine groups.

Observational Variables and Gains in Achievement

Among the indirect variables were observations and judgments made by teachers, diagnosticians, and parents. (See chap. 10.) Most of these variables correlated significantly with achievement as measured on the pretest and with the WISC IQs.

With respect to the relationship between these observational variables and gains in achievement, the variables "approach to reading" and "speech:quantity" correlated significantly with gains in reading achievement, the correlation coefficients being .17 and .20, respectively ($p < .05$). In the case of "speech:quantity," the above-average stanine group's mean was significantly higher than for the below-average group, but this was not true of the variable "approach to reading."

The diagnosticians' observations during the assessment of reading and spelling appeared to have some predictability with respect to gains in achievement. The functions involved are characteristics that could be influenced positively in the treatment process.

Direct Reading and Spelling Variables and Gains in Achievement

The preceding analyses showed that only a few indirect variables appear to be of value in providing differential prediction as to which pupils are most likely to make good progress in reading and spelling achievement in a remedial program. Many of these variables are of value in predicting the achievement levels for an undifferentiated group of students. The analyses of the entire cohort showed that the best single predictor of achievement on the posttest at grade 3-4 was the pretest in the same subject at grade 1-2. The developmental scores, as used in this particular study, represent that part of the posttests in reading and spelling that could not be predicted from the pretests.

The basic model underlying this study and its diagnostic procedures places a lot of emphasis on the reading and spelling processes through what has been labeled *function analysis*. The various indices coming out of this analysis have been studied, particularly their relationship to the developmental scores. This involved those 11 variables that emerged from the factor analysis of a much larger number of variables from the Dia-Gjessing test.

Some of the 11 variables correlated significantly with sex and scholastic aptitude. But sex and IQ showed very low, nonsignificant correlations with achievement gains of the dyslexic group. Nevertheless, the data for these 11 variables were studied for boys and girls separately, and they were corrected for differences in IQ. By comparing the means for the three stanine groups, above average (top 23%), average (middle 54%), and below average (lowest 23%), certain common characteristics for both sexes appeared.

The main findings across these 11 variables can be summarized quite briefly. Two variables emerged as being most powerful in differentiating between the high and the low gainers. These factors were complex phonological functions (factor 1) and complex orthographic functions (factor 11). Both of these factors differentiated significantly between the two extreme stanine groups in reading, but only the factor complex orthographic functions differentiated significantly in spelling.

Several of the nine remaining variables also differentiated among the three stanine groups, but none of them at a statistically significant level. They may, nevertheless, have some value for differential diagnosis as part of the entire 11-factor profile. Five variables fit this pattern: reversals (factor 7), severe reading problem (5), phonological cluster function (2), orthographic speed (9), and attentiveness (8).

The Classroom Situation, the Teachers' and Parents' Perceptions of the Children's Degree of Reading and Spelling Difficulties, and the Remedial Program, All Seen in Relation to Growth in Achievement

Classroom Averages and Gains in Achievement

In addition to the individually prescribed instruction for the dyslexics, there may have been other classroom factors that contributed to growth in school achievement. One such factor that was studied in some detail was the relationship between achievement gains and the average achievement level of the pupil's own class. The reason for studying this was the fact that classroom membership was found to correlate positively with the dyslexics' achievement level at various grade levels (Solheim, 1984). As discussed briefly in chapter 1, a high score on classroom membership was associated with higher achievement, and vice versa.

To study this relationship further, it was necessary to study achievement gains against the actual achievement score averages, without the corrections for differences in ability or any environmental factors that were made earlier to study the classroom membership factor. The variable used, then, was the mean achievement test score for each classroom, after the scores for the dyslexics had been excluded. Each dyslexic child's pretest score in reading, spelling, and mathematics was compared with the average for the classroom to which he or she belonged.

The question was whether the variation in classroom averages on the pretest was associated with growth in achievement. Table 14.6 shows the correlation coefficients between these means and gains in achievement for reading and spelling. The table also includes correlations between the classroom averages and the scores of the dyslexic children at grade 1-2 and grade 3-4, plus the correlations with "instructional pacing," a concept discussed below. The correlations with the factor previously defined as classroom membership are given in parentheses.

The data in Table 14.6 indicate, first, that the developmental scores for the dyslexic pupils did not correlate significantly with the classroom means in reading or spelling. It would appear, then, that the classroom averages are relatively neutral in relation to changes in school achievement from grade 1-2 to grade 3-4. It also means that the dyslexic pupils maintained their relative position from the pretest to the posttest independent of the classroom means.

Table 14.6 indicates, second, that the classroom means at the time of the pretest correlated positively with the dyslexic pupils' achievement levels at grade 1-2 and again at grade 3-4, especially in spelling. This implies that those dyslexia pupils who were in classrooms that had relatively high pretest means tended to do better than the pupils who were in classrooms with low mean achievement scores. And the ranks that were established at the time of the pretest at grade 1-2 appear to have been quite stable over time.

To what extent were the classroom averages affected by how the teachers paced their instruction in the literacy skills? The question of *instructional pacing* was studied by asking the teachers, in the middle of fourth grade, to evaluate their own pacing in teaching various skills on a 5-point scale from "very slowly" to "much faster than average." The bottom line in Table 14.6 shows the correlation between the level of instructional pacing and gains in literacy skills as well as actual achievement in grade 1-2 and again in grade 3-4. The correlations were not significant (although the correlation with reading did reach +0.14).

Table 14.6 also shows, in the far right column, that there was a significant positive correlation between the classroom averages and the level of instructional pacing, as judged by the teachers. The fact that classrooms in which the instructional pacing was the basis. This has, in fact, been also been found by others (e.g., Hansen, 1978). This finding was confirmed through additional analyses that showed a correlation, but less strong, significant even intercorrelation between instructional pacing, reading level of achievement, and language development. It would appear that this was a most important factor in achievement in the literacy skills at the classroom level. This pacing program, in part, to what we have called the "teacher variable." This we might call what may be called the "teacher variable."

Teacher and Pupil Efficacy of Instruction: A Closer Review of Gains in Achievement

In the "middle" of mind bogs are, at the end of the school the dyslexic children were well rated. Validity questions regarding reliability, reduced variabilities and school situations, then. The teacher's of 18 subject values indicated in relation to the class' achievement in reading and spelling; and other behaviors.

TABLE 14.6. Correlation of dyslexic children ($n = 18$) reading and spelling scores and gains in achievement with classroom mean scores and teachers' instructional pacing

Variable used to measure achievement	Reading			Spelling			Instructional pacing
	Gain	Grade 1–2 score	Grade 3–4 score	Gain	Grade 1–2 score	Grade 3–4 score	
Classroom means in reading, grade 1–2	−.01 (−.03)[a]	.11 (.06)	.04 (−.01)	.04 (−.02)	.18[b] (.29)[c]	.18[c] (.20)[c]	.23[c] (.24)[c]
Classroom means in spelling, grade 1–2		.03			.12	.08	.21[c] (.22)[c]
Instructional pacing, grades 1–3	.14		.14	−.02			

[a] Numbers in parentheses are correlations with "classroom membership."
[b] Significant at .05 level.
[c] Significant at .01 level.

instructional pacing was the fastest also had the highest mean scores has also been found by others (e.g., Hansen, 1979). Our findings were confirmed through additional analyses that showed these correlations remained significant even after correction for scholastic aptitude, sex, self-concept, level of aspiration, and language development. It would appear that instructional pacing is a significant factor in achievement in the literacy skills at the classroom level. This pacing probably represents, in part, what we have labeled classroom membership, or what may be called the "teacher variable."

Teacher and Parent Evaluations of the Relationship of a Variety of Factors to Gains in Achievement

In the middle of fourth grade and at the end of ninth, the dyslexia students' *parents* were asked a variety of questions regarding their child's reading and writing difficulties and school attitudes in grades 2, 4, and 9. These evaluations were analyzed in relation to the child's developmental scores. The *teachers* were asked similar questions.

The same rating scale was used to tabulate the parents' responses at the three different grade levels. These results were summarized earlier in this chapter. A main finding was that 64% of the parents thought their child had "severe" or "very severe" reading and spelling difficulties in the second grade, 20% thought so by the fourth grade, and only 9% thought so by the ninth grade. The scale showed a definite reduction in the use of these two most extreme categories.

To study the parent evaluations, a "discrepancy scale" was developed. This scale would express how the parents perceived their own child's development in reading and spelling from the second to the fourth grade. The scores obtained were different from the developmental scores, since the assumption was that parental judgment implied also an evaluation of the child's overall development in accordance with age and grade in school. Virtually every pupil will show some growth in achievement, even if relative rank within the class declines. Hardly any parent perceived that their child's rank in the class had declined. A review of the "discrepancy scale" data confirmed this assumption. Only in the case of four pupils (2.7%) did the parents judge problems in the fourth grade to be relatively more severe than in the second grade. We also found a significantly high positive correlation between parental evaluations and achievement test results at both the second and fourth grade levels ($p < .01$).

The parent evaluations and their relationship with the developmental scores were studied initially by determining the correlations for the dyslexia group as a whole. Second, the differences between the extreme developmental stanine groups were analyzed. The correlation between the discrepancy scores and the developmental scores in reading was a significant $+.22$ ($p < .05$). The correlation for spelling was also positive but not significant. The corresponding correlations between discrepancy scores between ninth and second grade and developmental scores were also positive but nonsignificant.

These relationships, although of rather modest magnitude, were illuminated further by comparing parent evaluations for the two extreme developmental stanine groups, that is, the 23% of pupils who showed the most relative gains with the 23% who showed the most relative declines in achievement. The study of the discrepancy scores showed that only 2.7% of the parents thought that their child had showed a relative decline in achievement, whereas 80% judged their child's relative rank in achievement to have improved. These numbers may be partly responsible for the relatively low correlations just described.

We will first look at the group with the low developmental scores. According to the parent evaluations, 76% of these pupils had "severe" or "very severe" problems with reading and spelling in second grade. This percentage dropped to 38% in fourth grade and to 13% in ninth grade. The corresponding percentages for the stanine group with high developmental scores were 56, 12, and 0%.

According to the parents, then, there were clear differences between these two extreme groups. It was interesting to note that the categories "insignificant" or "none" to describe the children's degree of reading difficulties in the fourth grade were checked for 64% of the positive gainers but only 14% of the negative gainers. The differences in spelling were not quite as pronounced. All in all, the parent evaluations were quite consistent with the test results.

With respect to the teachers' evaluations of reading and spelling, the analyses presented earlier showed that they demanded more reading and spelling skills than the parents. There was, nevertheless, a high correlation between the teachers' and the parents' evaluations at the ninth-grade level, $r = +.53$ ($p <$ .01). Teachers and parents did agree to a large extent about the pupils' relative ranks, although the parents used a more positive scale. (The difference in means does not, of course, affect the magnitude of the correlation coefficient.) The relationship between the teacher evaluations and the developmental scores in grade 9 was about the same as that described above for the parent evaluations at grade 4.

Although the three approaches to evaluating progress—parent evaluations, teacher evaluations, and testing (developmental scores)—showed a great deal of correspondence, the three approaches differed sufficiently with respect to their frames of reference that it would seem unreasonable to expect the same judgment with respect to the development of individual pupil's relative advancement or decline. Parents and teachers evaluated the pupils' reading and spelling difficulties against a functional standard, albeit with different levels of expectancy, while the developmental scores were based upon changes in each pupil's relative rank in relation to the cohort norms for grade 1-2 and grade 3-4.

The children's *school attitudes*, as reported by teachers and parents, were also studied in relation to the developmental achievement scores. The parents had been asked to rate this when the children were in grades 2, 4, and 9. The ratings from these three different points in time correlated significantly. The ratings also correlated significantly with the parents' evaluations of reading and spelling difficulties, yielding rather consistent ratings across variables and over time. The children with the least degree of learning problems appeared to enjoy school the most. When compared with the developmental scores, the reported school attitudes correlated significantly in grades 4 and 9 but not in grade 2. It appears, then, that the parents found school attitudes to improve as the children's achievement progressed. There was no such relationship between growth in achievement and school attitudes according to the teachers' ratings.

The Extent of Remedial Instruction and Gains in Achievement

On the questionnaire for the third grade, the teachers were asked to indicate the amount and type of remedial instruction that had been offered each dyslexic child. A variety of instructional arrangements had been employed. The teachers were also asked about the degree to which the child's parents had participated in the treatment plans.

With regard to the last question, the teachers confirmed that the parents had participated in the case of 67% of the pupils. How did this factor relate to the development of the two extreme stanine groups? There was a tendency, at least in reading, toward more parental cooperation for the higher gainers — 73% of parents participated versus 59% for the low gainers.

The remedial instructional plans used ranged from private tutoring in a pullout program to a variety of group plans. In general, the pupils who received the most help tended to show the smallest gains. Children in the stanine group with the lowest developmental scores received by far the most intensive instruction in terms of individual tutoring and team teaching, whereas those in the high stanine group were more likely to be recipients of group instruction.

This finding is a reminder that the effect of special education efforts cannot always be judged by the amount of remediation administered. Were this the case, one would have to conclude that the less help provided the greater the gains. Such an interpretation would, of course, be erroneous. One possible explanation for the lack of results from great efforts could be that these particular pupils received the wrong kind of help. This may indeed be the case for some of them. Another explanation could be that many of these students had very complex problems along with other difficulties, which prevented learning from taking place. This particular angle will be discussed later in conjunction with the discussion of growth by dyslexia type.

The great amount of effort carried out, especially on behalf of students with the most severe problems, was undoubtedly the result of an awareness by the teachers and the specialists that these students did have problems of considerable magnitude. Despite this strong effort, one is left with the feeling of having been unsuccessful with this group of students. In those cases where achievement gains were minimal, one must wonder what these pupils would have been like without this special help, not only with respect to reading and spelling but also to other school subjects, as well as school attitudes.

Clinical Dyslexia Groups and Gains in Literacy Achievement

The dyslexia sample's growth in literacy achievement has previously been analyzed in relation to a variety of direct and indirect variables. The division of the dyslexia sample into various types has also been described in previous chapters.

This section deals with the relationship between the four clinical dyslexia types and their developmental scores in reading and spelling.

To study these relationships, each of the four dyslexia groups was divided into three stanine groups, as was discussed earlier with regard to the entire dyslexia sample. The stanine scale used was based on a normalized distribution of the developmental scores for the dyslexia group only. (That would, of course, result in an overall mean of 5 and a standard deviation of 2.)

Table 14.7 shows the mean developmental scores in reading and spelling for the four dyslexia types by sex. The audiovisual group did particularly poorly in reading; this group's mean was significantly below the others ($p < .05$). The visual group also had a lower mean IQ reading than the auditory and "other" groups, and the difference was almost statistically significant.

There were also some rather large sex differences within the dyslexia groups. For the audiovisual dyslexia group, the mean for the boys in reading was virtually a full standard deviation below the total dyslexia group mean of 5, whereas the girls' mean was 4.86. Unfortunately, this group was very small, 11 boys and 7 girls, which makes the data difficult to interpret. It would appear safe to conclude, however, that the audiovisual and visual groups made much less progress in reading than the other two groups. There was a similar trend in spelling, but it was nowhere near as pronounced or significant.

These results are consistent with the underlying dyslexia theory (Gjessing, 1977), which states that the prognosis for gains in literacy achievement is particularly poor in audiovisual dyslexia and quite poor in visual dyslexia.

Each of the four dyslexia types was also divided into stanine groups according to developmental scores, to determine if there was accumulation at either extreme. These data are summarized in Table 14.8. The far right column shows the distribution of the total dyslexia sample which was predetermined on the basis of a normal distribution so that the three groups would contain 23, 54, and 23%. Within the four groups there was some variation from the normal split. The biggest deviation occurred in the group with audiovisual dyslexia, where only 1 child in 18 (5.6%) was in the top group whereas half were in the bottom stanine group. The remaining data were quite consistent with the summary data shown in Table 14.7.

Part of the work of classifying these dyslexic children also involved dividing each of the four types into two groups, the "pure" cases and the "complex" cases, again on the basis of Gjessing's model. A study was carried out to determine if the distributions across the dyslexia groups differed for these two subtypes within each dyslexia category. Two categories were already, by definition, already complex—audiovisual and other forms of dyslexia. This analysis, therefore, concentrated primarily on the auditory and the visual types.

Within the auditory dyslexia group, 40 of 73, or 55%, were considered pure types. The corresponding numbers for the visual group were 35 of 53, or 66%. The stanine groups showed different distributions for these splits. For the auditory group, the differences were so small that the splitting of the group into pure and complex types would seem to have no particular value for prognosis in read-

TABLE 14.7. Summary statistics of the developmental scores for the four clinical dyslexia groups by sex

Subject	Sex	Dyslexia type											
		Auditory			Audiovisual			Visual			Other		
		N	x	SD	N	x	SD	N	x	SD	N	x	SD
Reading	Boys	53	5.47	1.96	11	3.09	1.58	28	4.86	1.82	20	5.20	2.02
	Girls	19	5.05	2.04	7	4.86	2.27	25	4.48	1.90	16	5.56	1.63
	Total	72	5.36	1.97	18	3.78	2.02	53	4.68	1.85	36	5.36	1.84
Spelling	Boys	54	5.04	1.85	11	4.46	1.64	28	4.64	1.66	21	5.00	2.34
	Girls	19	4.95	2.59	7	5.43	1.62	25	5.32	2.02	16	5.13	1.89
	Total	73	5.01	2.05	18	4.83	1.65	53	4.96	1.85	37	5.05	2.13

TABLE 14.8. Stanine groups in reading and spelling within the four dyslexia types

Stanine achievement level	Dyslexia type				
	Auditory N (%)	Audiovisual N (%)	Visual N (%)	Other N (%)	Total (%)
Reading					
1–3	12 (16.7)	9 (50.0)	13 (24.5)	7 (19.4)	41 (22.9)
4–6	40 (55.6)	8 (44.4)	29 (54.7)	20 (55.6)	97 (54.2)
7–9	20 (27.8)	1 (5.6)	11 (20.8)	9 (25.0)	41 (22.9)
Total	72 (100.0)	18 (100.0)	53 (100.0)	36 (100.0)	179 (100.0)
Spelling					
1–3	15 (20.5)	5 (27.8)	12 (22.6)	10 (27.0)	42 (23.2)
4–6	40 (54.8)	10 (55.6)	31 (58.5)	17 (45.9)	98 (54.1)
7–9	18 (24.7)	3 (16.7)	10 (18.9)	10 (27.0)	41 (22.7)
Total	73 (100.0)	18 (100.0)	53 (100.0)	37 (100.0)	181 (100.0)

ing and spelling. The situation was a bit different for the visual dyslexia group. Here 60% of the pure cases fell in the lowest stanine group, and 75% of the highest stanine group were also pure cases, in contrast to the total 66% incidence figure. These data suggest that the prognosis for children with a pure form of visual dyslexia may be better than for those with a complex form.

The complex or confounding characteristics were primarily emotional. A relatively large number of students with a visual-emotional configuration were found in the lowest stanine group for developmental scores in reading and spelling. Of all the children diagnosed as having visual-emotional dyslexia, 45% scored in the lowest stanine group and 7.5% scored in the highest group in reading and spelling. The expected frequencies for both of these stanine groups were, of course, 23%.

A further analysis of the pupils with audiovisual dyslexia combined with emotional problems showed that 75% of them scored in the lowest stanine group and only 12% scored in the highest group, a distribution quite similar to that of visual dyslexia with emotional complications. The fourth dyslexia group, other forms, showed no differences between those whose learning problems were combined with emotional problems and the pure cases.

The analysis of the relationships between dyslexia types and growth in literacy achievement suggests that children who were judged clinically to have audiovisual dyslexia or to have any other type of dyslexia in combination with emotional problems were overrepresented among these who showed low developmental scores. A diagnosis of audiovisual or visual dyslexia implies a relatively poor prognosis for achievement of literacy skills. If the children with these types of dyslexia also have emotional problems, the prognosis is even poorer. The finding that emotional problems are particularly influential in combination with either of the two visual dyslexias is consistent with the underlying dyslexia theory (Gjessing, 1977).

TABLE 14.9. Mean developmental scores in reading and spelling for the seven Q-factor groups by sex

| | Group | | | | | | |
| | QI | | QII | | QIII | | |
Subject	Minus	Plus	Minus	Plus	Minus	Plus	Residual
Reading							
Boys	4.5	6.0	5.3	3.8	4.6	4.9	5.2
Girls	5.0	5.7	4.6	3.7	5.0	4.4	6.2
Total	4.6	5.8	5.0	3.7	4.7	4.7	5.5
Spelling							
Boys	4.9	5.0	5.6	4.6	4.2	4.2	5.3
Girls	5.1	5.3	5.4	4.7	5.7	5.0	5.4
Total	5.0	5.1	5.5	4.6	4.8	4.5	5.3

The Statistical Dyslexia Groups and Gains in Literacy Achievement

The analysis of gains in achievement that was done for the clinical groups was also done for the seven Q-factor groups identified in a Q-factor analysis. The mean developmental scores in reading and spelling for the seven groups by sex and by total are given in Table 14.9.

There were no significant sex differences between the pairs of means for any of the seven groups or either of the two school subjects. The subsequent discussion thus deals only with the combined means for both sexes. In reading, the QI-plus group attained the highest mean, the residual group the second highest, and the QII-plus group the lowest by far. The QII-plus mean was significantly lower than the means for QI-plus ($p < .05$), QIII-plus ($p < .05$), and the residual Q group ($p < .01$). In spelling, however, none of the combined means was significantly different from any of the others.

A comparison of these findings with the results from the clinical groups leads to some interesting observations. In review, the clinical groups would rank from high to low in terms of gains in achievement as follows: auditory, other forms, visual, and last, audiovisual dyslexia. When these results are compared with those for the statistical groups, one will find that one of the Q groups, which was seen as a variant of visual dyslexia, QI-plus, showed the largest achievement gain, whereas another Q group, which was also judged to be a variant of visual dyslexia, QII-plus, was clearly the poorest gaining group of all Q groups. The third group, judged also to be a variant of visual dyslexia, QIII-plus, showed about average gain in reading.

The Q-factor groups that were judged to be similar to the clinical auditory dyslexia group (the Q-minus groups) showed about average gains, with little variation in each. The residual Q group showed the second highest average gain in reading.

As was the case with the clinical groups, the Q groups were also studied with respect to additional, complicating factors. In the case of the clinical groups, emotional problems appeared to be the most critical ones. How did this relate to the results for the seven Q-factor groups?

Starting with the Q-plus groups (visual dyslexia), the QIII-plus group had the highest incidence of emotional problems in addition to dyslexia, 52% of the group members. This incidence was the highest for all Q-factor groups. Within the low stanine group for the QIII-plus group, the incidence of emotional difficulties was 67%. The QII-plus group also had a significant incidence of emotional problems (44%), but there was no accumulation of these cases in either extreme stanine group.

The group with the highest mean developmental score, QI-plus, had a very low incidence of pupils with emotional problems in addition to dyslexia, only 15%.

Among the Q-minus groups, which were judged to be variants of auditory dyslexia, the 31% of children in group I-minus and 32% in II-minus had emotional problems in addition to dyslexia. This was about average for the entire dyslexia sample. There were no differences between the low and high stanine groups for any of the Q-minus groups.

The QIII-minus group resembled the QI-plus group in that it contained relatively few children with emotional difficulties, only 15%. The mean growth for this group, however, was relatively low.

Finally, the residual group, which had somewhat above-average mean gains in reading achievement, revealed a 43% incidence figure for emotional problems on top of dyslexia. The incidence of emotional problems among the pupils in the high and low stanine groups was the same.

At this point it would appear possible to draw some conclusions, taking this multitude of findings into account. First, the various Q-factor groups varied considerably with respect to growth in achievement. This variability appeared to be inconsistent with the findings from the clinical groups, where the auditory dyslexics showed the greatest gains. The various Q groups were judged to be variants of auditory and visual dyslexia, but there was no tendency for either of those sets of groups to do better than the other. All three Q groups that were judged to be basically cases of auditory dyslexia showed about-average gains on the developmental scores in reading, whereas the clinical auditory dyslexia group showed the greatest gains.

Even though the QIII-minus group contained very few children with emotional complications, the group growth in achievement was no better than that of the other Q-minus groups. The reason may be that emotional problems do not compound learning disabilities in cases of auditory dyslexia. This seemed also to be the case with the clinically based auditory dyslexia group. Another possibility would be that the QII-minus group is affected by more inhibiting factors than the other Q-minus groups. One such factor would be what has been described as orthographic speed. (See Figure 11.5) The inhibiting effect of very low orthographic speed was confirmed in the case of the QII-plus group, which did extremely poorly on this variable had by far the lowest developmental scores of all Q-factor groups.

In contrast to the three Q-minus groups, there was a relatively large amount of variation in achievement growth among the three Q-plus groups, considered to be variants of visual dyslexia. The relatively poor scores of the QII-plus group was just discussed. It looked as if poor performance on the factor orthographic speed was particularly important in explaining overall poor performance, although this group also contained a strong emotional element. But the emotional element was strongest for the QIII-plus group, which showed relatively good developmental scores. This was most likely the result of high performance on factors 1 and 11, complex phonological functions and complex orthographic functions. (See Figure 11.5) The significance of these two variables was documented in Chapter 11. It is also worth noting that the QIII-plus group also performed well on orthographic speed (factor 9), which was just described as an important inhibiting factor for growth in reading achievement. High performance on the direct factors 1, 9, and 11 combined appears to have compensated for the strong emotional element in this group.

The group with the highest developmental mean in reading, QI-plus, warrants close scrutiny. It had a very low incidence of emotional problems, but that is hardly the sole explanation. Figure 11.3 showed that this group did very well on the direct factors 1 and 11, complex phonological functions and complex orthographic functions. On the whole, the QI-plus group had the best results of all groups on these two variables.

The clinical analyses suggested that an emotional element was a strongly inhibiting factor in visual dyslexia. The Q-factor analysis also showed that emotional elements were important in visual dyslexia; they were strong in the case of QII-plus and particularly strong in the case of QIII-plus. The presence of emotional elements in the Q groups coincides with the findings of the clinical analysis, although the emotional elements did not seem to affect growth in achievement to any great degree.

Finally, let's look closer at the residual group, which showed the second highest mean developmental score in both reading and spelling. There was a considerable emotional element involved with this group, since 43% of the children were considered to have emotional problems of some sort. The incidence of emotional problems was the same for the high as for the low stanine groups for developmental scores. Figure 11.9 showed that this group differed greatly with respect to one direct variable, severe reading problems (factor 5). Their relatively rapid growth in achievement was probably the result of fairly good scores on complex phonological functions (factor 1) and complex orthographic functions (factor 11). There did not appear to be, within this group, the imbalance between the audio-phonological and the visuoorthographic skills that some researchers see as a major factor in the development of modality-related dyslexia (Aaron, 1982; Gjessing, 1977).

The subgroups of dyslexia have been described and discussed in Chapter 11 and here on the basis of clinical and statistical analyses. In both chapters comparisons have been made between the two approaches to grouping. With respect to literacy skills, the comparisons in Chapter 11 were made on the basis of *test scores* from the group tests in reading and spelling at the end of first grade (Table 11.9). In this chapter, however, the comparisons were made on the basis of the *developmental scores*, which assessed gains in literacy skills from grade 1-2 to grade 3-4. The developmental scores did not express achievement per se, but rather relative gains in achievement in comparison with the gains achieved by the members of the Bergen cohort who had no learning disabilities. This latter approach has certain advantages over the analysis of test scores only for the two grade levels — growth was studied in more detail and the regression effect was reduced.

This research project has clearly documented that it is not only possible but very useful to draw comparisons between clinically and statistically based group analyses within the same representative sample of children. There are many possibilities for analyzing differential effects as well as for cross-validating findings and interpretations.

Summary and Discussion of the Growth and Efficacy Data

This chapter started out by reviewing some studies that could reasonably be used for comparison with our data with respect to follow-up and growth data. The results of the present study were then reviewed in relation to gains in literacy achievement and the effects of the remedial programs. The outcomes were evaluated by parents and teachers. Test results obtained at the end of first grade and the beginning of second (grade 1-2) were compared with results from the end of third grade and the beginning of fourth grade (grade 3-4). A developmental scale was developed, the results of which were compared with the evaluations by parents and teachers as well as with the literacy (direct) and the nonliteracy (indirect) variables.

When making comparisons with other studies one must take into consideration the fact that there is a great deal of variability in sample selection, assessment methods, remedial methods, and statistical analyses. Monroe's 1932 study analyzed the gains in reading achievement for three different groups of children, each group receiving a different degree of remedial instruction. Over a period of 7 months the groups showed mean gains of 1.39, 0.79, and 0.14 years in grade equivalent (GE) units. The first group showed considerable gain over the 7-month period, the third group showed rather minimal growth, and the second group was in between. (It may be inaccurate to say that the middle group showed "average" gain, even though they gained about 0.7 year in 0.7 year. This is the nature of the GE scale. It is a decimalized scale, but the units vary in magnitude, being largest in the primary grades (Karlsen, 1980). Since remedial readers achieve much below grade level to begin with, a 1.0-year gain in 1 year might even be interpreted as above average for this chronological grade level.) The growth for the Bergen dyslexia sample appeared, nevertheless, to correspond to that of Monroe's second group. But it must be kept in mind that there was a great deal of variability within this sample.

Kline and Kline (1975) evaluated the results from two groups of children with reading disabilities. The first group received special help in a clinic. Within this group, 95.7% showed some progress. For 17.5% the progress was judged to be very positive. For the second group, which received no help, the corresponding percentages were 44.8 and 3.4%. Within the two groups, the clinic group and the school group, the percentages of children who showed no progress were 4.3 and 49%, respectively.

Satz (1978) reported follow-up data over a 3-year period during which no remediation took place. Several groups were followed. Within the group that had exhibited severe reading reading disabilities, 6.9% showed enough progress to be within the average range; the corresponding incidence for the group with moderate reading disabilities was 17.7%.

The parents of the dyslexic children in the Bergen sample judged their children to have more positive progress from grade 2 to grade 4 to grade 9. The percentage of parents who thought their child had severe or very severe reading disabilities at these three grade levels was 64, 18, and 9%, respectively. (Only 14 of the 64% who had problems in second grade were reported to have severe or very severe problems in the ninth grade.)

The third-grade teachers thought that 83% of the dyslexic children had received at least some benefit from the remedial efforts initiated in the second grade. Nevertheless, the teachers in the ninth grade still considered 20% of the dyslexic pupils to have severe or very severe reading difficulties.

On the basis of the most severe judgments in the ninth grade—the teachers' incidence figure of 20%—the incidence of severe or very severe reading disabilities within the total Bergen cohort of over 3,000 was still about 2% for the ninth grade, after the special remedial programs that had been initiated as part of the Bergen Project. The corresponding incidence figure for the second grade was estimated at about 5%.

The evaluations made by the teachers and the parents also covered school attitudes, factors of considerable importance when assessing the totality of the lives of dyslexic pupils. The figures presented here represent the incidences of negative school attitudes. (The term used in Norwegian, *mistrivsel*, has no English equivalent, although the word *misthriving* may convey the concept of people who do not enjoy or do well in their environment.) The incidence of negative school attitudes in the second grade was reported by the parents of 18% of the children. By the fourth grade this figure had dropped to 4%, whereas it went back up to 13% in the ninth grade. The teachers reported the same incidence figure in the ninth grade.

The school attitude statistics for the fourth grade were considered quite satisfactory. The increase in negative attitudes in the ninth grade may, in part, be the result of the normal increase in negative attitudes often associated with the onset of puberty. The fact that the special remedial programs were discontinued after fourth grade was undoubtedly also a major factor in the increase in negative attitudes. Many of these pupils needed the professional and emotional support that was built into the project's special remedial program.

Growth in literacy skills achievement from grade 1–2 to grade 3–4 was analyzed by means of a developmental score, expressed as a stanine scale, using the cohort data as the norm. A score below the middle stanine range of 4 to 6 was indicative of a relative regression in rank, while a stanine score of 7, 8, or 9 represented a relative advancement in rank. Although the combined learning disability group (dyslexics plus retarded) split pretty much 50/50 around the mean of 5, the stanine score distribution for the group deviated markedly from the normal curve that represented the cohort. The learning disabled distribution was bimodal. Whereas 23% of the cohort scored above the average range, that is, stanines 7 to 9, and the same percentage was below average, that is, stanines 1 to 3, these figures for the learning disabled sample were 40.4 and 43.9%, respectively. Only 15.7% scored in the middle three stanines, whereas 54% of the cohort scored within this range (4–6).

This biomodal distribution was characteristic of the retarded group as well as the dyslexic, although more so for the latter, since only 14% of children in this group fell in the mid-range, but 23.5% of the retarded fell in the middle three stanines.

Growth in achievement was also analyzed against the test scores obtained in grade 1–2 and again in grade 3–4. On the first test, 96% of the dyslexic children scored at stanines 1 to 3 in reading. The corresponding number for mathematics was 57.3%. These incidence figures for the retarded group were 88.3 and 97.1%, respectively. Despite the much higher scholastic aptitude level among the dyslexics, a slightly higher percentage of them were below average in reading than the retarded group. The opposite was the case, of course, in mathematics.

By the end of the third grade and 2 years of remedial treatment, 20.9% of the pupils who were at the end of first grade had obtained reading test scores of stanines 1 to 3 scored within the average range, that is, stanines 4 to 6. Among those who scored 1 or 2 initially, 35.3% moved up to stanine 3 or higher. Within the retarded group, 23.3% went from stanines 1 to 3 to 4 or higher by the end of third grade.

Again, *specific* literacy skills deficiencies were documented for the dyslexia group. They not only performed more poorly than the retarded group at the end of first grade, they gained less in literacy skills in the next 2 years of remedial and regular instruction. These two groups received very similar treatments, but it was more beneficial for the retarded than for the dyslexic. This finding confirms the very serious nature of specific reading disabilities and also the fact that good scholastic aptitude will not automatically compensate for this problem.

It is almost impossible to draw any valid conclusions with respect to the efficacy of the remedial program employed in this project. The main reason is that we did not, for ethical reasons, leave a relevant comparison group untreated. In addition, there were the perennial problems of all research projects of this kind, such as the regression effect, which we tried to keep to a minimum.

It is also problematic to draw parallels with other studies of prognosis and efficacy in the case of dyslexia. The Bergen Project occupies a place somewhere between a prognostic follow-up study (e.g., Schonhaut & Satz, 1983) and a more typical efficacy study (e.g., Kline & Kline, 1975; Monroe, 1932).

If this project is considered an efficacy study, the results were, on the average, quite similar to those of Monroe's group 2. This group was carefully diagnosed at a clinic but was treated in school by educators of varying degrees of specialization. Monroe's group 2 received pretty much the same treatment as provided for the children in the Bergen Project.

Monroe's group 3 had also gone through the same diagnostic work-up as group 2, but no systematic treatment was provided by the school. Monroe found big differences between the achievement test results for these two groups. At the time of the follow-up, group 3 had regressed markedly in comparison with their nonhandicapped peers, whereas group 2 showed a growth rate similar to the norm after remediation was initiated. It would seem reasonable to assume that what happened to Monroe's group 3 would have happened to the dyslexic pupils in the Bergen Project if a remedial program had not been initiated.

The study by Kline and Kline (1975) reported a larger mean difference between treated and untreated dyslexia groups. Their treated group was taught in a clinic, similar to Monroe's group 1. The results of this type of treatment were very favorable, quite similar to those of Monroe. The treatment program in Bergen was not as intensive, nor were the results as good.

The Bergen Project yielded a variety of positive results, the parent evaluations being the most enthusiastic. With respect to growth in reading achievement, parents' judgment was that only 9% of the dyslexics could be described as having severe or very severe reading difficulties by the ninth grade. The teachers judged this incidence figure to be about 20%. On the basis of these evaluations, it was concluded that three of every five children with severe reading disabilities had achieved functional literacy by the ninth grade.

The reading test results showed that of those children who had scored at stanine 1, 2, or 3 at the end of first grade, 21% had moved into the average range by scoring stanine 4 or higher at grade 3–4. Schonhaut and Satz (1983) found that the transition from severe reading disability to "functional reading ability" occurred in only 7% of cases. His definition of functional reading ability was similar to ours. Even though direct comparisons between these projects are quite hazardous because of differences in cultures, languages, educational systems, and so on, it nevertheless appears from our data that systematic diagnostic-prescriptive remedial programs are effective.

Despite our relatively good results we are left with a considerable problem. Significant progress can be documented for only some of the children. Despite all our efforts, a good proportion of the dyslexic children studied still have severe reading disabilities. What to do with these children will be discussed in Chapter 15.

Gain in achievement was correlated with a large number of directly measured variables, indirectly measured variables, and variables. Very few of these correlated to any significant degree with gains in achievement as measured on the developmental scale. One finding worth mentioning here relates to the discrepancy between WISC Verbal IQ (VIQ) and WISC Performance IQ (PIQ). There was a tendency for children with a small difference between these two IQs to do better than those with a large difference. The *direction* of the IQ difference was not correlated with gains in reading achievement.

The results of the comparisons between VIQ and PIQ did suggest that problems with literacy skills achievement increased as the discrepancy between these two IQs increased. This finding lends some support to the "balance theory" as a partial explanation of some dyslexia problems (Aaron, 1982; Gjessing, 1977). On the other hand, which of these two IQs was higher did not seem to be significant.

We found an inverse relationship between the number of hours of remedial work provided and achievement gains; that is, the pupils who were given the most instruction gained the least. One might conclude from this that the less help pupils were given, the more they gained. This paradoxical finding was, however, most likely the result of teachers spending a disproportionate amount of time and effort on the children who had the most severe problems. The effort on behalf of the children with the greatest problems did not result in proportionate gains.

The clinical analyses showed the largest gains in literacy skills achievement for the auditory dyslexia group and the next largest for the group "other types." Audiovisual dyslexia showed the smallest gains. The combination of emotional difficulties and dyslexia seemed to affect audiovisual and visual dyslexics the most.

Q-factor analysis showed a fair amount of variability in mean gains for the various groups. The group that showed the poorest gain on the achievement tests and the Q-factor group with the largest achievement gains both appeared to resemble most closely the clinical visual dyslexia group. The addition of emotional problems to the learning disability appeared to be more detrimental for the visual Q groups also. Among the Q groups identified as variants of auditory dyslexia, the group that most resembled audiovisual dyslexia (QI-minus) showed the poorest gains in achievement.

In general, there was a fair degree of correspondence between the clinical and the statistical subgroups. Some literacy subskills, as well as emotional problems, seemed relatively strongly associated with achievement. These were complex phonological functions (factor 1), complex orthographic functions (factor 11), and orthographic speed (factor 9). Our conclusion was that an analysis of clinically and statistically identified groups from the same cohort yields valuable insights and should be encouraged in future research on subtypes of dyslexia.

Part V The Bergen Project's Contribution to Research and Its Applied Educational and Clinical Value

CHAPTER 15

Summary, Conclusions, and Discussion of the Entire Project

H.-J. Gjessing

The Bergen Project was a developmental study that focused on children with school learning problems. It could be described as a research project as well, since it had theoretical as well as applied goals. The scientific objectives were twofold: to find research strategies that allowed for observations and examinations of personal and environmental factors based on individual processes and functions, and to acquire traditional quantitative results and products.

Goals, Design, and Previous Published Reports

The project encompassed four phases:

Phase 1. The initial group testing in the classrooms,
Phase 2. Individual clinical examinations of children with specific school learning disabilities (dyslexics) and children with general school learning disabilities (retarded),
Phase 3. Additional individual clinical examinations by medical researchers,
Phase 4. Follow-up studies.

The project lasted about 10 years. A number of interim, brief reports have been published in Norwegian, Swedish, and Danish, as well as in English. The "final report" was a series of three book-length comprehensive reports, all published in Norwegian. A considerable amount of data have still not been published, although many of them have been statistically analyzed. It is quite possible that additional analyses may be carried out later by individual members of the research team on this project.

The first of the three final reports (Gjessing, Nygaard, Solheim, & Aasved, 1982) dealt with the theoretical and professional premises of the project. Discussed in this report are such topics as interaction statistical analysis, which is particularly germain when studying extreme groups; self-concept; learning disabilities, underachievement, and sensory deficits, so often associated with reading difficulties.

Report II (Solheim et al., 1984) dealt primarily with the findings from the entire cohort of Bergen children who entered first grade in 1976 ($n > 3,000$), all of whom participated in the study. These data were all based on group assessments done in the various classrooms.

Finally, Report III (Gjessing et al., 1988) analyzed the volume of assessment results, tests, and observations of individuals as well as groups. Working with literally hundreds of variables made it possible to examine a multitude of relationships and interactions. It became necessary to delimit and organize such an analysis. This was done by dividing the data into dependent and independent variables. School achievement (reading, spelling, and math) variables were the dependent criterion variables, while the other characteristics (background data, linguistic-cognitive factors, socioemotional factors) were the independent or predictor variables. These predictor variables constituted the pool of data that could be drawn from to "explain" school achievement.

This book is the only comprehensive report of the Bergen Project in English. It deals primarily with the findings of the entire project, but it also sheds considerable light on the comparison groups, on the entire normative cohort, and on the retarded sample from the same cohort.

Main Objectives and Findings of the Cohort Assessments

The main purpose of phase 1 was to collect extensive group data on the entire cohort, beginning with a study of variability in three school subjects: reading, spelling, and mathematics.

Our findings were quite consistent with previous research in this area—individual differences in school achievement among peers are of considerable magnitude. But the qualitative information is only part of the picture; it attains additional meaning as we relate the data concretely to what the school expects on specific tests. Consider, for example, the individual differences in reading rate at the third-grade level. It varies from 4 to 5 to more than 130 words per minute, with rates at all stages in between. On the basis of such normative information an attempt was made to differentiate between functional and nonfunctional reading ability, considering what may be minimum requirements for this grade. It was concluded that about 10% of the pupils were doing very poorly, 4 to 5% were clearly lacking functional and reading ability.

During phase 1 attempts were also made to look at many correlates of achievement to determine what some of the antecedents may be for the tremendous variability.

Regression data revealed that the best predictors of achievement were linguistic-cognitive in nature. This factor explained anywhere from 26 to 42% of the variance, depending on the school subject.

The socioemotional factor thought to be an important factor and considered second, contributed rather minimally, explaining only 1.2 to 2.7% of the variance.

The background factor, which included age, sex, and parental occupation, explained from 6 to 9% of the variance. This contribution is rather modest in light of the fact that this factor was placed first in the regression equation.

In addition to individual differences, variability among classroom averages was also looked at. Mean growth in achievement from first to fourth grade was studied, controlling for variability in initial achievement. Classroom averages showed relatively stable ranks over 2 years, the correlation being closed to .80. But within these rather stable averages there were some changes. Some classroom averages changed rather significantly. From the total pool of 145 classrooms we compared the 16 classrooms with the highest positive gain with the 16 with the smallest gain. These classroom averages were the basis for the factor referred to as *classroom membership*. In Norway it is customary for a teacher to stay with the same class over several years, so that most of the children in our study had been taught by the same teacher from the first through the third grade, the time span for which classroom membership was studied.

Classroom membership contributed significantly to the explained variance by anywhere from 6 to 17%, depending on the criterion variable or combination of variables studied. Some statistics revealed systematic differences among the various classrooms independent of the linguistic-cognitive abilities of the pupils; in fact, the interclass variability could not be explained by factors that we could control for in this entire study. This factor could be thought of as the teacher variable.

Summary of the Group Data

The pupil characteristics that contributed the most to the large individual differences among the Bergen cohort were controlled for by means of regression analysis. As already stated, the linguistic-cognitive factor set contributed the most. It would seem particularly important, therefore, to take these factors into consideration when providing educational opportunities and stimulation for the children.

The background factors of age, sex, and socioeconomic status (SES) made relatively modest contributions to the explained variance in school achievement. In other words, knowledge of children's ages, sex, and SES are very limited bases from which to predict success in school. It may be surprising that there is such a low correlation between SES and school achievement, since the American research generally indicates very substantial correlations between these two variables, but the Bergen data are quite consistent with previous research in other Scandinavian countries (Gjessing, 1958a; Malmquist, 1958).

The most parsimonious explanation for the lack of correlation between SES and school achievement is probably the fact that culturally and socioeconomically Norway is a relatively homogeneous society. The main sources of variability in school achievement can certainly not be ascribed to socioeconomic or home factors, but are more likely the results of pupil variability in linguistic-cognitive abilities and the extent to which the school is capable of utilizing and challenging these abilities.

The contribution of the socioemotional factors, as assessed in this project, to the prediction of school achievement was very modest, perhaps remarkably and surprisingly so. It is difficult to place this finding in perspective, since there is extremely limited research evidence in this field in the Scandinavian research literature.

These findings all relate to the group data obtained on one cohort of school children, analyses for smaller groups and individual children showed relationships that differed considerably from the central tendencies. These relationships have been studied in considerable detail through interactional and multivariate analyses based on the individual data for the dyslexic and retarded pupils. Some relationships were also significant at the classroom level. For example, there was an interaction between the socioemotional factors and level of linguistic-cognitive functioning. Among children with relatively low linguistic-cognitive functioning, there was significant positive correlation between school achievement and such socioemotional factors as self-concept, level of aspiration, classroom behavior, and peer status.

The classroom membership factor functioned basically independently with respect to the explained variance, possibly because it was calculated after controlling for the three sets of variables studied—the linguistic-cognitive, the socioemotional, and the background factors. With some reservations the classroom membership factor was viewed as being related to the classroom milieu as such; it was the contribution of each classroom "atmosphere" to pupil achievement. No additional empirical data were collected that could shed more light on this factor, and no teacher data were collected relating to either static or dynamic characteristics. The findings do raise some important as well as sensitive issues with respect to the participating teachers. There is no doubt that these data are of considerable interest and significance regarding the role of teachers.

Results Relating to the Dyslexics and the Retarded

Two target groups within the cohort were studied intensively. The first group consisted of children with severe learning difficulties in the literacy skills of reading and writing, which was labeled the *dyslexic* group. The second group of children had low general scholastic ability; for the sake of brevity these children have been referred to as *retarded*. Criteria were developed to identify the children in each of these groups. The dyslexics were selected on the basis of their very low levels of functioning in reading and spelling, despite adequate or even above-average levels of school ability; they were clearly underachievers with respect to the literacy skills. The label dyslexia was used simply to mean school achievement in reading and spelling that was significantly below expectancy. No medical criteria were applied for inclusion in this group. The criterion for inclusion in the retarded group was simply low scores on an IQ test—an average score at least 2 standard deviations below the cohort mean on two tests, which is below IQ 70.

Socioemotional Status

Comparisons between the two target groups and the remainder of the cohort revealed numerous negative characteristics of the target groups. According to the teacher evaluations, the target groups had poor self-concepts, lacked self-confidence, and exhibited social nonconformity, which resulted in poor acceptance by peers. The last was expressed directly in the peer evaluations, which showed the two target groups to have low peer status on the average. The dyslexic children also indicated a lower sense of well being in school than other pupils. Negative socioemotional characteristics were present in both target groups, but were more pronounced for the retarded group than for the dyslexics.

A number of comparisons were also made with respect to certain aspects of self-concept between the target groups and appropriate control groups. For example, the dyslexia group rated much lower than the control group on "feelings of subject matter mastery," indicating awareness of low achievement status by the end of third grade. But this, again, is merely an average; there were many exceptions. In fact, the two score distributions with regard to this factor overlapped to a large extent. About the only thing one can say for certain is that more children in the dyslexic group perceived themselves as being less competent in school than their matched peers, a perception that is, of course, consistent with the facts.

This particular finding prompts a number of questions relating to value judgments with considerable psychological and educational overtones. Why do some dyslexic children report positive self-concepts with regard to success in school? Why do children with learning difficulties exhibit such varied reactions to this experience? How do the experiences of schooling really affect children? What would be a desirable educational objective in this respect—a "positive" or a "realistic" self-concept? These educational issues are certainly difficult to explain or answer.

The target groups showed slower educational growth in reading and spelling than the cohort as a whole, but there was much variability. Some of the dyslexics showed above-average growth in achievement after remediation was initiated, whereas others continued their pattern of slow growth. It is interesting to note that even though children with similar characteristics are given appropriate remedial instruction, they vary considerably with respect to the outcome of this instruction. Some develop very positively educationally as well as psychologically, others continue at the same rate, and others again show negative development.

How can these different growth patterns be explained? Are there common characteristics among the high gainers that differentiate them from the very slow gainers? Attempts were made to analyze these issues with the use of multivariate techniques and interaction analysis, with special emphasis on the dyslexic group. The findings will be summarized later in this chapter.

Theory of Dyslexia and Its Assessment

Definition of Dyslexia

The construct dyslexia was given a rather broad, pragmatic, and reality-oriented definition: *Dyslexia* refers to an inordinate amount of difficulty with the learning of literacy skills (reading and/or writing) which cannot be assumed to be caused *primarily* by intellectual, sensory, or motor deficits. In most cases, emotional problems have not played a primary, causative role. The literacy achievement levels must be significantly below expectancy based on the person's intellectual level and past educational opportunities.

A qualitative "function analysis" that considers all factors in a totality will often reveal unique patterns of reading and writing characteristics (Gjessing, 1977).

In conclusion, our definition of dyslexia deviates somewhat from the typical definition. We emphasize the differential diagnostic value of qualitative differences in reading and spelling behavior. We do not require average or higher intellectual ability. We do not exclude cases with other problems in addition to an achievement deficit. We do, however, maintain the requirement of a significant achievement-ability discrepancy, especially for research purposes. We make no assumptions or restrictions with respect to etiology. On this last point our opinion is at variance with most of the medical writers, but we confine our definition to what we can observe and what is supported by hard data.

The Dyslexia Model

Our clinical diagnostic investigations utilized a unique typological model that had evolved from previous practical experiences with the diagnostic study of children with learning disabilities. The model differentiates between the types of dyslexia related to the sensory modalities (auditory, visual, and audiovisual dyslexia) and nonmodality-related forms of dyslexia (emotional, educational, and a miscellaneous group of rare types).

This model has several noticeable characteristics:

It is based on typology. It functions with subcategories that differ to the extent that they require differential treatment and should be studied as separate entities.

It is polythetic. The polythetic typology model was used to group those children with the most common traits and characteristics. (See Chapter 10). This approach yields subgroups that have no absolute criteria for inclusion, in contrast to a monothetic approach, where group membership is based on a unique set of traits and characteristics.

It is hypotheticodescriptive. This approach starts with results from practical clinical experiences and systematic analysis of behavior during the reading and writing process. This does not preclude the model being supported by clinical-neurological and cognitive theories and models.

It is based on specific symptoms and categorization of behavioral characteristics during the reading and writing process, based on principles of interaction analysis and what we have called *function analysis*. This means essentially that specific errors and types of errors in reading and spelling can be determined and understood within their context and the totality of the reading or spelling process. One must not only study the records of errors, but also how children approach the literacy skills when they are so engaged. The products of literacy behavior and the observations of this behavior must then be seen within the interactional context of nonliteracy variables, such as sensory deficits, speech problems, and neurological and socioemotional variables.

We have differentiated between dyslexia types related to sensory modalities (auditory, visual, and audio-visual) and nonmodality-related types (emotional and educational). Grouping according to sensory modalities is, as analyzed in Chapter 8, commonly done in the international research literature, although at times different labels are used. But the subgroups emotional and educational dyslexia are quite common. The reasons for this vary. Some researchers do not consider these learning disabled children dyslexic, despite a pronounced discrepancy between the level of scholastic aptitude and the relatively low achievement in the literacy skills. The reason for the avoidance of the dyslexia label is generally a lack of medical etiology. Other researchers may overlook the cases of emotional and educational dyslexia: Such a diagnosis is rarely made until a child has attended school for several years, and it often requires prolonged contact with a child before a reliable differential diagnosis can be made.

Function Analysis

The term *function analysis* was coined to describe a clinical diagnostic approach for the study of reading and writing difficulties. It has many things in common with what in the American literature has been labeled *informal reading inventory, miscue analysis*, or the *individual diagnostic conference* (Karlsen, 1980). Function analysis considers records of errors in oral reading and spelling from dictation, as well as behavioral observations while the child performs these tasks. It differs from most approaches by its strong emphasis on behavioral observations. This provides a considerably more detailed diagnosis for use in remediation.

How a person functions with respect to the literacy skills is, of course, the result of underlying processes. Function analysis is, therefore, an indispensable requirement for an understanding of these processes. Within the context of the analysis of reading and spelling difficulties this behavior is viewed as the final expression of the many underlying and interacting elements that may change and vary, depending on the total context (Gjessing, 1980a). Such an approach renders almost meaningless the simple counting and categorizing of reading and spelling errors without consideration for their context and the patterns of interaction of underlying processes.

A number of different recording systems have been developed to analyze reading and spelling errors, depending on the purposes of the analysis. Basically, these procedures can be classified as being *selective, quantitative,* or *function analytical.* The selective approach tends to select and focus on particularly significant errors, such as reversal errors. The quantitative method classifies all errors, but each error is analyzed in isolation and grouped according to a rather mechanical classification scheme. Function analysis is built on certain hypotheses regarding the processing of the written word. These hypotheses are the outgrowth of clinical observations and certain theoretical models.

In our dyslexia model and its attendant function analysis, different symptoms relating to the written word are interpreted in light of the underlying processes. Some of these symptoms are rather unequivocally characteristic of a certain type of dyslexia, whereas other errors cannot be easily classified: They must be viewed within the total configuration of symptoms. We are talking about not only such direct symptoms as reading and spelling errors and behavior during reading and writing, but also indirect symptoms (correlates of reading and spelling difficulties) such as delayed language development, mixed dominance, incidence of dyslexia among relatives, and so on.

Tests Used for Function Analysis

To apply our dyslexia model in a clinical setting, we designed a series of experimental tests (Gjessing, 1979). This test battery includes extensive and detailed subtests relating to the processes involved in reading and writing behavior.

In addition to the diagnostic tests, materials were developed for treatment and teaching according to the results and the combinations of problems identified by the diagnostic tests (Gjessing et al., 1980).

The diagnostic test battery was factor analyzed *after* its initial application with the children in the Bergen Project identified as having serious learning problems. The test was originally based on practical clinical experience and theoretical insight. It was assumed that a factor analysis at the initial development stage would be of limited relevance, because it would in all likelihood reject items and eliminate certain nuances that would make the test more streamlined for large-scale testing, but would obliterate some refinements of utility with only a handful of children. The factor analysis was done a posteriori to get some insight into the validity of this theoretical-clinical approach to test construction.

Our data base was the result of the diagnostic test. The factor analysis covered the direct variables associated with reading and writing behavior and all the error analyses from reading and writing observations. There was a total of 74 variables. A principal-components factor analysis resulted in 11 factors, each containing variables that made meaningful interpretation possible.

The factors were arranged in a certain order on the basis of our dyslexia model. The early ranks were assigned to those factors assumed to differentiate most sharply between pupils with auditory dyslexia and those with visual dyslexia, where it was assumed that auditory dyslexics would score relatively low and the visual dyslexics would do quite well. The later ranks were assigned to those factors that would yield the opposite results. The factors in the middle were assumed to not differentiate between these two main groups, at least not at this relatively early stage of schooling. The ranks and labels of the 11 factors that came out of the factor analysis are as follows:

1. Complex phonological functions.
2. Phonological cluster functions.
3. Phonological assimilation.
4. Orthographic error detection.
5. Severe reading problems.
6. Semantic literacy functions.
7. Reversals.
8. Attentiveness.
9. Orthographic speed.
10. Phonological dependence.
11. Complex orthographic functions.

Numerous variables accounted for factors 1 and 11. These two factors were therefore labeled "complex," but their main characteristics related to phonological (reading) and orthographic (spelling) functions. The general impression otherwise is that most of the subtests of the diagnostic battery were represented rather unifactorially. The insignificant overlap among factors other than 1 and 11 would seem to suggest that the diagnostic test used had identified many specific literacy skills.

Another question of interest would be if the different subtests/dimensions of the diagnostic test clustered as predicted from the theory of dyslexia on which the test was based. The general impression is clearly that the statistical analysis supported the validity of Gjessing's diagnostic reading test.

All of the 11 factors could, of course, be considered to be new, complex variables. Each pupil's factor score could then be based on these variables. Since these factor scores could conceivably be used for diagnostic purposes, scores for each factor were derived by adding the standard scores for each set of variables represented in each factor. These sums were then converted to ordinary standard z scores (mean $= 0$, SD $= 1$). The pupils' z scores for each of the 11 variables would then represent new profiles of test results.

These profiles were analyzed and the mean profiles were calculated for the four types of dyslexia. The clinical analyses, based on the dyslexia model, had resulted in a four-way classification of dyslexia: auditory, audiovisual, visual, and other types. The last group encompassed what had previously been labeled emotional dyslexia, educational dyslexia and other, rare types of dyslexia, all of them being the nonmodality-related types of dyslexia.

The four final dyslexia groups were compared across the mean z scores for the 11 factors, to determine if the statistically based variable combinations yielded profiles consistent with what was expected from the clinical analyses. A positive outcome of such a comparison would have to be interpreted as a mutual validation of the clinically and statistically based interpretations of the different variables. This would also confirm that a clinically based analysis could be used to classify children with specific learning difficulties into instructional subgroups.

It turned out that the four dyslexia groups had clearly distinct profiles across the 11 factors. These profiles corresponded well with the patterns that had been predicted from the definitions of the groups.

Review of Typological Dyslexia Models

For comparison purposes, a number of other dyslexia models were reviewed. The Gjessing model was published in 1953, but it was several years before much thinking along this line appeared in the international research literature. It was not until the late 1960s that such an approach to this problem found supporters in the Anglo-American literature. While relatively few typological dyslexia studies were published by the early 1970s, there are by now so many that it is not possible to give a detailed analysis of each of them here.

To arrive at a relatively brief but comprehensive summary of the available research, the studies were categorized into two main groups. The first group was those that had as their central categories the audiophonological versus the visuo-spatial types, as had the Gjessing model. The second group was those that had not based their theories primarily on the sensory input channels.

The various theories were summarized under these two main rubrics by listing the investigator's name, date of publication, subgroup designations, primary data base with respect to reading and writing behavior (direct symptoms: literacy skills variables) or more general cognitive, linguistic, or neurological variables (indirect symptoms: nonliteracy skills variables). Each investigator's professional affiliation was also indicated, that is, psychology or medicine.

A large number of the typologies reviewed contained subgroups that were analogous to the first three categories of the Gjessing model (Table 8.1). This is particularly true of those investigators who placed their main emphasis on the direct variables (D)—reading and writing behavior specifically. But even those who based their typology on more indirect variables (ID)—cognitive and linguistic test results—have quite often, partly or completely, arrived at the same categories. The basic auditory-versus-visual division is found among psychologists as well as physicians and people using either statistical or clinical approaches.

The audiophonological syndrome (A) has been given a variety of designations by various investigators, as has the visuospatial-based syndrome; the terminology varies probably more than the underlying concepts. Currently some writers speculate that these two main types have their bases in the left and right hemispheres, respectively, rather than being based on sensory modalities.

Research Problems Associated With Dyslexia

A major objective of the Bergen Project was to consider the many problems of research methodology that are peculiar to empirical research related to dyslexia, and those that relate more generally to clinical research. Statistically, one must often deal with grossly skewed distributions; clinically, the human judgment factors are often difficult to handle in empirical research of the kind reported here.

The reliability and the relevance of clinical and statistical analyses were considered in detail. Clinical judgment can conflict directly with test results. Most clinicians know firsthand cases in which test results, if allowed to dominate their conclusions and recommendations, would have been highly misleading. Some of the most obvious examples come from the assessment of intelligence.

This brings up a major dilemma in research, especially research that relates to human behavior – the contrast between the subjective and the objective reality as it is being perceived. Within the context of the research reported here, this contrast relates to clinical practice versus clinical research. One is confronted by a paradox: The theoretical research basis for a certain "objective" reality is often perceived as inadequate or insufficient in clinical practice.

Considerations of these various viewpoints resulted in our adopting an eclectic, integrated approach. Such an approach appears to be quite well accepted in principle. The problem is to apply it within a single research project. This approach is demanding because of the need for personnel with theoretical as well as practical backgrounds, but also because the idiographic, qualitative, clinical approaches lack status with respect to topics and fields that have generally been perceived as "nomothetic territory." One could, of course, choose to skip this issue entirely, as has been done by most, or one can try to justify a nomothetic or an idiographic alternative. One could also, as was done in the Bergen Project, justify and apply the integrated alternative, despite an awareness of its complexities.

From the very beginning we were critical of attempts to simplify the set of complex issues that are represented by dyslexia, an approach often taken by researchers in the past. One of the main issues relates to the homogeneity-heterogeneity of dyslexia, that is, is dyslexia a single syndrome or does it have many forms (manifestations) and are we talking about one or many causes of or conditions leading to dyslexia? These issues have been discussed in detail, particularly as related to the points of view expressed by Wiener and Cromer (1967) and by Applebee (1971). Like us, these researchers could see no other approach for further developments in dyslexia research than to accept the very complex and interactional nature of dyslexia, "something which everyone must accept, but few will act accordingly." (Applebee, 1971, p. 98) This viewpoint necessitates a systematic search for relevant and appropriate procedures for subgroupings within the general symptom complex commonly referred to as dyslexia.

Research Results Relating to the Total Dyslexia Group

Within the entire Bergen cohort of over 3,000 pupils, less than 300 were classified as dyslexics. This dyslexic cohort was first studied as a total group, and later according to dyslexia type subgroups. Despite the many weaknesses involved in attempts to search for correlates or causative factors in dyslexia within a total dyslexia sample, we did this nevertheless in order to take a closer look at our enormous data base from this vantage point and to compare our findings with those in the research literature.

The many variables were classified as *direct* (relating to literacy skills variables) and *indirect* (nonreading variables). The first analyses related to the direct variables, the Gjessing Diagnostic Reading Test (Dia-Gjessing) and the many group test variables. The relationships between the direct and the indirect variables were then analyzed (see Table 10.1). Finally, the data from all of these variables were compared with the available normative information.

The analyses and comparisons among the direct (literacy skills) variables yielded results that could be of considerable importance for our understanding of reading and writing processes. First, we had the comparisons between the individual tests (Dia-Spelling) and the group tests for silent reading and spelling. Dia-Gjessing provides separate assessments for spelling (Dia-Spelling), oral reading (Dia-Oral reading) and silent reading (Dia-Silent reading). The correlational analyses revealed differences and similarities among the variables that were interpreted as reasonable and informative and that were consistent with the clinical observations (Gjessing, 1978).

Comparisons of the direct and indirect variables resulted in a considerable range of findings. Among the measured indirect variables, the strongest relationships with the direct variables were found for the areas of perception, memory, and language. The systematic observations of the teachers and the school psychologists (observed indirect variables) showed the highest positive correlations with the literacy skills. Such observations appear to be at least as good overall predictors of learning disabilities as many of the more elaborate formal assessments that were made.

Table 10.6 presents the summary data for the total dyslexia group, the total norm group (cohort), and boys and girls within both groups. Several significant sex differences were revealed. The verbal variable that differentiated most sharply between boys and girls was word pronunciation. This subtest also differentiated sharply between the total dyslexia group and the entire cohort. The variable melody reproduction also differentiated very sharply between the boys and the girls within the total dyslexia ($p < .001$), whereas the same variable did not correlate with the literacy skills variables.

Within the total dyslexia sample the girls performed more poorly than the boys quite consistently on a number of main indirect variables. This was particularly true in the area of scholastic aptitude (IQ). But the girls tended to outperform the boys in the literacy skills. Generally speaking, there were larger differences between scholastic aptitude and school achievement for the boys with dyslexia than for the girls. Among the dyslexics of higher scholastic aptitude there was a preponderance of boys.

One major objective was to determine the extent to which various indirect variables, independent of each other, contributed to achievement in the literacy skills for the total dyslexia sample. The intercorrelations among these variables were also determined. But because of the strong emphasis on the subcategories of dyslexia, there was relatively little emphasis on the multivariate prediction of school success for this sample.

Nevertheless, a stepwise regression analysis was carried out with the Dia-Total (summary score for reading and spelling) as the criterion variable. The first two variables in the regression equation were the language tests "word pronunciation" and "syntax." These two variables explained 20% of the variance for Dia-Total. Two additional language tests, "auditory discrimination" and "melody reproduction," made insignificant contributions to the prediction. The Bender Gestalt test added 7.7% to the variance, VADS an additional 3.3%, and "hand asymmetry" 4.6%. In other words, five of these seven variables appeared to have predictive value, explaining all together around 35% of the variance in Dia-Total. Adding the rather time-consuming WISC-R to the regression equation at this point would have added a mere 0.2% to the explained variance. (Had this test been placed first in the regression equation, it would have explained 6.8% of the variance.)

An earlier correlation study had identified the most significant observational variables, which were entered into the regression analysis at this point. Their contributions were very strong, even though they were introduced into the regression equation behind the various language tests and WISC. This was particularly true of observations that had been labeled "reading style," "phonetic dependence," "concentration," "achievement drive," and "reaction to problems." These added about 22% to the explained variance. By adding the teacher observation variables, it was possible to explain about 63% of the variance, or a multiple correlation of $R = .79$ between Dia-Total and the variables that had been entered into the regression equation.

Results of the Typological Subgrouping of the Dyslexia Group

All of the dyslexic children were classified according to type of dyslexia, based on the four-category model, by means of analysis of the clinical data. The variables involved in this study were then analyzed by subgroup and by sex, when relevant. This subdivision made it possible to identify a number of intergroup differences and interactions that did not appear in the total dyslexia group.

Interscorer Agreement

The various professionals involved were asked to categorize each pupil according to type of dyslexia, these placements being made independently. The extent of this agreement varied from 62.1 to 93.4%, depending on which group of evaluators did the classification.

The primary reason for doing this analysis was to determine the interrater reliability of the diagnostic test (Dia-Gjessing). The underlying concern was, of course, the particular dyslexia model involved. These analyses showed that the use of a battery of tests based on this model can bring out systematic differences

among children with dyslexia with sufficient accuracy to classify these children
with a relatively small error element. This does not, of course, necessarily imply
that this is the best scheme for classifying children according to type of dyslexia.

Comparisons Among the Clinical Subgroups

The data from the four dyslexia subgroups were compared for the various direct
(reading and spelling) and for the indirect (nonreading) variables. The visual dyslexia group performed significantly better than the auditory and audiovisual
groups in spelling (Dia-Spelling) and oral reading (Dia-Oral reading). There was
also an interesting interaction between spelling and oral reading for the auditory
and visual groups. As the theory had predicted (Gjessing, 1977), the visual dyslexics performed significantly better in spelling than in oral reading, whereas the
opposite was true of the auditory dyslexics. This particular interaction would
appear to be of considerable importance for our understanding of the processes
involved in reading and spelling, and it can be utilized in the diagnosis of reading
and spelling difficulties.

With respect to the indirect variables, the following findings would appear to
be of considerable interest:

It is part of the underlying theory that "musicality" is a trait of significance
for differential diagnosis. Clinical and classroom observations had indicated
that the inability to reproduced a melody by singing was characteristic of children with auditory dyslexia (Gjessing, 1977). Our data supported this observation (Table 11.3). A more careful interaction analysis showed this characteristic to be true only for boys. This finding was also independent of scholastic aptitude (IQ). There were several other linguistic-phonological characteristics on which children with auditory dyslexia had much greater difficulties
than children with visual dyslexia, including such variables as "word pronunciation," "listening comprehension," "articulation," and "quality of spoken language" (Table 11.2). These findings were consistent with the underlying theory
(Gjessing, 1977).

The international dyslexia research indicates considerable interest in the
general ability test Wechsler Intelligence Test for Children (WISC). A number of
different hypotheses were explored with respect to this test, especially differences among the four dyslexia groups with respect to WISC-Total IQ, discrepancies between WISC-Verbal IQ and Performance IQ, and some schemes for
analyzing the various WISC subtests (e.g., Bannatyne, 1971). Although there
were significant differences among the dyslexia groups with respect to WISC-
Total IQ, the groups did not differ with respect to discrepancies between Verbal
IQ and Performance IQ. The last finding is at variance with what is often discussed in the literature, but the Bergen data gave no support for the notion that
the difference between Verbal IQ and Performance IQ is of diagnostic usefulness.
Nor did the data support the Bannatyne findings regarding a three-way split of the
WISC subtests into conceptual, spatial, and sequential abilities; such a split
seemed to have no utility for differential diagnosis.

Koppitz (1977) has claimed differential usefulness for the VADS test. Within the four dyslexia groups only one subtest appeared to have differential diagnostic characteristics. This subtest was Aural-Written, on which the auditory dyslexics performed significantly below the visual dyslexics.

With regard to laterality, it has often been assumed that among children with learning disabilities there is a higher-than-normal incidence of lefthandedness and mixed eye-hand dominance. It has also been found almost universally that there is a higher incidence of lefthandedness among boys than girls; this was also the case in the Bergen cohort. There was also a higher incidence of mixed laterality and uncertain laterality among the pupils with visual dyslexia compared with the other three dyslexia groups. It was consistent with the underlying theory in this project that there would be a higher incidence of lefthandedness, mixed dominance, and unclear dominance among the visual dyslexics compared with the auditory dyslexics (Gjessing, 1977).

Furthermore, it was also noted in this project that there was a particularly high incidence of lefthandedness among the children who were classified as retarded.

Statistically Based Subgroups

The total dyslexia group of 181 children (14 were eliminated because of missing data) could be divided into subgroups by means of statistical analyses. Extensive preliminary analyses were carried out to evaluate Q-factor and cluster analysis and how the resultant subgroups corresponded with the clinically based subgroups. These two statistical approaches resulted in subgroups that overlapped to a considerable extent. They also overlapped with the clinically based groups. Most of the statistical subgroups had a preponderance of pupils who had been classified as auditory or visual dyslexics in the clinical approach, that is, they appeared to represent groups whose main problems were related to either auditory or visual functions. The results from the two statistical approaches were fairly similar to those of the clinical analyses.

For the sake of brevity, the comparison between the clinical and statistical subgroups was limited to the Q-factor analysis. This seems reasonable, since cluster analysis yielded very similar results.

As in the preliminary explorations, the final Q-factor analysis resulted in three main factors (factors I, II, and III), and within each factor were two contrasting groups, one with a positive loading and one with a negative. These were referred to as the Q-plus and Q-minus groups. The QI-plus group was those with high positive loading on factor I, and so forth. Those children who did not fit into any of the six groups (n = 30) were separated into a seventh (residual) group. The factor I groups consisted of 26 (minus) and 40 (plus) pupils, the factor II groups contained 22 and 25, respectively, and the factor III groups had 13 and 25 pupils. To avoid group selection on the basis of differences in school ability, the data were corrected for differences in IQ.

Six of the seven Q-factor groups could be divided into two main types of dyslexia, auditory and visual, with three variants on each type. The seventh group (the residual group) was not modality related. These groups are described briefly here.

The three Q-minus groups were variants of auditory dyslexia. The QII-minus and the QIII-minus groups fit pretty much the predicted profile for auditory dyslexia, but they differed especially with respect to spoken language characteristics. The QII-minus group had significant speech problems, problems often associated with auditory dyslexia, whereas the QIII-minus group had no particular problems with oral language. They differed also with respect to orthographic speed, which was quite high for the QII-minus group and very low for the QIII-minus group.

The QI-minus group did not have the expected profile of low phonological functioning and high visuoorthographic ability. Of the three Q-minus groups, the QI-minus group functioned at the lowest level educationally; these children had extremely limited reading ability, often resorting to guessing.

The three Q-plus groups were variants of visual dyslexia. The profiles of the QII-plus and QIII-plus groups coincided greatly with the predicted profile, with good performance in the phonological skills and poor functioning in the visuoorthographic area. The QII-plus group had very slow orthographic speed, which was not the case for the QIII-plus group.

The QI-plus group differed considerably from the predicted profile. The children performed unexpectedly well in the visuoorthographic area and in several important nonreading areas, notably general scholastic ability. They appeared to have mastered the beginning phonics skills of the primary grades, but may develop problems as the demand for decoding flexibility and reading rate increases.

A more detailed discriminant analysis of the 11 factors that came out of the factor analysis indicated three that were particularly powerful in differentiating among the six modality-related groups. These factors were complex phonological functions, orthographic speed, and complex orthographic functions. The next three factors in order of ability to differentiate among groups were phonological dependence, phonological cluster functions, and orthographic error detection.

The Q residual group differed from the first six by not being sensory modality related. It would correspond to the three types originally labeled emotional dyslexia, educational dyslexia, and other types of dyslexia; these three groups were collapsed into one in the project, and labeled simply other forms of dyslexia.

Agreement Between Clinical and Statistical Subgroups

Of particular interest was a determination of the extent to which the statistically determined groups agreed with the dyslexia typology. The validity of these two approaches has often been discussed in the theoretical literature, but there do not appear to be any data from this field that could contribute to some empirically based ideas.

The Bergen data revealed that within each of the Q-factor groups there was a definite accumulation of pupils from either the auditory dyslexia group or the visual dyslexia group, according to the clinical classification (see Table 11.13).

In the first Q-factor group (QI-minus), 20 of the 26 pupils belonged to the clinical group auditory dyslexia and none were in the visual dyslexia category. If we limit our comparisons between the clinical and statistical classifications to pupils belonging to the clinical visual or auditory dyslexia groups, the correspondence within the QI-minus group would be 100%. This correspondence supported the conclusion that this group represented a variant of auditory dyslexia.

A similar situation existed with respect to the fourth Q-factor group (QII-plus). Of the 25 pupils, 16 belonged to the clinical visual dyslexia group and was classified as having auditory dyslexia. Here again, the comparison is limited to auditory and visual dyslexics only, the correspondence is 100%.

Group overlapping for the remaining Q-factor groups varied from 67% (QIII-plus) to 90% (QII-minus) if the analysis is again limited to auditory and visual dyslexics only. There was, then, a considerable degree of overlap in group membership between the clinical and statistical methods of grouping.

It must be emphasized that the overlap, which is merely summarized here, reflects overestimates, since it was based only on the clinical groups auditory and visual dyslexia. Furthermore, the discussion was limited to pupils belonging only to the six distinct Q-factor groups.

The correspondence between the two methods of grouping for the remaining two clinical dyslexia groups, audiovisual and other forms of dyslexia, was by no means as clear-cut (see Table 11.12). But even with some disagreement between the two approaches to grouping, the correspondence is certainly far from random. This finding, coupled with the high interrater reliability for the clinical groups, would indicate that the distinction phonological/auditory versus orthographic/visual is certainly a viable point of departure for a subdivision of children with dyslexia. There was also a distinct impression that the results of the differential instruction given these children supported the subgroup classifications.

These data provide good documentation as to the usefulness of hypothetically derived clinical subgrouping and also of a nonhypothetical, empirical, and statistically derived subgrouping based on the same sample, as done in this project. It lays a foundation for comparative studies, new hypotheses, and more nuances, and provides a mutual validation that cannot be arrived at by the use of only one of the two approaches.

Ophthalmological Investigations

The Bergen Project included medical research with the learning disabled children, covering ophthalmology and pediatric neurology.

With respect to eye conditions, the entire cohort of over 3,000 children was given screening tests for visual problems. In addition, the children with learning problems were given much more extensive and detailed clinical examinations and, when indicated, treatment. This was also true of other children in the rest of the cohort who were identified as having visual problems.

Involving the total cohort in the screening proved particularly helpful, since the learning disabled children were found to have visual characteristics that for all

intents and purposes were the same as for the normal children. Among the dyslexics there was a slightly higher incidence of manifest strabismus, convergent as
well as divergent, as well as of latent convergent strabismus. These problems as
well as a number of other visual characteristics occurred with about equal frequency in all four dyslexia subgroups.

The total dyslexia group was also divided into three groups according to level
of reading achievement, based on growth from grade 1-2 to grade 3-4. These
groups did not differ with respect to any of the numerous visual characteristics
studied; that is, the type or degree of visual difficulty was not related to the extent
to which the children had reading and spelling difficulties.

Perhaps the most important finding in this area was that most of the pupils who
were identified in the screening testing as having visual problems belonged to the
normal group. For example, 123 children were identified by screening as having
manifest or intermittent strabismus. Of these, only 16 were classified as dyslexics.

Follow-up testing of the 55 dyslexic pupils whose screening results were questionable yielded some interesting results. Their visual problems related to refraction and manifest and latent strabismus, and the children were evenly distributed
across the four dyslexia groups and the three achievement level groups. Later
follow-up revealed that the pupils with minor acuity problems or with latent
strabismus who had been prescribed glasses (lenses or prisms, respectively), did
not use them 5 years later. Among the 16 children who had worn glasses at least
part of the time, only one reported that the glasses were beneficial, but this pupil,
too, felt no need for the glasses.

On the basis of the statistical analyses and intensive individual examinations it
would seem reasonable to conclude that children with dyslexia do not differ from
other children with respect to a variety of visual characteristics. Most children
with visual problems are not dyslexic.

These findings are quite consistent with past research. It is nevertheless possible that a visual handicap can present an additional burden in individual cases of
dyslexia.

Neurological Examinations

Neurological examinations were undertaken relatively late in the project, at the
fifth-grade level. They involved 164 (70%) of the 235 learning disabled children,
i.e. 70% of the total learning disability group. [The 30% attrition (71 children)
was caused by a variety of factors, but a major one seemed to be that the parents
simply got tired of the many special examinations involved in this project. A very
common excuse from the parents was that in their opinion their child no longer
had reading and spelling difficulties to any appreciable degree.] The dyslexics
and the retarded were analyzed as one group.

The examinations in the neurological area were quite extensive and involved
standard neurological tests. One subgroup of around 100 children with learning

disabilities were also examined with computer tomography (CT) and electroencephalography (EEG). The criteria used to select this particular sample were (a) definite signs of neurological dysfunction in the clinical examinations and/or (b) unsatisfactory progress in the remedial programs in reading and spelling.

The neurologists who carried out these examinations noted the following variables as differentiating best between dyslexics and controls:

1. Reading and writing difficulties among first-degree relatives (parents, siblings).
2. Fine motor coordination (copying designs, handwriting, cutting a circle with scissors, follow-the-finger test, diadochokinesis, tongue movements, head-tongue dissociation).
3. Gross motor coordination (physical education skills, balance).
4. Fine sensation (agnosia, graphesthesia).
5. Right-left discrimination.
6. Speech functions (age of clear speech, vocabulary, articulation).
7. School achievements (language and mathematics) and ability to concentrate.
8. Behavior and emotional problems (age at bladder control, general behavior, and ability to sustain social contact during the examination).
9. Sex (higher frequency of dyslexia in boys than in girls).

On the basis of our results the following conclusions may be drawn:

1. In severe cases of learning disability a neuropediatric examination is indicated to diagnose possible signs of minimal brain dysfunction.
2. Reading and writing problems may involve different causative factors.
3. A possibly associated brain lesion can be localized in different parts of both brain hemispheres.
4. Dyslexics of normal intellectual ability score higher than those of low intellectual ability in fine motor functions, fine sensation, and some other functions.

Evaluation by Parents and Teachers

The comments of the parents of the learning disabled children regarding the treatment and progress made by the children from second to fourth grade and from fourth to ninth were extremely positive. Whereas 64% of parents felt that their child had severe or very severe problems in the second grade, only 18% felt that way by the fourth grade. By the ninth grade, the percentage had dropped to 9%.

The teacher evaluations by the end of third grade indicated that 83% of the pupils had benefited to some extent from the programs initiated at the beginning of second grade. Nevertheless, the teachers in the ninth grade rated 20% of the dyslexics as still having severe or very severe learning problems.

To place this 20% incidence figure in perspective, the ninth-grade teachers were asked to evaluate also the initial cohort of about 3,000 students, to determine the incidence of learning problems in a "normal" population. These data suggested that about 2% of the original cohort had severe or very severe learning

problems by the ninth grade. At the end of second grade the corresponding incidence figure was about 5%.

The parent and teacher evaluations also dealt with the children's feelings of
well being in school, an issue considered of considerable importance and one
given much emphasis in this project. Only the data on the children who did not
thrive in their school environment will be dealt with in this summary.

By the end of second grade the parents of the dyslexic children reported
that 18% of them did not enjoy school; by the fourth grade this percentage
was reduced to 4% but by the ninth grade it had risen to 13%. This increase in
percentage of children who have generally negative feelings toward school in
the ninth grade may be accounted for in part by the negative feelings often
expressed by normal children during puberty. It appeared that many of the
dyslexic pupils continued to need the emotional and educational support of the
remedial program. Data from other sources suggest that having 13% of ninth
graders express negative feelings about school may be a relatively small incidence (Sandven, 1968).

Test Results

Growth in school achievement was assessed at the time of transition from first to
second grade (grade 1-2) and again from third to fourth grade (grade 3-4). A
"growth score" scale was developed, based on the cohort norm and expressed in
stanines, so that an above-average score would represent more than average
growth between the two assessments and a below-average score would indicate a
loss in rank.

The mean for the total learning handicapped group (retarded and dyslexic) was
quite similar to the norm, with about a 50-50 split between those who made more
than average gain versus those whose gain was less than the norm. But the score
distributions were much more variable than the norm; in fact, they were bimodal. Within the lowest three stanines (1-3) was 43.9% of the total learning handicapped group, compared with the cohort norm of 23%. The top three stanines
(7-9) contained 23% of the cohort and 40.4% of the total learning handicapped
sample. The middle three stanines (4-6), which normatively contain 54% of the
population, contained only 15.7% of the combined learning handicapped group.

These bimodal distributions were much more pronounced for the dyslexia
group than for the retarded group, since 14% of the dyslexics and 23.5% of the
retarded scored within the middle three stanines (4-6).

A more detailed analysis of the achievement test scores indicated that 96% of
the dyslexics scored at stanines 1 to 3 in reading at grade 1-2. The corresponding
percentage for the retarded was 88%. Despite relatively good and at times very
good scores in scholastic aptitude (IQ), a higher percentage of the dyslexics
than of the retarded scored at the low end of the reading test distribution. The
exact opposite situation, and to a much higher degree, was true in the area of
mathematics.

By grade 3-4, 21% of the total learning handicapped sample who in grade 1-2
had scored stanine 1, 2, or 3 had moved into the average range or higher; that is,

they now scored at least at stanine 4. The data for the total learning handicapped sample showed that by grade 3-4, 35.3% had stanine scores of 3 or higher. Among the retarded group, 23.3% went from stanine scores 1 to 3 in grade 1-2 to stanine scores of 4 or higher in grade 3-4. The corresponding percentage for the dyslexic group was 20.7.

These data give rather clear documentation about the severity of the literacy skills problems of children with dyslexia. They scored appreciably lower than the retarded at the time of the initial testing (grade 1-2), and their achievement growth was significantly slower than the retarded. These two groups of learning handicapped pupils received basically the same type of remedial instruction, but the retarded progressed more rapidly than the dyslexics. This finding is indicative of the very severe nature of the dyslexia problem, and shows that good scholastic aptitude does not necessarily compensate.

It is impossible to draw any definitive conclusions regarding the efficacy of the remedial instruction carried out within this project. The main reason is that because of ethical considerations no relevant comparative control group was selected from which the experimental treatment was withheld. One cannot in good conscience withhold treatment from children for 9 years, unless the experimental method is completely unknown, which was not the case here. In addition, there were other research methodological problems that have been common to all special education efficacy studies, not the least of which is the regression effects. We tried to keep these at a minimum in this study.

There are also drawbacks to comparing the results from one study with the diagnostic and treatment data from another with respect to dyslexia. The Bergen Project occupies a middle ground between a purely prognostic follow-up study (e.g., Schonhaut and Satz, 1983) and the more typical efficacy study (e.g., Kline & Kline, 1975; Monroe, 1932).

If our project is viewed as an efficacy study, the results on the average seem to be quite similar to those reported by Monroe (1932) for her group 2. That group consisted of children who had been carefully diagnosed in her clinic and then treated in a normal school setting by professional personnel who had varying degrees of specialized training. The group received treatment that was quite similar to that offered in the Bergen Project. Monroe's group 3 went through the same diagnostic process as group 2, but the schools provided no systematic treatment. Follow-up data revealed large differences in school achievement between these two groups. Group 3 had regressed significantly in comparison with the norm, whereas group 2 had developed at the same rate as the normative group after the special treatment was initiated.

It seems reasonable to assume that the same situation would have occurred in the Bergen Project if one group had been selected to receive no special instructional program.

Growth in Achievement of the Clinical and Statistical Subgroups

Growth in school achievement was studied not only for the total group but for subgroup memberships as well. The two kinds of subgroups studied were the four clinical groups and the seven Q-factor groups. The findings in this area were quite extensive; they will be summarized rather briefly here.

Among the clinical groups, those with auditory dyslexia and those with "other" forms of dyslexia made considerably better progress than those with visual or audiovisual dyslexia. There was a relatively high incidence of emotional problems among the children with audiovisual and visual dyslexia.

Q-factor analysis also revealed significant variations among groups. Those in the visual Q-factor groups appeared to exhibit emotional difficulties. With respect to scholastic achievement, the group that overlapped mainly with the clinical audiovisual dyslexia group (QI-minus) showed the least amount of progress.

Generally speaking, there was considerable agreement between the results for the clinical and the statistical subgroups. Among the 11 main achievement factors identified by the earlier factor analysis, three were strongly correlated with achievement: complex phonological functions (factor 1), complex orthographic functions (11), and orthographic speed (9). As a group, these represented various phonetic skills.

These types of analysis and group comparisons according to clinical and statistical methods within the same sample of dyslexic children appear to yield information that should be useful in the study of the typology of dyslexia.

Implications of the Findings for Special Education in General

The Use of Interaction Analysis in Special Education Efficacy Studies

As a result of the generally discouraging results reported from various special education efficacy studies in the 1970s (Gjessing, 1974a), we developed the following hypotheses relating to the interactional effects of special education programs:

1. There are, within the special education groups (retarded and learning disabled), pupils who profit appreciably from special education programs and who depend on such programs for their educational development.
2. There are, within these special education groups, pupils who receive no effect, positive or negative, from special education programs.
3. There are also, within these special education groups, pupils who respond negatively, and whose educational progress appears to be hampered by such programs (Gjessing et al., 1982).

These hypotheses, and the challenges they present from a research as well as a practical point of view, were among the central issues explored by the Bergen Project.

Among the learning disabled pupils, some have made remarkable progress in comparison with their peers, some have made no progress, and some have regressed (Solheim et at., 1984; Chapters 6 and 14 of this book).

One cannot establish a clear-cut cause-and-effect relationship with regard to the effect or lack of effect of the special education programs. But clearly, looking only at main effects and mean scores for the learning disabled as a group may obscure the issue more than it clarifies it. To get at the underlying variability, which is very important (we are dealing with the futures of many individuals), we must look closely at the interaction effects, as was done in the Bergen Project.

Our findings may not be particularly surprising to people with practical experiences in educational settings. It nevertheless seems important to have empirical confirmation from an extensive and representative sample of children. The results of the Bergen Project would lend substantial evidence against the tendency of recent years to dismantle organized special education, which is based on an individualized diagnostic-prescriptive approach.

The Use of Scholastic Aptitude Data for Prognostication

One generally finds achievement expectancy tied to scholastic aptitude. The logical extension of this would be to base predictions of progress in achievement for the learning disabled on their scores on scholastic aptitude (IQ) tests. Extensive data along this line were collected for the two target groups with learning difficulties, group 1 with average or above-average ability (dyslexia), and group 2 with relatively low scholastic ability (retarded). The average results were contrary to the common prediction; from grade 1-2 to grade 3-4, the second group showed the most growth.

A closer look at variability in achievement within the two groups provides a more differentiated picture. Although group 1 had the lower mean, it had a much larger standard deviation; that is, pupils who gained the most and those who gained the least tended to be in group 1. Again, we are back to a recurring theme—one must look at the interaction among variables. This is important for several reasons. High ability does not necessarily mean that serious problems with literacy skills acquisition cannot develop. Above-average school ability does not necessarily compensate for a predisposition for dyslexia. This is clearly documented by the specificity of dyslexia and its strong resistance to treatment. Despite the fact that the dyslexic children received a great deal of special attention over and above what they would normally get in their schools, from the standpoint of both instruction and emotional support there still remained a significant group that appeared not to have benefited much from the special help. If learning disabled children do not receive even more special help than was offered in this project, quite a few will remain functionally illiterate, despite good mental ability. Our schools' inadequacy in dealing with this particular problem has certainly been clearly and unequivocally documented. On the other hand, the results also indicate that a majority of children who have severe learning problems at the end of first grade have been able to overcome their problems in learning the literacy skills.

The data from the Bergen Project also shed considerable light on the problems of the second target group, the mentally retarded. Their prognosis for learning the literacy skills was on the average somewhat better than for the children with specific learning problems. Some persons have long maintained that the schools should pay as much attention to the retardeds' problems in learning the literacy skills as to the same problems among children with average or above-average mental ability (e.g., Gjessing, 1977). But this belief may have been based on principles of equality and humanistic considerations rather than on empirically based optimism. The Bergen data give this a sound, empirical base. From a prognostic viewpoint, the reading and writing difficulties of retarded children should be given at least as much attention as is given the same difficulties in other children. This finding has considerable consequences not only for special education but also for research on children's difficulties when learning reading and writing.

The Importance of Socioemotional Factors

In the prediction of achievement by the use of regression analyses, socioemotional factors contributed rather marginally when entered into the regression equations after the very powerful linguistic-cognitive component. Not even if the socioemotional variables were entered first in the equations did they play a relatively significant role. (These factors did appear to play a somewhat more important role at grade 3-4 than at grade 1-2.) But by doing separate analyses for retarded and dyslexic children, some interesting interactions were discovered. Children of low linguistic-cognitive functioning who had relatively good ratings on the socioemotional scales did better in school achievement than those who rated low in both areas. This would seem to indicate that in the case of low cognitive functioning, good socioemotional status will, to some extent, compensate for lack of cognitive ability when it comes to school achievement.

One might thus conclude that the significance of socioemotional factors, as measured in this project, should be neither overestimated nor underestimated when considered in relation to literacy skills difficulties, at least in the primary grades. The research data presented here do not support the notion that remedial therapeutic intervention in the socioemotional area done in *isolation* would have an appreciable effect on school achievement. On the other hand, the quality of the socioemotional environment appears to compensate for inadequate linguistic-cognitive development. This suggests that children with learning disabilities ought to be given broadly based support, stimulation, and remediation.

The Importance of Classroom Membership

Classroom membership, defined simply as belonging to a certain classroom, having a certain teacher, was a particularly important factor to study, not only in and of itself but also because in the primary grades in Norway the classrooms remain intact, *with the same teacher*, for the first three years. The growth data given here include the cumulative effect of the child's being in the same class with the same teacher from the beginning of first grade through the end of third.

Classroom membership and growth in school achievement were highly positively correlated for all pupils, including those who had learning difficulties. As a group, the children with learning difficulties, general as well as specific, gained more in achievement if they were members of classes whose achievement progress was quite rapid, than if they belonged to classes whose school progress was relatively slow (Table 14.6).

Empirical documentation of this finding is particularly important, since one often finds in the professional literature the opinion that the opposite is likely to be true, that is, that it is to the advantage of children with learning difficulties to attend classes that progress relatively slowly in the school subjects. Relatively rapid growth is probably symptomatic of certain qualities. It could result from better environmental backgrounds of the pupils, or from better qualified teachers, but probably interplay between these two variables is most important. The fact that classroom membership was an extremely powerful determinant of school achievement needs to be explored in more depth to explain this somewhat unexpected finding.

Discussion of the Results Specifically Related to Dyslexia

Dyslexia Typology and Its Relevance

One major objective of the very detailed analysis of the dyslexia data was to evaluate the subcategories of dyslexia derived from an underlying theory with a variety of empirical data. This was assumed possible from extensive clinical experience. The basis of the research was a clinical-hypothetical dyslexia typology model for diagnosing literacy skills problems that uses "function analysis," a special observational method for observing children during the reading process.

This research project yielded empirical data that documented the basic principles of a dyslexia typology and the appropriateness of the proposed dyslexia model and the method of function analysis. This conclusion is based on several main findings, summarized here.

An a posteriori factor analysis of the battery of diagnostic tests of reading and writing difficulties revealed a very interesting factor structure. The diagnostic tests were shown to have differential diagnostic properties that coincided for the most part with those predicted from the theory. The systematic qualitative observations underlying the typological model were supported by the empirical data.

Independent evaluations by experienced clinicians showed very high interrater correlations when the dyslexia cases were classified on the basis of the underlying theory. This interrater reliability confirms empirically that the premises and criteria of the differential diagnostic capabilities of this model can be applied to evaluate achievement problems in reading and writing and yield rather unequivocal and objective results when used by qualified diagnosticians.

A purely statistical classification scheme, Q-factor analysis based on the scores obtained by the dyslexia sample on the diagnostic test battery for reading and writing difficulties resulted in clusters of pupils that reflected the clinical dyslexia model of audiophonologic versus visual-spatial characteristics and difficulties. Q-factor analysis also yielded further differentiations of the two modality-related clinical groups by identifying three variants of each of the main categories.

Further comparisons of the group memberships of the dyslexia pupils within the clinically based and the Q-factor analysis-based subcategories revealed good correspondence. This was especially true when the comparison was limited to the two main categories, audiophonological dyslexia and visual-spatial dyslexia.

The points just summarized appear to give, as a whole, considerable support to the view that a *typological* analysis would be a highly defensible point of departure for further dyslexia research. It is particularly desirable to compare clinical and statistical analyses of data collected on one group of dyslexics. This could easily lead to further refinement of dyslexia types.

Interaction Analysis as a Research Method

The Bergen team has asserted, and will continue to assert, that the many components involved in the dyslexia syndrome are very complex and that their influence varies for the different forms of dyslexia. The dyslexia model used here led to the confirmation of a variety of interactions.

The subgrouping of the dyslexia sample led to results and information regarding interactional relationships that would not have emerged if this sample had been studied as a single group. The more distinct and typical characteristics of the various dyslexia subgroups, as described earlier on the basis of practical clinical experiences, are reflected in the statistical interaction analyses, but not as strongly and unequivocally as had been expected from the preliminary earlier clinical dyslexia materials (Gjessing, 1976).

This brings up the issue of how one chooses a research method, certainly a central issue in dyslexia research. Some earlier clinical studies did in contrast to the Bergen data, not involve a representative cohort of peers from a specific, defined area. They were the typical referral data found in a clinic, with considerable variation in ages of the clients, who had been referred from a variety of people, mostly teachers, parents, and physicians.

The differences in the degree to which the Bergen data and the referral data exhibited various characteristics, particularly the indirect nonreading variables, were believed to be the result of differences in selection procedures. The earlier material came from the most extreme, and for the schools and the parents, most perplexing cases of reading and spelling difficulties, covering a very wide age span. The Bergen data covered the total range of reading and spelling difficulties within a cohort of peers. It is certainly reasonable to assume that the more typical characteristics of the different dyslexia subgroups found through practical clinical observation in a clinic sample would be more pronounced than when data is gathered from a normative sample in which all degrees of learning disabilities are represented.

That the variability in the degree to which children with learning disabilities exhibit certain characteristics is the result of sample selection (e.g., a referral sample compared with a representative sample) is an important finding. The indirect (nonreading) variables appear to play a much lesser role in a representative sample than in a clinic sample, and they yield more "significant results" in a referral sample. This finding should lead to considerably more caution when drawing general conclusions from a clinic sample, particularly conclusions relating to etiology.

A Theory Relating to Causation

It has been proposed here that the dyslexia syndrome represents a complex pattern of interacting and contributing causative factors. Nevertheless, we do maintain that the most basic and dominating problem in a clear majority of dyslexia cases is the *lack of balance* between orthographic-spatial and phonological-sequential processing. (See, for example, Figure 8.1 relating to the reading process.) This has been observed and described for decades (Gjessing, 1953) and described more theoretically in the 1970s (Gjessing, 1977). In the Anglo-American literature, a similar theory has been formulated by Aaron (1982), who has done empirical research with a basis in neurology to support his theory. This approach also finds considerable support in more recent research relating to the differential roles of the two hemispheres in the reading process, research that is quite unrelated to the much earlier theories of Orton.

Both clinical and statistical data from the Bergen Project regarding the validity of grouping dyslexics into visual and auditory types support such a balance theory. The data also support the used of the WISC-verbal–WISC-performance discrepancy, since the persistence of dyslexia problems appears to increase as this discrepancy increases. Which WISC score is higher seems to be unimportant—it is the magnitude of the difference (plus or minus) that appears to be the deciding factor.

This support for a "balance theory" may mean that a processing imbalance is an important etiological factor and is not necessarily pathological in nature. If this theory is correct, it would have considerable consequences for the treatment of dyslexia. It certainly contradicts the theory of overcompensation, in which only the learner's strength is thought to be capitalized on and the weaker areas of linguistic-cognitive functioning are largely ignored. Assuming the correctness of this balance theory, one would try to strengthen areas of weakness so that the dyslexic learner would achieve the necessary balance in his or her linguistic-cognitive processing system. One would not, of course, ignore the motivational value of compensation, but would emphasize the learners' strengths as well.

Prognosis and Effect Associated With Dyslexia

The earlier discussion of the development over time of children with dyslexia differentiated between prognostic research and efficacy studies. The prognostic studies did not involve systematic and controlled remedial efforts, whereas the efficacy studies involved varying degrees and types of treatment. The Bergen Project falls somewhere between these two approaches. In this project the students with dyslexia were followed from the first to the ninth grade. Over this time span the study was primarily prognostic. In grades 2 and 3 there was much intervention in the form of diagnostic testing, consultations, and very concrete individually prescribed remediation. But there was no untreated control group of dyslexic children; ethical considerations did not allow for such an experimental design.

Carefully executed prognostic studies (e.g., Shonhaut & Satz, 1983) show rather discouraging results with regard to the educational development of children with dyslexia. Group results such as these are quite typical. (Data relating to variability and interaction are rarely presented.) Some efficacy studies, however, have yielded encouraging results, especially those that have employed individually prescribed remedial programs in a clinical setting and based on thorough clinical diagnostic studies. But developmental studies, particularly efficacy studies, are highly problematic with respect to research methodology. It is important that this be pointed out again, before the data from the Bergen Project are discussed.

In brief, the teacher evaluations and the test results revealed moderately positive results. About three out of five pupils who at the end of first grade had serious or very serious reading difficulties had overcome their difficulties or at least had them appreciably reduced by the ninth grade. However, it was also estimated that by the end of compulsory school attendance (ninth grade), there was a core of about 2% of the total Bergen cohort with a significant literacy skills deficiency. This appears to be considerably better than what would have been the case without the diagnostic and remedial intervention, although no empirical statistical data have been collected that verify this impression. This conclusion was drawn as the result of the evaluations by teachers and parents and the achievement tests. The parents viewed the outcome in a particularly positive way. The conclusion drawn, of course, depends on which set of data is given priority.

The teachers' evaluations and the achievement test results are undoubtedly more objective than the parents' opinions. On the other hand, there is reason to believe that the parent evaluations are important expressions also of the feelings and experiences of the children themselves, because of the very extensive involvement of the parents in the Bergen Project. It went much beyond parental involvement in the typical school situation. The expressions of the parents, therefore, in our opinion are descriptive of the total educational and psychological situation in which these students found themselves at the end of compulsory schooling. This situation appeared to be much more positive than what is ordinarily found for Norwegian students at that age (Sandven, 1968).

In addition to its effects on school achievement, the intervention program appeared to have a considerable positive attitudinal and mental hygienic effect. A survey of school attitudes among the dyslexic pupils in the fourth grade, as reported by the parents, indicated negative school attitudes among only 4% of them. From a global view, these results indicate relatively positive developments of the dyslexic pupils, certainly more positive than most prognostic longitudinal studies forecast. We assume that this is the result of the very broad spectrum of assessments used, but it may be primarily the result of the very thorough and detailed educational and psychological intervention program and the close cooperation between the schools and the homes over an extended period of time. On the other hand, one has to remember that despite this broadly based intervention there remained a 2% core of students who had great problems with reading and writing at the end of the ninth grade. This is a challenge to which neither researchers and clinicians working with the practical effects of dyslexia nor our schools can remain indifferent.

Future Research Strategies and Challenges

There are many new developments in the field of dyslexia research, especially in cognitive psychology, neuropsychology, and medicine, that show a great deal of promise. A few ideas regarding dyslexia research will be mentioned here; these ideas transcend the many detailed issues currently being investigated.

Future dyslexia research should, to the degree possible, encompass representative samples from carefully defined populations. Some recent studies based on referral samples are of interest. They can be used to generate hypotheses, but they do not yield the proper data from which to generalized, compare, or develop treatment strategies. Because of uncertainty with respect to sampling, they contribute relatively little to the cumulative body of systematic research that is needed at the present time. The study of referral (clinic) samples will hardly qualify for anything but preliminary work, regardless of quality.

Future dyslexia research should be based on interdisciplinary teamwork. One could argue, of course, that we have had examples of this since shortly after World War II (e.g., Robinson, 1946). This may be correct, but the way the teamwork was executed was not particularly satisfactory. The interdisciplinary approach has suffered from lack of common objectives, theory, and methodology. Most of the more recent studies show relatively thorough diagnostic workups as these relate to indirect (nonreading) variables, which are generally studied in conjunction with dyslexia, but neglected or missing detailed analyses of the direct (reading and spelling) variables. One must acknowledge the heterogeneity of the dyslexia problem with respect to not only etiology but also the development of the literacy skills. A thorough analysis of reading and writing behavior is necessary, regardless of the researchers' affiliations and points of view.

Dyslexia researchers should attempt to develop a common set of diagnostic tests and prescriptive materials, much of which can be used internationally. This is, of course, an enormous undertaking. Tests and materials need to be more specific than what is available today. Interactional research is promising and challenging, but its potential contributions require appropriate assessment instruments.

Dyslexia researchers should also coordinate their statistical procedures. This is the last link in the chain of requirements of good research principles for innovation in this field. But good and appropriate statistical treatments of the data will be of little help if the more basic requirements for good research have not been met, such as, for example, good sampling, integrated cross-disciplinary teamwork, and qualitatively satisfactory assessment instruments. Without these basic elements, statistical refinements are of no help.

In the real world, these recommendations relating to research methodology may appear to be unrealistic. For several professionals from widely different disciplines to coordinate their research efforts is very demanding, often conflicting with personal needs and ambitions. Be that as it may, the real world requires that the complexity of the dyslexia problem be acknowledged and that the problem be tackled with research of very high caliber. The words of Applebee may be an appropriate finish for this book: "Despite its complexity, to continue with models which have proven worthless is just as foolish as, on the other hand, giving up any attempts to find a solution." (Applebee, 1971, p. 112). The same can be said for research procedures.

Sample Selection Procedures and Grouping of Pupils

H.D. Nygaard

This appendix describes how, on the basis of the group testing in grade 1-2, the various target groups were selected for further individual diagnostic assessment and remedial instruction. Some additional groups and also control groups were selected for use as study and comparison groups in specific situations. The characteristics of the various groups are presented in tabular form.

After a brief overview of the various groups, the tests used in the selection process are discussed and the selection criteria are described. Finally, comparisons are made among the groups on the relevant variables.

Purposes and Bases for Grouping

As described in chapter 6, there were two main target groups for this project: target group 1, children with specific learning disabilities (dyslexic), and target group 2, children with general learning disabilities (retarded). Two smaller groups were also studied: low ability underachievers, (retarded children with additional learning disabilities) and the PPT group, (children selected by the school in cooperation with school psychology services). These four groups constituted the entire sample of children with learning disabilities studied in the Bergen Project. These children were subjected to extensive individual diagnostic testing for the purpose of getting better insights into their problems, on the basis of which the most appropriate instructional programs could be initiated.

To determine if the target groups were, indeed, selected according to the criteria, and to control the results in special instances, we defined some additional comparison groups. Table A.1 gives an overview of the various study groups and the number of cases involved. The table also summarizes the data for the various control groups and their sizes.

The "total cohort" at the beginning of first grade was 3,090. The cohort studied in this report refers to the 2,962 pupils who had just started second grade when the target groups were selected. This cohort was the parent population from which all groups were selected and which is referred to when the size of a group is described as a percentage of the total cohort of about 3,000.

TABLE A.1. Overview of the learning disability groups and the various control groups

Group		Girls	Boys	Total
			Number	
Learning disability groups	A.			
a. Target group 1: specific learning disabilities		70	125	195
b. Target group 2: general learning disabilities		16	19	35
c. Low ability underachievers (combination 1 and 2)		3	10	13
d. PPT group: selected by school and psychologist		8	8	16
	Total	97	162	259
Comparison groups for the target groups	B.			
a. Overachievers: contrasted with target group 1		105	149	254
b. High ability: contrasted with target group 2		51	37	88
c. Average: stable average scores		60	47	107
Control groups: special groups for the analysis of	C.			
a. Socioemotional factors		64	107	171
b. Eye-examination data		21	72	93
c. Neurological data		22	19	41
d. Reading and spelling tests		64	66	130
e. Language test		21	22	43

Of this cohort, 259 children (8.7%) went through the second phase of the selection procedures and were considered cases of specific or general learning disabilities.

The learning disability groups and the comparison groups, parts A and B in Table A.1, as well as most of the control groups in part C, were identified from test results in reading and spelling, plus a school ability (IQ) test. These tests were administered at the transition between grades 1 and 2. The school ability test used was Sandven's "Modenhetsprøve," a Norwegian intelligence test developed in the 1950s. Reading was assessed with a silent reading test, developed for the project by Gjessing. Spelling was assessed in the dictated mode, using a test developed for use in all related Scandinavian projects. Each of these group tests was designed to be taken in one school period, and it was taken by the entire Bergen cohort.

The tests were administered twice, at the end of first grade (May-June), and again at the beginning of second grade (September). Retesting was done to avoid selection errors due to statistical artifacts, such as regression effects and poor test reliability, as well as errors arising from the test situation itself.

Selection Procedures and Group Descriptions for Phase 2

The groups listed in parts A and B of Table A.1 will be described in the order in which they appear in the table. The groups listed in part C are described in the appropriate chapters.

TABLE A.2. Summary statistics and correlations between school ability test and achievement tests in grades 1 and 2 ($n \approx 3,000$)

	Grade 1				Grade 2			
Tests	Ability	Reading	Spelling	Mathematics	Ability	Reading	Spelling	Mathematics
Mean (X)	35.1	72.9	30.1	61.8	38.4	90.7	30.8	65.5
Standard deviation (SD)	7.3	37.9	6.8	18.0	7.5	40.9	6.7	17.7
Number of items	59	149	40	89	59	149	40	89
Grade 1: Ability								
Reading	.47							
Spelling	.44	.67						
Mathematics	.54	.53	.55					
Grade 2: Ability	.75[a]	.46	.45	.55				
Reading	.44	.89[a]	.67	.53	.44			
Spelling	.44	.63	.84[a]	.54	.47	.65		
Mathematics	.54	.51	.54	.82[a]	.58	.54	.55	

[a] The correlations are test–retest reliability coefficients. (All coefficients are significant, $p < .01$).

In the selection of the learning disability groups and the comparison groups, extensive use was made of the intercorrelations among the various test scores. In particular, this pertains to the correlations between the school ability tests and the achievement tests, as well as the test–retest correlations. Table A.2 summarizes the relevant correlation coefficients and summary statistics. The results of the mathematics test are included for comparison. Table A.2 gives a tabulation of the main statistics used in conjunction with the selection procedures, which will be described here. All correlations are positive and significantly different from zero ($p < .01$).

The correlations between the school ability test and the achievement tests are of about the same magnitude in first and second grade; they are generally higher with mathematics. The test–retest correlations (underlined) are, of course, the highest. They are .75, .89, .84, and .82 for school ability, reading, spelling, and mathematics, respectively. These correlations are sufficiently high for the test scores to be considered relatively stable over time. All correlations are, however, far from perfect ($r = 1.00$), even for the test–retest results. As far as test reliability is concerned, it would have been desirable to have higher test–retest correlations, especially for the school ability test.

Since there is a close relationship between correlation and regression, a considerable regression effect was anticipated. This effect would reveal itself as a tendency for the pupils with extreme tests scores to achieve scores closer to the mean at the time of retesting. The effect would be revealed whether we use two different tests or administer the same test twice. We corrected for this effect to some extent by administering all tests twice. The selection criteria for underachievers were supplemented by a statistical regression analysis.

This much having been said about the test results and the correlations, we can now describe the criteria used in selecting the various groups mentioned in sections A and B of Table A.1.

Learning Disability Groups

"Target group 1," specific learning disabilities, was selected on the basis of five criteria that, in turn, were based on the results of the tests of reading, spelling, and school ability. These criteria are listed here in the order in which they were applied:

1. Underachievement.
2. Low achievement.
3. Consistent scores.
4. Subject areas (reading and spelling).
5. Teacher recommendation and parental consent.

"Target group 2" general learning disabilities, was selected on the basis of three criteria that, in turn, were based on the results of the school ability test:

1. Low score on the ability test.
2. Consistent scores.
3. Teacher evaluation and parental consent.

Target Group 1: Specific Learning Disabilities

The following is a more detailed description of the five criteria.

*Underachievement**

There is generally a great deal of correspondence between the results of a school ability test and achievement test scores (see Table A.2). But for certain pupils there may be a considerable disparity between these two. When achievement test scores are appreciably lower than what are predicted from the ability test, we have a case of "underachievement." The statistical determination of underachievement was done with regression analysis, using the most common definition of underachievement in the international literature (Nygaard, 1976, 1981, 1982; Thorndike, 1963).

The most important aspect of the concept of underachievement is that it directs attention to the relationship among different pupil attributes. In this case, one must compare school ability and school achievement.

---

*The concept of "underachievement" is quite problematic (cf. Nygaard, 1981, 1982). But the concept is retained here in the meaning described, since it is, among other things, relatively well known and commonly used in research internationally.

Regression analysis is based on the correlation between a predictor variable and a criterion variable. In this project, the predictor variable was operationally defined as the pupil's score on the school ability test, the criterion variable being defined as the achievement test score. Two separate analyses were made, one using the reading test as the criterion variable, the other using the spelling test results. From the correlations between the predictor variable and the criterion variables, based on the data for the total cohort (Table A.2), regression lines were drawn to determine the predicted achievement test score when the school ability test score was known. The discrepancy between this predicted score and the obtained score was the basis for the determination of underachievement. The criterion for a classification of underachievement was a discrepancy of -1 standard deviation for reading and -1.5 standard deviation in spelling. These criteria will be discussed further, after a discussion of low achievement.

Linear regression was used in all analyses. Analyses that controlled for curvilinearity yielded little additional information, although there was some effect for extreme school ability scores. It was particularly noticeable in the relationships with reading and mathematics. Since the curvilinearity existed only for the upper end of the school ability distribution, it had very little influence on the selection of pupils for target group 1.

Low Achievement

A pupil was classified as a "low achiever" on the basis of achievement test scores independent of school ability scores. The pupil simply had to obtain an achievement test score that was low within the frequency distribution of such scores for the entire cohort.

Initially we did not intend to use low achievement as one of the selection criteria for target group 1. Gjessing's definition of dyslexia, which was used in this study, sets no limits with respect to school ability or school achievement; it considers only the relationship between them.

Because of lack of the necessary resources, however, it became necessary to add low achievement as a criterion; we simply could not include all under-achievers in the very extensive evaluation undertaken in this project. Priority was given to underachievers who had the biggest problems, that is, those who were also low achievers. The upper limit for the classification of low achievement was 0.75 standard deviation below the cohort mean in reading and 1.0 standard deviation in spelling. The reason for this differential is explained below. When achievement test scores are distributed normally, these selection criteria will identify the lowest 23% and 16% in reading and spelling, respectively.

The Criteria for Underachievement and Low Achievement

The use of different criteria for defining underachievement and low achievement in reading and spelling was related to two separate issues. First, there were statistical reasons. Second, we wanted to make certain that, from the very beginning, we included every child who appeared to have reading disabilities. This would, among other things, make it easier to compare our results with previous research that has concentrated mainly on reading disabilities.

The statistical issues need further elucidation. The frequency distributions for the total cohort were more negatively skewed in spelling than in reading. The results of the school ability test, however, were more symmetrical, approximating a normal curve. The distribution of children in the bivariate chart for ability versus reading had a somewhat different shape than the bivariate chart for ability versus spelling, even though the correlations were of comparable magnitude. This resulted in a very large group of low achievers who were also underachievers in *spelling* if we used the same statistical criterion for both. This initial criterion was 1 standard deviation below each pupil's predicted score (−1.0 SD) as it related to the cohort data. The skewness of the cohort data resulted in a disproportionately large number of students falling between −1.0 SD and −1.5 SD below the predicted spelling score. By using the criteria for underachievement at −1.5 SD and −1.0 SD for low achievement, we were able to select a group without a large accumulation of cases at the lower end, but still with fairly large variability both in school ability and spelling.

The criteria of −1.5 SD for underachievement and −1.0 for low achievement were considered acceptable for spelling, since they resulted in sufficiently large samples.

Figure A.1 shows the parallel situation with regard to school ability and reading in first grade. Setting the criterion at −1.0 SD for both underachievement and low achievement, resulted in a fairly large accumulation of reading scores with relatively little variability. A stricter criterion, such as −1.5 SD, would have resulted in a disproportionate reduction in the number of students selected, while at the same time reducing the variability in both reading and school ability. Raising the upper limit from −1.0 SD to −0.75 SD resulted in a more reasonable and acceptable distribution. This resulted in the inclusion of more pupils, which was considered desirable.

In the case of both reading and spelling, the additional criteria of consistency of test scores, teacher evaluation, and parental consent contributed to a reduction of the number of pupils who were finally selected.

Stability of Test Scores

The rationale for repeating the selection instruments was described earlier. This third selection criterion, stability of the test scores, utilized the retest data as follows: The first two selection criteria, underachievement and low achievement, were applied to the test results from first grade (May-June) and the test results from second grade (September) independent of each other. Only those pupils who qualified both times were included for further evaluation.

This approach made it possible to control for the most critical effects of regression and other sources of error in the test results. The net effect was that only

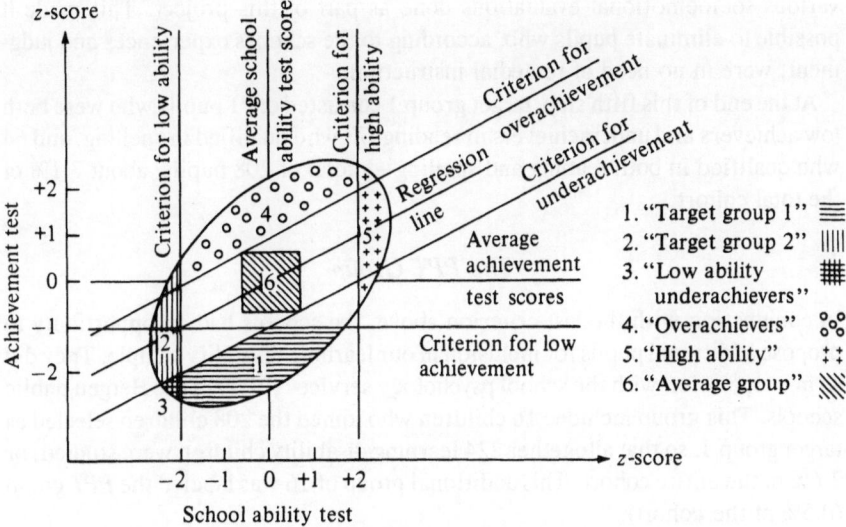

FIGURE A.1. Group model. Illustration of the characteristics of the two target groups and the comparison groups on the school ability test and an achievement test at a given point in time. (Selection was based on several such analyses.)

those pupils were selected whose low scores remained stable over the summer vacation, from the end of first grade until the beginning of the second.

Subject Areas

The two literacy skills of reading and spelling were analyzed separately. After the application of the third criterion, target group 1 consisted of three groups: Pupils with stable learning problems in reading ($n = 172$) pupils with spelling problems ($n = 93$), and pupils with difficulties in both areas ($n = 77$), for a total of 342 children, or about 11.5% of the total cohort.

Target group 1 at this point was then relatively large, especially in light of previously estimated incidence figures of 3 to 5% for Norway (Gjessing, 1977). But the fifth and last selection criterion reduced the 11.5% incidence figure appreciably.

Teacher Recommendation and Parental Consent

The first four selection criteria for target group 1 were basically statistical in nature. The criteria for underachievement and low achievement in reading were sufficiently broad to include quite a few pupils. The last and final selection criterion was for the teachers to evaluate the children selected thus far, and for the parents to consent to having their child participate in the project. The teachers used past assessments of the pupils, and they were given access to the various socioemotional evaluations done as part of this project. This made it possible to eliminate pupils who, according to the school's experiences and judgment, were in no need of remedial instruction.

At the end of this fifth step, target group 1 consisted of 71 pupils who were both low achievers and underachievers in reading, 73 who qualified in spelling, and 64 who qualified in both reading and spelling–a total of 208 pupils, about 7.1% of the total cohort.

The PPT Group

In conjunction with the last criterion above, the schools had an opportunity to propose additional pupils for inclusion in our learning disability sample. They did so in cooperation with the school psychology services (PPT) of the Bergen public schools. This group included 16 children who joined the 208 children selected as target group 1, so that altogether 224 learning disability children were studied, or 7.6% of the entire cohort. This additional group of 16 was labeled the *PPT group* (0.5% of the cohort).

Target Group 2: General Learning Disabilities

Low School Ability Test Scores

The school ability (IQ) test used as a criterion for underachievement was also used as a criterion for selection to target group 2. Low ability was defined as a score 2 standard deviations below the cohort mean or lower. In a normal distribution of school ability scores, one would expect to identify about 2% of the cohort with this criterion (≤ -2 SD).

Stability in School Ability Test Scores

The school ability test was given twice, as described previously. In order to be included in target group 2, a pupil had to reach the criterion (≤ -2 SD). One would expect about 2% of the pupils to score at or below -2 SD on a normally distributed ability test. With a cohort of about 3,000, about 60 should be selected. A slight degree of negative skewness, however, resulted in a somewhat higher number. On the other hand, the prerequisite of test–retest stability resulted in an appreciable reduction because of regression effects and other causes of instability. Only about 40 pupils (1.3%) fell in this group. (Actually, it was 40 out of 2,759, 1.4%, because of missing data, as explained below.)

An additional 30 or so pupils were selected for a variety of reasons. Some who took the test only once (test or retest) and scored below -2 SD were included. A few obtained extremely low scores on one of the tests, but did not satisfy the criterion of test score stability. The reason for including these additional pupils was that application of the third criterion would result in an evaluation of these somewhat ambiguous data and would, in turn, eliminate some of the pupils from this target group.

Teacher Recommendation and Parental Consent

As was done for target group 1, the last and final criterion for inclusion in target group 2 was an evaluation by the children's teachers as to the accuracy of the test scores. The parents also had to give their consent for their child to participate in this project. Altogether 25 pupils were rejected by these criteria, resulting in a final target group 2 with 48 children, or 1.6% of the cohort. This group now was of a size consistent with expectations based on statistical criteria.

Of the 48 children in target group 2, 8 had test results in both reading and spelling that satisfied the criteria for low achievement in both of these areas. This was probably not too surprising for this group. It was probably of more significance that 13 pupils satisfied the criteria for both target group 1 and target group 2. This group will be referred to as "low ability underachievers," and is described below.

Low Ability Underachievers: Low School Ability and Specific Difficulties in Spelling

When dyslexia and underachievement were defined for this project, no lower limits were set for the school ability test or for the achievement tests. It was, therefore, possible for pupils scoring below −2 SD in school ability to also score proportionately lower in achievement. Such pupils would qualify for both of the first two target groups according to the original criteria. As just mentioned, 13 children qualified.

Since these pupils qualify as having specific learning problems, it would seem most reasonable to place them in target group 1. But doing so would result in certain problems of interpretation when comparing target groups 1 and 2. It seemed most appropriate, therefore, to separate these children out as a group of their own. This resulted in a reduction by 13 children in each of target groups 1 and 2, the final number of cases in these groups becoming 195 and 35, respectively. (See Table A.1.)

It turned out that the 13 low ability underachievers qualified as underachievers only in spelling, not in reading. The reason why none was selected in reading is most likely statistical, caused by the difference in negative skewness in the two achievement tests.

Summary Regarding Selection of the Learning Disability Groups

Distribution of the Pupils in Various Groups

The different groups described above constituted the total learning disability sample. This sample had the following consistency: Target group 1 had 70 girls and 125 boys, a total of 195 children. Target group 2 had 16 girls and 19 boys, 35 altogether. The low ability underachievers, the special group of 13 children who qualified in both groups 1 and 2, consisted of 3 girls and 10 boys. The PPT group that was selected by the school psychologists consisted of 8 boys and 8 girls, a total of 16. This total sample of children with learning disabilities consisted of 97 girls and 162 boys (259 children, or 8.7% of the total cohort).

Sex Differences

Among children with reading and writing difficulties, one consistently finds a preponderance of boys. This sex difference is found in research in which the investigator selects a sample on the basis of predetermined criteria, and also in situations where the sample is "clinical," that is, based on referrals because of evidence of learning difficulties (Bakwin, 1973; Gjessing, 1977; Myklebust & Boshes, 1969; Thorndike, 1963).

On the other hand, the selection method does seem to play an important role with regard to sex differences. When the selection criterion is low achievement in a school subject in which boys usually score lower than girls, one will obviously get more boys when selecting from an undifferentiated population. A similar situation exists with regard to underachievement, albeit this is a bit more complex. One possible method of dealing with these sex differences would be to analyze the data for boys and girls separately (Noss, 1977; Thorndike, 1969).

This issue was considered from the very beginning of the Bergen Project (Nygaard, 1982b). We decided that the various groups were to be selected without regard for sex of the subjects. This decision was based on several considerations. First, teaching was not differentiated by sex, nor were educational objectives and requirements. The children took the same tests in conjunction with this project. In addition, special education is not differentiated by sex, but is organized according to the child's needs and the demands and expectations associated with age and grade levels.

The results from this project indicated appreciable sex differences, especially in spelling and school ability, both favoring girls. The statistical selection criteria resulted in a disproportionately large number of underachieving and low-achieving boys in spelling. The most pronounced sex difference is in the category low ability underachievers, which consisted of 3 girls and 10 boys.

If one were to assume that the sex differences resulted from the fact that boys generally develop more slowly than girls, the selection procedures, based on an undifferentiated total group, would lead to more unreasonable results than was the case. This statement is justified by the fact that there was more total variability among the test results for boys than for girls. This difference in variability was evidenced also by the fact that there was a preponderance of boys in the category overachievers (Table A.1).

For the reasons described here, it appeared most reasonable to view the entire cohort of pupils as one when selecting the children for the various learning disability groups as well as for the various comparison groups. This did not preclude the possibility that the data could be analyzed by sex, or that statistical controls for sex difference could be introduced later on.

Additional Groups to Control for Selection Criteria for Target Groups 1 and 2

A contrast group was selected for each of the two target groups. These were "overachievers," to contrast with the underachievers (target group 1) and "high ability children," to contrast with the low ability children (target group 2), plus an "average group." (See Table A.1.) The purpose was to determine, by contrasting these groups, the adequacy of the selection criteria for the original target groups. Contrast groups were also used to study change over time (Chapter 2).

Overachievers: A Contrast Group to Target Group 1

When regression analysis is used to identify a group of underachievers, one can also easily identify the contrasting group, children whose school achievement is appreciably higher than what might have been predicted from the school ability test.

It was considered necessary to contrast the overachievers and underachievers in the same school subjects, that is, the overachievers were identified as such in reading, spelling, and combination reading and spelling, just as was done for target group 1.

The main criterion for reading was stable overachievement, that is, on both the first test (grade 1) and the retest (grade 2) the pupil had to score at least $+1.25$ SD higher than the expected reading score based on the school ability test. In spelling, the criterion was at least $+1.0$ SD. The use of these criteria resulted in groups of sizes 128, 87, and 46 for reading, spelling, and the combination of these two, respectively. Of these 261 pupils, 7 had school ability test scores below -2 SD, thus also qualifying them for target group 2. The group overachievers was reduced by these 7 cases, resulting in group sizes of 127, 82, and 45 for reading, spelling, and the combination group, respectively, or 254 children (Table A.1). No attempt was made to get the teachers' recommendation with respect to overachievement, as was done in the case of the two target groups.

High Ability: A Contrast Group to Target Group 2

A contrast group for target group 2 (low school ability) was identified as pupils who had high test and retest scores on the school ability test. For this group to be of about the same size as the earlier selected group 2, the selection criterion was set at $+1.5$ standard deviation or more above the cohort means on the two tests. Altogether 88 pupils were identified as belonging to this group, 51 girls and 37 boys (Table A.1).

The Average Group: A Group With Consistent Average Scores

This group was the result of an attempt to determine if some pupils consistently obtained average scores across a variety of achievement and ability tests. This group would have average scores comparable to the cohort means. Again, the tests in reading, spelling, and school ability were used. In addition, the scores on the mathematics test were used to stabilized this group even further. Thus eight test scores were used to define this group. An attempt to find pupils who scored exactly at the mean for all eight tests resulted in a count of 0 (out of 3,000). The size of such a group would, of course, vary with how broadly one defines "average." By setting the outer limits at $+0.75$ SD and -0.75 SD, 131 pupils (4.4%) were identified. The interval ±0.75 SD seemed to be an acceptable definition of average, since it would ordinarily identify the middle 55% of all pupils in any one test, assuming normal distributions. Of the 131 pupils selected, 24 were part of a norming group for some language tests, so they were eliminated. The final average group, then, consisted of 107 pupils, which seemed like a reasonable size for comparison purposes (Table A.1).

Recapitulation and Evaluation of the Selection Procedures and Group Comparisons

The group selection procedures reviewed so far relate to the learning difficulty groups and some comparison groups, altogether seven groups, as enumerated in Table A.1, sections A and B.

Figure A.1 presents these groups graphically, showing their relative positions on the basis of results of the school ability test and an achievement test. (The PPT group is not shown on this figure.) The ellipse-shaped area in Figure A.1 is a scatterplot showing the results of a school ability test along the horizontal (x) axis and of a school achievement test along the vertical (y) axis.

The units along both axes are z scores, based on the results from the total cohort of about 3,000. These are standard scores that use the standard deviation as the unit, expressed as deviations from the mean. A z scale has a mean of zero ($\bar{X} = 0$) and a standard deviation of one (SD = 1). This means that $z = +1.00$ is 1 standard deviation above the cohort mean, while $z = -1.00$ corresponds to a point on the distribution 1 SD below the mean. Since the scales are the same for both tests, direct comparisons are possible. When test scores are normally distributed, 68% of the pupils will fall within the area delineated by $\pm 1z$.

The regression line is used to predict the most likely score to expect on the achievement test when the ability test score is known. The regression line and the means and standard deviations for the two tests have been used to draw the conceptual diagram for the various groups, using the statistical criteria specified for each one.

Figure A.1 gives a graphic conceptualization of the groups selected and the criteria used in their selection at a specific point in time and for a specific school subject. It was done twice (test and retest) for two school subjects (reading and spelling).

Target group 1 and its contrasting group, overachievers, were so classified on the basis of deviations from the predicted scores on the achievement tests. The limits for overachievement and underachievement have been drawn, therefore, as lines parallel with the regression line at a distance corresponding to the criterion for the degree of deviation required for inclusion in these groups. The two resulting segments of the ellipse illustrate the placement of the overachievers and underachievers in relation to the total cohort.

Low achievement, a criterion for target group 1, relates back to the cohort mean and standard deviation on the achievement test. A horizontal line (parallel with the x axis) at a distance from the cohort mean corresponding to the selection criterion cuts out a segment of the ellipse that encompasses the low achievers.

TABLE A.3. Means and standard deviations[a] for school ability and achievement tests for the learning difficulties groups and the comparison groups

Groups	School ability $\bar{z}$	SD	Reading $\bar{z}$	SD	Spelling $\bar{z}$	SD	Mathematics $\bar{z}$	SD	N
1. Target group 1	−0.45	0.81	−1.37	0.28	−2.01	1.14	−0.97	0.99	195
2. Target group 2	−2.72	0.49	−1.29	0.45	−1.34	0.98	−2.00	0.58	35
3. Low ability underachievers	−2.72	0.51	−1.56	0.25	−3.58	0.54	−2.29	0.55	13
4. Overachievers	−0.29	0.71	1.12	0.71	0.79	0.45	0.36	0.77	254
5. High ability	2.03	0.27	1.09	0.70	0.86	0.43	0.97	0.43	88
6. Average	−0.02	0.34	−0.13	0.34	0.03	0.36	0.08	0.35	107
7. PPT group	−0.71	0.86	−1.07	0.37	−0.78	0.76	−1.04	1.11	16

[a] Some distributions are so highly skewed as to make the usual interpretations of standard deviations problematic.

Target group 2 and its contrasting group, high ability, both relate back to the cohort mean and standard deviation on the school ability test. By drawing vertical lines (parallel with the y axis) at a distance from the school ability test cohort mean corresponding to the criteria for high and low ability, segments of the ellipse become delineated that encompass the two ability groups as they relate to the total cohort.

The average group took in those pupils who obtained average scores on both test and retest on the school ability test as well as on three achievement tests, reading, spelling, and mathematics. Altogether eight different test scores had to be within the average range for a pupil to qualify for this group. Figure A.1 shows the group formed on the basis of one pair of test scores – school ability and one achievement test. The middle square delineates intercepts that fall within the average range on both tests.

Figure A.1 shows the relationship between two tests at one specific point in time. It simply illustrates the main principles used in the selection of the various study groups and comparison groups from the total cohort of about 3,000. The numerals 1 through 6 in Figure A.1 represent the following six groups: 1, target group 1; 2, target group 2; 3, low ability underachievers; 4, overachievers; 5, high ability; and 6, average group. The PPT group could not be placed in Figure A.1.

Table A.3 presents means and standard deviations for all tests of school ability, reading, spelling, and mathematics for all seven groups. The statistics in this table are all in z scores. The raw scores for test and retest were combined and new distributions were generated that were then converted to z scores for the total cohort of about 3,000.

When test data are normally distributed, the z scores for different tests will be comparable. But some caution must be used when interpreting the data in this study, since many of the distributions could not be described as normal. This was particularly true with respect to reading and spelling and with respect to some of the extreme groups. The latter problem is also significant when comparing extreme groups on certain variables because of regression effects.

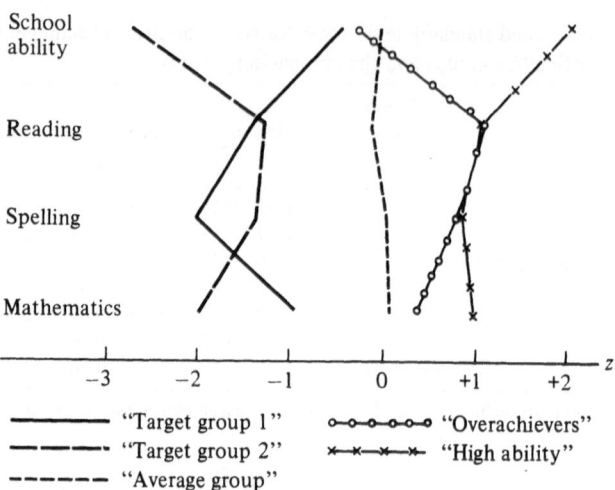

FIGURE A.2. Profiles of means for tests of school ability, reading, spelling, and mathematics for the two target groups and three comparison groups (grades 1 + 2).

The primary purpose of the following analyses relates to the selection criteria for the various groups. In this connection it was of interest to compare groups on single variables and on profiles based on several tests. Certain methodological problems arise here with the regression effects as they relate to the criteria for the various groups. This situation is particularly precarious when profiles based on several tests are analyzed.

Nevertheless, the results shown in Table A.3 have been presented as profiles in Figure A.2. The low ability underachievers and the PPT group have not been included. In this figure the horizontal axis is a z scale. On the basis of z scores, the means for the four tests have been plotted vertically for each of the five groups described. School ability means are on top, followed by the means of reading, spelling, and mathematics.

From the original definitions of the groups, one should have a fairly good notion as to the shape of these profiles. The cross-group differences for each test can readily be interpreted by going horizontally across the figure for each test. For example, on the school ability test we find target group 2 and the high ability group at opposite ends. Target group 1, overachievers, and the average group one would expect to find close to the middle, since they would have scores fairly evenly distributed on both sides of the mean. But in the case of target group 1, some of the pupils with the highest scores were deleted in the selection process because they did not comply with the low achievement criterion. Teacher recommendation and parental consent appeared to have a similar effect. Figure A.2 shows that especially target group 2, but also to some extent the overachievers, had school ability means somewhat below the cohort mean. The fact that the mean for overachievers was slightly below the cohort mean can be ascribed to the fact that the achievement tests had a considerable ceiling effect, which resulted in negatively skewed distributions.

From Table A.3 it is apparent that target group 1 and overachievers do not differ much in school ability. But both groups differ significantly from the average group. This implies, as was also shown in Table A.3, that target group 1 and overachievers both had school test means significantly lower than the average group mean; they were also, of course, lower than the cohort mean. Target group 2 had a mean significantly lower than all the others. In light of the selection criteria and the summary statistics obtained, it would appear that the results of the school ability test pretty much comply with the theoretical model.

The data pertaining to the low ability underachievers and the PPT group refer back to the information provided in Table A.3. Again, the results appear consistent with the selection criteria. The low ability underachievers scored very low on all tests, but especially in spelling. The PPT group scored generally low in all areas without any one particularly low mean.

With regard to the achievement test results of the five groups depicted in Figure A.2, a comparison among the various means gets a bit problematic. This is particularly true of the extreme groups, where there is a considerable regression effect, especially for target group 2 and the high ability group. But it is nevertheless of interest to look at the similarities and differences among the various results, especially as they would most likely be perceived by the teachers.

According to the selection criteria, one would expect to find clear differences between target group 1 and overachievers in reading as well as in spelling. Tests of significance confirmed this. The mathematics test was not involved in any selection process. Since these two groups are equivalent with respect to school ability, it would seem reasonable to assume that this would also be the case in mathematics. But the data in Table A.2 show that the correlation between mathematics and school ability is of about the same order as that with reading and spelling. Since these two groups are extreme groups with respect to reading and spelling, the data pertaining to these groups are subject to regression effects. It is not surprising, therefore, that the mathematics data occupy a middle position, as shown in Table A.3 and Figure A.2. All paired comparisons for the five groups shown in Table A.3 are significant. It would seem important to mention that some of the mathematics items were dependent on reading if the pupils did not ask for help, a factor that may have influenced the results. Some of the unevenness among the means in reading and spelling shown in Figure A.2 was most likely the result of different selection criteria with regard to underachievement, overachievement, and low achievement.

The contrasting groups target group 2 and high ability group also had achievement test results that differed appreciably, one being consistently below the cohort means and the other consistently above. One interpretation of Figure A.2 could bed that target group 2 is overachieving and that the high ability group is underachieving. But this apparent discrepancy between school ability and achievement may be the result of regression effects; this finding is consistent with other research on this topic.

The results of the achievement tests and their relationship to the cohort data are of some interest. For example, the average group, compared with all the other groups shown in Table A.3, differs from all groups on all achievement variables.

As can also be seen in Figure A.2, the two groups overachievers and high ability scored significantly above the average group, whereas target groups 1 and 2 scored significantly lower. The two extreme groups with respect to school ability, target group 2 and high ability, differed significantly from the average group despite the regression effects.

In the above analysis, the primary interest was to analyze the actual, obtained results of the individual tests as they relate to the conceptual definitions of the various groups. The data were consistent with the anticipated results.

Final Summary and Comments

An annual cohort of about 3,000 children in Bergen, Norway, was tested and grouped using certain statistical criteria based on the test–retest results of a school ability test, a reading test, and a spelling test. Two of these groups were the main target groups for the research project. Target group 1 consisted of pupils with specific learning disabilities and target group 2 consisted of pupils with general learning disabilities, that is, low school ability (IQ).

Target group 1 had pupils whose results on the reading and spelling tests were markedly lower than what was predicted from the results of the school ability test. They were clearly underachievers in reading and spelling ($n = 195$).

Target group 2 consisted of pupils with extremely low scores (-2 standard deviations below the cohort mean or lower) on the school ability test. It was predicted that these children would have reading and spelling scores consistent with the results of the school ability test ($n = 35$). Statistical calculations and tests of significance indicated that these children, as a group, had achievement characteristics that complied with this prediction.

A group of low ability underachievers was also defined, which complied with the criterion for target group 2 but, in addition, were underachievers in spelling ($n = 13$).

A fourth group, the PPT group, consisted of pupils selected by the school in cooperation with the school psychology services. This group had the most difficulties in mathematics and reading ($n = 16$).

These four learning disability groups altogether comprised 259 pupils, or 8.7% of the total Bergen cohort.

In the additional analyses of these learning difficulties groups and various control and comparison groups, it was of central importance to keep in mind how the groups were defined. It was particularly important to be aware of the many correlations associated with the various tests for school ability and achievement, because target group 2 was defined within an extremely limited range of school ability whereas target group 1 was defined within highly limited ranges on tests of reading and spelling.

References

Aaron, P.G. (1982). The neurology of developmental dyslexia. In R.N. Malatesha & P.G. Aaron (Eds.). *Reading disorders. Varieties and treatment.* New York: Academic Press.

Aaron, P.G., & Baker, C. (1982). The neuropsychology of dyslexia in college students. In R.N. Malatesha & L.C. Hartlage (Eds.), *Neuropsychology and cognition, Vol. 1*, Norwell, MA: Kluwer Academic Publications.

Aasved, H., Lothe, W.E., Bertelsen, T., & Odland, M. (1984). Öyeundersökelse av elever i förste klasse i Bergensskolene. [Eye examinations of first graders in Bergen, Norway.] In R. Solheim et al. (Eds.), *Bergen-prosjektet. Utviklingsforlöp og laereproblemer hos elever i de tre förste skoleår. II. Sökelys på småskolealderen.* Bergen-Oslo-Tromsö: Universitetsforlaget.

Ackerman, P.T., Peters, J.E., & Dykman, R.A. (1971). Children with specific learning disabilities: WISC profiles. *Journal of Learning Disabilities, 4*, 150–166.

Allport, G.W. (1937). *Personality: A psychological interpretation.* New York: Holt.

Allport, G.W. (1940). The psychologist's frame of reference. *Psychological Bulletin, 37*, 1–28.

Allport, G.W. (1946). Personalistic psychology as science: A reply. *Psychological Review, 53*, 132–135.

American Academy of Pediatrics, American Academy of Ophthalmology and Otolaryngology, & American Association of Ophthalmology (1973). The eye and learning disabilities. *Journal of Learning Disabilities, 6*, 332–333.

Applebee, A.N. (1971). Research in reading retardation. Two critical problems. *Journal of Child Psychiatry, 12*, 91–113.

Aschehoug og Gyldendals store norske leksikon [Norwegian encyclopedia]. (1980). Oslo: Kunnskapsforlaget.

Asher, S.R., Renshaw, P.D., & Hymel, S. (1982). Peer relations and the development of social skills. In S.G. Moore & C.R. Cooper (Eds.), *The young child. Review of research. Vol. 3.* Washington, DC: National Association for the Education of Young Children.

Bailey, K.D. (1973). Monothetic and polythetic typologies and their relation to conceptualization, measurement and scaling. *American Sociological Review, 38*, 18–33.

Bakker, D.J. (1970). Temporal order perception and reading retardation. In D.J. Bakker & P. Satz (Eds.), *Specific reading disability: Advances in theory and method.* Rotterdam: Rotterdam University Press.

Bakker, D.J. (1979). Hemispheric differences and reading strategies: Two dyslexias? *Bulletin of the Orton Society, 29*, 84–100.

Bakwin, H. (1973). Reading disability in twins. *Develomental Medicine and Child Neurology, 15*, 184–187.

Balow, B., & Blomquist, M. (1965). The long-term effect of remedial reading instruction. *The Reading Teacher, 18*, 581–586.

Bander, R., & Grinder, J. (1975). *The structure of magic I. A book about language and therapy.* Palo Alto, CA: Science and Behavior Books.

Bander, R., & Grinder, J. (1976). *The structure of magic II.* Palo Alto, CA: Science and Behavior Books.

Bannatyne, A. (1971). *Language, reading and learning disabilities.* Springfield, IL: Charles C. Thomas.

Baron, F. (1979). Orthographic and word-specific mechanisms in children's reading of words. *Child Development, 50*, 60–72.

Bateman, B. (1965). An educator's view of a diagnostic approach to learning disorders. In J.A. Hellmuth (Ed.), *Learning disorders.* Seattle: Special Child Publications.

Bateman, B.D. (1968). *Interpretation of the 1961 Illinois test of Psycholinguistic Abilities.* Seattle: Special Child Publications.

Beck, S. (1953). The science of personality: Nomothetic or ideographic. *Psychological Review, 60*, 353–359.

Bellack, A.S., & Hessen, M. (1980). *Introduction to clinical psychology.* New York: Oxford University Press.

Belmont, L., & Birch, H. (1966). The intellectual profile of retarded readers. *Perceptual and Motor Skills, 22*, 787–816.

Bender, L. (1938). *A Visual-Motor Gestalt Test and its clinical use.* Research Monograph No. 3. New York: American Orthopsychiatric Association.

Bender, L. (1946). *Instructions or the use of Visual Motor Gestalt Test.* New York: American Orthopsychiatric Association.

Bender, L. (1970). Use of the Visual Motor Gestalt Test in the diagnosis of learning disabilities. *Journal of Special Education, 4*, 29–39.

Bender, L. (1957). Specific reading disability as a maturational lag. *Bulletin of the Orton Society, 7*, 9–18.

Benton, A.L. (1978a). Some conclusions about dyslexia. In A.L. Benton & D. Pearl (Eds.), *Dyslexia: An appraisal of current knowledge.* New York: Oxford University Press.

Benton, A.L. (1978b). Developmental dyslexia: Neurological aspects. *Advances in Neurology, 7*, 1–41.

Benton, C.D. Jr. (1968). Management of dyslexias associated with binocular control abnormalities. In A.H. Keeney & V.T. Keeney (Eds.), *Dyslexia: Diagnosis and treatment of reading disorders.* St. Louis: C.V. Mosby.

Benton, C.D. Jr., McCann, J.W. Jr., & Larsen, M. (1965). Dyslexia and dominance. *Journal of Pediatric Ophthalmology, 2*, 53–57.

Bergstrom, K., Bille, B., & Rasmussen, F. (1984). Computer tomography of the brain in children with minor neurodevelopmental disorders. *Neuropediatrics, 15*, 115.

Berner, C.E., & Berner, D.E. (1953). Relation of ocular dominance, handedness, and the controlling eye in binocular vision. *Archives of Ophthalmology, 50*, 603–608.

Bettman, J.W. Jr., Stern, E.L., Whitsell, L.J., & Gofman, H.F. (1967). Cerebral dominance in developmental dyslexia. *Archives of Ophthalmology, 78*, 722–729.

Betts, E.A. (1946). *Foundations of reading instruction.* New York: American Book.

Billingslea, F.Y. (1948). The Bender-Gestalt: An objective scoring method and validating data. *Journal of Clinical Psychology, 4*, 1–27.

Birch, H.G. (1962). Dyslexia and the maturation of visual function. In J. Money (Ed.), *Reading disability: Progress and research needs in dyslexia*. Baltimore: Johns Hopkins University Press.

Birch, H., & Belmont, L. (1964). Auditory-visual integration in normal and retarded readers. *American Journal of Orthopsychiatry, 34*, 852–861.

Birch, H., & Belmont, L. (1965). Auditory-visual integration, intelligence and reading ability in school children. *Perceptual and Motor Skills, 20*, 295–305.

Birch, H., & Lefford, A. (1963). Intersensory development in children. *Monographs of the Society for Research in Child Development, 28* (Whole No. 89).

Bishop, D.V.M., Jancey, C., & Steel, A.McP. (1979). Orthoptic status and reading disability. *Cortex, 15*, 659–666.

Bishop, Y., Fienberg, S., & Holland, P. (1975). *Discrete multivariate analysis; theory and practice*. Cambridge, MA: MIT Press.

Black, F.W. (1974). Self-concept as related to achievement and age in learning-disabled children. *Child Development, 45*, 1137–1140.

Blalock, H.M.Jr. (1968). The measurement problem: A gap between the languages of theory and research. In H.M. Blalock, & A.B. Blalock (Eds.), *Methodology in social research* (pp. 5–27). New York: McGraw Hill.

Bloom, B.S. (1976). *Human characteristics and school learning*. New York: McGraw-Hill.

Bloomfield, L., & Barnhart, C.L. (1961). *Let's read: A linguistic approach*. Detroit: Wayne State University Press.

Bö, O.O. (1972). The extent of the connection between cerebral dominance of speech functions (auditory and vocal), hand dominance, and dyslexia. *Journal of Educational Research, 16*, 61–88.

Boder, E. (1968). Developmental dyslexia: A diagnostic screening procedure based on three characteristic patterns of reading and spelling. In *Claremont reading conference, Thirty-Second Yearbook*. Claremont, CA: Claremont Graduate School.

Boder, E. (1973). Developmental dyslexia: A diagnostic approach based on three atypical reading-spelling patterns. *Developmental Medicine and Child Neurology, 15*, 663–687.

Boersma, F.J., & Chapman, J.W. (1981). Academic self-concept, achievement expectations, and locus of control in elementary learning-disabled children. *Canadian Journal of Behavioral Science, 13*, 234–245.

Brod, N., & Hamilton, D. (1971). Monocular-binocular coordination vs. hand-eye dominance as a factor in reading performance. *American Journal of Optometry, 48*, 123–129.

Bronfenbrenner, U. (1974). Developmental research, public policy, and ecology of childhood. *Child Development, 45*, 1–5.

Bruininks, R.H., Rynders, J.E., & Gross, J.C. (1974). Social acceptance of mildly retarded pupils in resource rooms and regular classes. *American Journal of Mental Deficiency, 78*, 377–378.

Bruininks, V.L. (1978a). Peer status and personality characteristics of learning disabled and nondisabled students. *Journal of Learning Disabilities, 11*, 29–34.

Bruininks, V.L. (1978b). Actual and perceived peer status of learning disabled students in mainstream programs. *Journal of Special Education, 11*, 51–58.

Bryan, T.H. (1974a). An observational study of classroom behaviors of children with learning disabilities. *Journal of Learning Disabilities, 7*, 26–34.

Bryan, T.H. (1974b). Peer popularity of learning disabled children. *Journal of Learning Disabiities, 7*, 361–368.

Bryan, T.H. (1976). Peer popularity of learning disabled students: A replication. *Journal of Learning Disabilities, 9,* 49–53.

Bryan, T.H. (1978). Social relationships and verbal interactions of learning disabled children. *Journal of Learning Disabilities, 11,* 107–115.

Bryan, T.H., & Bryan, J. (1975). *Understanding learning disabilities.* Sherman Oaks, CA: Alfred.

Bryan, T.H., & McGrady, H.J. (1972). Use of a teacher rating scale. *Journal of Learning Disabilities, 5,* 199–206.

Bryan, T.H., Wheeler, R., Falcon, J., & Henek, T. (1976). Come on dummy. An observational study of children's communications. *Journal of Learning Disabilities, 9,* 661–669.

Camp, B., & Dolcourt, J. (1977). Reading and spelling in good and poor readers. *Journal of Learning Disabilities, 10,* 300–308.

Carlsen, R. (1971). Where is the person in personality research? *Psychological Bulletin, 75,* 203–219.

Chapman, J.W., & Boersma, F.S. (1979). Academic self concept in elementary learning disabled children. *Psychology in the Schools, 16,* 201–206.

Chassan, J.B. (1961). Scholastic models of the single case as the basis of clinical research design. *Behavioral Science, 6,* 42–50.

Clark, M.M. (1970). *Reading difficulties in schools.* Baltimore: Penguin Books.

Coff, L.A. (1978). the validity of the Visual-Aural Digit Span Test as predictor of word recognition and spelling for learning-disabled children. San Diego: California School of Professional Psychology. *Dissertation Abstracts International, 38A,* 6517A–6518A.

Cole, M., & Kraft, M.B. (1964). Specific learning disability. *Cortex, 1,* 302–313.

Coltheart, M., Masterton, J., & Byng, S. (1985). Types of errors in surface dyslexic reading. In K. Patterson, J. Marshall, & M. Coltheart (Eds.), *Surface dyslexia.* London: Erlbaum.

Coltheart, M., Patterson, K.E., & Marshall, J.C. (Eds.) (1980). *Deep dyslexia.* London: Routledge & Kegan Paul.

Critchley, M. (1970). *The dyslectic child.* London: Heinemann Medical Books.

Critchley, M., & Critchley, E. (1978). *Dyslexia defined.* Sussex, England: Charles C. Thomas.

Cronbach, L.J. (1957). The two disciplines of scientific psychology. *American Psychologist, 12,* 671–684.

Cronbach, L.J. (1975). Beyond the two disciplines of scientific psychology. *American Psychologist, 30,* 116–127.

Cronbach, L.J., & Snow, R.E. (1977). *Aptitudes and instructional methods.* New York: Irvington.

Cullen, J.L., Boersma, F.S., & Chapman, J.W. (1981). Characteristics of third-grade learning disabled children. *Learning Disability Quarterly, 4,* 244–230.

Dalby, M. (1973). Laeseretardation—neurologiske aspekter [Reading retardation—neurological aspects]. *Nordisk tidsskrift for tale og stemme, 33,* 54.

DeFries J.C., & Decker, S.N. (1982). Genetic aspects of reading disability: A family study. In R.N. Malatesha & P.G. Aaron (Eds.), *Reading disorders. Varieties and treatments.* New York: Academic Press.

DeHirsch, K., Jansky, J., & Langford, W.S. (1966). *Predicting reading failure: A preliminary study.* New York: Harper & Row.

Delacato, C.H. (1966). *Neurological organization and reading.* Springfield, IL: Charles C. Thomas.

Denckla, M.B. (1972). Clinical syndromes in learning disabilities: The case for "splitting" vs. "lumping." *Journal of Learning Disabilities, 5*, 401–406.

Deutsch, M. (1965). The role of the social class in language development and cognition. *American Journal of Orthopsychiatry, 35*, 78–88.

Dixon, J.W., & Brown, M.B. (1983). *BMDP statistical software 1983. Printing with additions.* Berkeley: University of California Press.

Doehring, D.G. (1983). What do we know about reading disabilities? Closing the gap between research and practice. *Annals of Dyslexia, 33*, 175–183.

Doehring, D.G., & Hoshko, I.M. (1977). Classification of reading problems by the Q-technique of factor analysis. *Cortex, 13*, 281–294.

Doehring, D.G. Hoshko, I.M., & Bryans, B.N. (1970). Statistical classification of children with reading problems. *Journal of Clinical Neuropsychology, 1*, 5–16.

Doehring, D.G., Trites, R.L., Patel, P.G., & Fiedorowicz, C.A.M. (1981). *Reading disabilities. The interaction of reading, language, and neuropsychological deficits.* New York: Academic Press.

Dorland's illustrated medical dictionary, 26th edition. (1981). Philadelphia: W.B. Saunders.

Downing, J. (1973). *Comparative reading: Cross national studies of behavior and processes in reading and writing.* New York: Macmillan.

Drake, W.E. (1968). Clinical and pathological findings in a child with a developmental learning disability. *Journal of Learning Disabilities, 1*, 9–25.

Duffy, F.H., Denckla, M.B., Bartels, P.H., & Sandini, G. (1980). Dyslexia: Regional differences in brain electrical activity by topographic mapping. *Annals of Neurology, 7*, 412–420.

Duffy, F.H., Denckla, M.B., Bartels, P.H., Sandine, G., & Kiesling, L.S. (1980). Dyslexia: Automated diagnosis by computerized classification of brain electrical activity. *Annals of Neurology, 7*, 421–428.

Duffy, F.H., & Geschwind, N. (1985). *Dyslexia. A neuroscientific approach to clinical evaluation.* Boston: Little, Brown.

Dunlap, E.A. (1965). Role of strabismus in reading problems. *Transactions of the Pennsylvania Academy of Ophthalmology and Otolaryngology, 18*, 9–15.

Dunlop, D.B., & Dunlop, P. (1974). New concepts of visual laterality in relation to dyslexia. *Australian Journal of Ophthalmology, 24*, 110–112.

Dunlop, D.B., & Dunlop, P. (1976). A new orthoptic technique in learning disability due to visual dyslexia. In I.S. Moore, J. Mein, & L. Stockbridge (Eds.), *Orthoptics past, present and future.* New York: Intercontinental.

Dunlop, D.B., Dunlop, P., & Fenelon, B. (1973). Vision—laterality analysis in children with reading disability: The results of new techniques of examination. *Cortex, 9*, 227–236.

Dunlop, P. (1979). Orthoptic management of learning disability. *British Orthoptic Journal, 36*, 25–35.

Eames, T.H. (1948). Comparison of eye conditions among 1,000 reading failures, 500 ophthalmic patients, and 150 unselected children. *American Journal of Ophthalmology, 31*, 713–717.

Eames, T.H. (1955). The influence of hypermetropia and myopia on reading achievement. *American Journal of Ophthalmology, 39*, 375–377.

Eames, T.H. (1959). Reading failures and non-failures. *American Journal of Ophthalmology, 47*, 74–77.

Edfeldt, A.W. (1981, April). *A general model for the reading process.* Research bulletins from the Institute of Education, University of Stockholm, 9(2).

Edfeldt, A.W. (1982). *Läsprocessen* [The reading process]. Lund, Sweden: Liber.

Elvenes, J. (1986). *Leseprosessen. Vansker og metoder* [The reading process. Problems and methods]. Oslo, Norway: Gyldendal.

Engleman, L., & Harligan, J.A. (1983). K-means clustering. In W.J. Dixon (Ed.), *BMDP Statistical Software*. Berkeley: University of California Press.

Ericson, B. (1981, December). Reading disabilities and emotional disturbances. *Uppsala Reports on Education, 11*.

Fernald, G., & Keller, H. (1921). The effect of kinesthetic factors in development of word recognition in the case of non-readers. *Journal of Educational Research, 4*, 357–377.

Fester, C.B., & Skinner, B.F. (1957). *Schedules of reinforcement*. New York: Appleton-Century-Crofts.

Fisher, K.W. (1980). A theory of cognitive development: The control and construction of hierarchies of skills. *Psychological Review, 87*, 477–531.

Flax, N. (1973). The eye and learning disabilities. *Journal of Learning Disabilities, 6*, 328–332.

Fletcher, J.M., & Satz, P. (1980). Developmental changes in neuropsychological correlates of reading achievement: A six-year longitudinal followup. *Journal of Clinical Neuropsychology, 2*, 23–37.

Forman, B.D., & McKinney, J.D. (1975). Teacher perceptions of the classroom behavior of learning disabled children. *Learning Disability Quarterly, 4*.

Fowler, M.S., & Stein, J.F. (1980). New evidence for visual ambilaterality in some dyslectics. *British Orthoptic Journal, 37*, 11–15.

Freud, S. (1953). *On aphasia*. New York: International Universities Press.

Fries, C. (1963). *Linguistics and reading*. New York: Holt, Rinehart & Winston.

Frostig, M. (1961). *The Marianne Frostig Developmental Test of Visual Perception*. Palo Alto, CA: Consulting Psychologists Press.

Fuller, G.B., & Friedrich, D. (1974–1975). Three diagnostic patterns of reading disability. *Academic Therapy, 10*, 219–231.

Gagné, R.M. (1970). *The conditions of learning* (2nd ed.). New York: Holt, Rinehart & Winston.

Galaburda, A.M. (1983). Developmental dyslexia: Current anatomical research. *Annals of Dyslexia, 33*, 41–53.

Galaburda, A.M., & Kemper, T.L. (1979). Cytoarchitectonic abnormalities in developmental dyslexia: A case study. *Annals of Neurology, 6*, 94–100.

Galaburda, A.M., Sherman, G.F., Rosen, G.D., Aboitiz, F., & Geschwind, N. (1985). Developmental dyslexia: Four consecutive patients with cortical anomalies. *Annals of Neurology, 18*, 222.

Gardner, E.F., Rudman, H.C., Karlsen, B., & Merwin, J.C. (1983). *Stanford Achievement Test*. San Antonio, TX: The Psychological Corporation.

Garrett, M.K., & Crump, W.D. (1980). Peer acceptance, teacher preferences and self-appraisal of social status among learning disabled students. *Learning Disability Quarterly, 3*.

Gates, A.I. (1927). *The improvement of reading*. New York: Macmillan.

Gates, A.I. (1947). *The improvement of reading* (3rd ed.). New York: Macmillan.

Gergen, K. (1971). *The concept of self*. New York: Holt.

Geschwind, N. (1983). Biological associations of left-handedness. *Annals of Dyslexia, 33*, 29–40.

Geyer, J.J. (1972). Comprehensive and partial models related to the reading process. *Reading Research Quarterly, 7*, 541–587.

Giebink, J., & Birk, R. (1970). The Bender Gestalt Test as an effective predictor of reading achievement. *Journal of Clinical Psychology, 26,* 484–485.

Gjessing, H.J. (1953). Lese- og skrivevansker [Reading and writing difficulties]. *Skole og samfunn,* 8.

Gjessing, H.J. (1958a). *En studie av lesemodenhet ved skolegangens begynnelse* [A study of reading readiness at the beginning of school]. Oslo, Norway: J.W. Cappelen.

Gjessing, H.J. (1958b). Lesevansker hos barn [Reading difficulties in children]. *Tidsskrift for den norske laegeforening, 5,* 187–190.

Gjessing, H.J. (1966). Samnordisk specialpedagogisk forskning [Joint Scandinavian research in special education]. In K.G. Stukat & R. Engstrom (Eds.), *Rapport från konferens i Göteborg, April 1966.* Gothenburg, Sweden: Lärarhögskolan.

Gjessing, H.J. (1969). Integrering av funksjonshemmede. Hva vil det kreve? [Integrating the disabled. What will it take?]. *Spesialpedagogikk, 3,* 2–10.

Gjessing, H.J. (1974a). Om sanering av spesialundervisningen og om alternative tilbud. Bakgrunnsstoff for en ny forskningsstrategi [Reorganizing special education and alternative options. Background for a new research strategy]. *Skolepsykologi, 4.*

Gjessing, H.J. (1974b). *Introduksjonsskriv til Norges almenvitenskapelige forskningsråd* om forskningsmidler [An introductory document to the Norwegian research council for research regarding funding of research]. University of Bergen, Institute of Educational Psychology.

Gjessing, H.J. (1976). *En retrospektiv analyse av 188 protokoller for barn med spesifikke lese- og skrivevansker, henvist fra Skolepsykologisk kontor i Drammen* [A retrospective anaysis of the protocols of 188 children with specific reading and writing disabilities, referred to the school psychology services in Drammen, Norway]. Mimeographed. Bergen, Norway: University of Bergen.

Gjessing, H.J. (1977). *Lese- og skrivevansker. Dyslexi. Problemorientering. Analyse og diagnose. Behandling og undervisning* [Reading and writing disabilities. Dyslexia. Issues. Analysis and diagnosis. Treatment and education.]. Bergen-Oslo-Tromsö: University Press.

Gjessing, H.J. (1978). Bergen-prosjektet i hovedtrekk [An overview of the Bergen Project]. In *Bergen-prosjektet — Et nordisk forskningssamarbeid om laereproblemer hos barn: I. Prosjekt-beskrivelse.* NU-rapport B, 7. Copenhagen: Nordiska Ministerrådet.

Gjessing, H.J. (1979). *Pröver for analyse av lese- og skrivevansker* [Tests for the analysis of reading and writing disabilities]. Bergen: Universitetsforlaget.

Gjessing, H.J. (1980a). Function analysis of reading and writing behavior. A methodological approach to improved research in reading disability. In R.M. Knights & D.J. Bakker (Eds.), *Treatment of hyperactive and learning disordered children. Current research.* Baltimore: University Book Press.

Gjessing, H.J. (1980b). Reading disability: Diagnosis based on psychoeducational analysis of the learning function. In *1980 Claremont Reading Conference 44th Year-book* (pp. 77–93). Claremont, CA: Claremont Graduate School.

Gjessing, H.J. (1982a). Spesifikke laerevansker: Pedagogisk-psykologisk diagnose med basis i funksjonsanalyse [Specific learning disabilities: Educational-psychological diagnosis based on function analysis]. In T. Höien (Ed.) *Lesevansker — diagnostisering — undervisning.* Stavanger-Oslo-Bergen-Tromsö: Universitetsforlaget.

Gjessing, H.J. (1982b). Prosjektets forskningsstrategiske og forsknings-metodiske utgangspunkt [The project's research strategy and methodology base]. In H.J. Gjessing, H.D. Nygaard, R. Solheim, & H. Aasved, *Bergen-prosjektet I: Laerevansker som samspillsproblem.* Bergen-Oslo-Tromsö: Universitetsforlaget.

Gjessing, H.J. (1983). *Praktisk indføring i funktionsanalytisk specialundervisning. Et forsøgs-og studieeksemplar* [Practical introduction to function analysis in special education. An experimental study proposal]. Translated and adapted to Danish conditions by B.H. Schmidt. Brodky, Denmark: County Schools.

Gjessing, H.J. (1986a). *Teacher power: Building school successes for dyslexic students.* Part I. Translated from the Norwegian by J. Boyd Todd. Pomona, CA: The Attic Press.

Gjessing, H.J. (1986b). *Parent power: Building school successes for dyslexic students*, Part II. Translated from Norwegian by J. Boyd Todd. Pomona, CA: The Attic Press.

Gjessing, H.J., Dahl, E., Jenssen, I.J., Rosmer, B., & Stegane, N. (1980). *Praktisk veiledning om lese- og skrivevansker* [Practical guidance regarding reading and writing disabilities]. Oslo: Tiden Norsk Forlag, Laeremiddelhuset.

Gjessing, H.J., Nygaard, H.D., Solheim, R., & Aasved, H. (1982). *Bergen-prosjektet I: Laerevansker som samspillsproblem* [Learning disabilities in the classroom]. Bergen-Oslo-Tromsö: Universitetsforlaget.

Gjessing, H.J., Nygaard, H.D., Solheim, R., et al. (1988). *Bergen-prosjektet III: Studier av barn med dysleksi og andre laerevansker* [Studies of children with dyslexia and other learning disabilities]. Oslo, Norway: Universitetsforlaget.

Goldberg, H.K. (1959). The ophthalmologist looks at the reading problem. *American Journal of Ophthalmology, 47*, 67–74.

Goldberg, H.K. (1968). Vision, perception and related facts in dyslexia. In A.H. Keeney & V.T. Keeney (Eds.), *Dyslexia, diagnosis and treatment of reading disorders.* St. Louis: C.V. Mosby.

Goldberg, H.K., & Arnott, W. (1970). Ocular motility in learning disabilities. *Journal of Learning Disabilities, 3*, 160–162.

Goldstein, H., Moss, J.W., & Jordan, L.J. (1965). *The efficacy of special class training and the development of mentally retarded children.* (Cooperative Research Project No. 619.) Washington, DC: U.S. Office of Education.

Goodman, H., Gottlieb, J., & Harrison, R.H. (1972). Social acceptance of EMR's integrated into a non-graded elementary school. *Journal of Mental Deficiency, 76.*

Goodman, K.S. (1967). Reading; A psycholinguistic guessing game. *Journal of the Reading Specialist, 6*, 126–135.

Goodman, K.S., & Gollasch, F.V. (1980). Word omissions: Deliberate and non-deliberate. *Reading Research Quarterly, 16*, 6–31.

Gorsuch, R.L. (1983). *Factor analysis* (2nd ed.). Hillsdale, NJ: Lawrence Erlbaum.

Gouge, B.M. (1976). A reliability and validity study of the VADS test for screening learning disabilities of second graders with teachers as examiners. *Dissertation Abstracts International, 36.*

Gough, P.B. (1972). One second of reading. In J.F. Kavanagh & I.G. Mattingly (Eds.), *Language by ear and by eye* (pp. 331–358). Cambridge, MA: MIT Press.

Gray, W.S. (1922). *Remedial cases in reading: Their diagnosis and treatment.* Supplementary Educational Monographs, No. 22. Chicago: Chicago University Press.

Gray, W.S. (1926–1970). Annual summary of investigations relating to reading. In *Elementary School Journal* (1926–32), *Journal of Educational Research* (1933–1970).

Griffin, D.C., Walton, H.N., & Ives, V. (1974). Saccades as related to reading disorders. *Journal of Learning Disabilities, 7*, 310–316.

Hagberg, B. (1975). Minimal brain dysfunction—Hvad innebär det för barnets utveckling och anpassning? [Minimal brain dysfunction—What does it imply for the child's development and adjustment?]. *Läkartidningen, 72*, 3296–3300.

Hagtvedt Vik, G. (1976). Reading disabilities in Norwegian elementary grades. In L. Tarnopol & M. Tarnopol (Eds.), *Reading disabilities. An international prospective*. Baltimore: University Park Press.

Hallgren, B. (1950). *Specific dyslexia. (Congenital word-blindness). A clinical and genetic study*. Doctoral dissertation. Stockholm: University of Stockholm.

Handlon, J. (1960, January). A metatheoretical view of assumptions regarding the etiology of schizophrenia. *AMA Archives of General Psychiatry*, 43–60.

Hansen, M. (1979). Interaction between reading test results and elementary reading programs. *Scandinavian Journal of Educational Research*, *23*, 79–89.

Harris, A.J., & Sipay, E.R. (1981). *How to increase reading ability* (7th ed.). New York: Longman.

Harris, A.J., & Sipay, E.R. (1981). *How to increase reading ability* (8th ed.). New York: Longman.

Harris, T.L., & Hodges, R.E. (1981). *A dictionary of reading*. Newark, DE: International Reading Association.

Hartmann, T. (1977). Noen saeregenheter ved kasusstudier som psykologisk forskningsmetode [Some unique features of case studies as psychological research method]. In M. Kragh (Ed.), *Konsekvenser av ulike vitenskapsteoretiske syn for klinisk psykologisk forskning*. Oslo: Norsk Almenvitenskapelig Forskningsråd.

Heber, R.A. (1961). A manual of terminology and classification in mental retardation. *American Journal of Mental Retardation, Monograph Supplement*.

Helveston, E.M., Billips, W.C., & Weber, J.C. (1970). Controlling eye-dominant hemisphere relationship as factor in reading ability. *American Journal of Ophthalmology*, *70*, 96–100.

Helveston, E.M., Weber, J.C., Miller, K., Robertsen, K., Hohberger, G., Estes, R., Ellis, F.D., Pick, N., & Helveston, B.H. (1984). Visual function and academic performance. *American Journal of Ophthalmology*, *99*, 346–355.

Hempel, C.G. (1952). *Typological methods in the national and social sciences*. Proceedings, American Philosophical Association. Eastern Division 1, 65–86.

Henry, S.A., & Wittman, R.D. (1981). Diagnostic implications of Bannatyne's recategorized WISC-R scores for identifying learning disabled children. *Journal of Learning Disabilities*, *14*, 517–520.

Hermann, K. (1955). *Om medfödt ordblindhed* [On congenital wordblindness]. Dissertation, Copenhagen: University of Copenhagen.

Hermann, K. (1959). *Reading disability*. Springfield, IL: Charles C. Thomas.

Hermann, K. (1967). *Om medfödt ordblindhed* [On congenital wordblindness] (3rd ed.). Copenhagen: Munksgaard.

Hermann, K. (1969). *Reading disability*. Copehnhagen: Munksgaard.

Hiebert, B., Wong, B., & Hunter, M. (1982). Affective influences on learning disabled adolescents. *Learning Disability Quarterly*, *5*, 334–343.

Hier, D., LeMay, M., Rosenberger, P., & Perlo, V.P. (1978). Developmental dyslexia. *Archives of Neurology*, *35*, 90–92.

Hinshelwood, J. (1896). The visual memory for words and figures. *British Medical Journal*, *2*, 1543–1544.

Hinshelwood, J. (1900). Congenital word-blindness. *Lancet*, *1*, 1506–1508.

Hinshelwood, J. (1917). *Congenital word-blindness*. London: Lewis.

Höien, T. (1980) *Ikonisk persistens og dysleksi* [Iconic persistence and dyslexia]. Stavanger, Norway: Rogalandsforskning.

Höien, T., & Jansen, M. (1986). *Leseinnlaering, leseprosess og lesemetoder (Learning to read, the reading process and reading methods).* Stavanger-Oslo-Bergen-Tromsö: Universitetsforlaget.

Holmes, J.A. (1953). *The substrata-factor theory of reading.* Berkeley: California Book.

Holowinsky, I.Z. (1980). Qualitative assessment of cognitive skills. *Journal of Special Education, 14,* 155–163.

Hooper, S.R., & Hynd, G.W. (1985). The relationship between the K-ABC and the VADS with reading disabled children: Validity of the K-ABC. *Journal of Psychoeducational Assessment, 3,* 77–97.

Hovland, O.J. (1977). *Manual for Koppitz' VADS Test* (The Visual Aural Digit Span Test, Norwegian translation). Unpublished. University of Bergen: Psychological Institute.

Howden, M.E. (1970. *A nineteen-year follow-up study of good, average and poor readers in the fifth and sixth grades.* Unpublished doctoral dissertation. Eugene, OR: University of Oregon.

Huelsman, C.B. Jr. (1970). The WISC subtest syndrome for disabled readers. *Perceptual and Motor Skills, 30,* 535–558.

Hunter, E., & Johnson, L. (1971). Developmental and psychological differences between readers and non-readers. *Journal of Reading Disabilities, 4,* 572–577.

Hynd, G., & Cohen, M. (1983). *Dyslexia: Neurological theory, research, and clinical differentiation.* New York: Grune & Stratton.

Iano, R., Ayers, D., Heller, H.D., McGettingen, J.F., & Walker, V.S. (1974). Sociometric status of retarded children in an integrated program. *Exceptional Children, 31,* 267–271.

Ingram, T.T.S. (1969). The nature of dyslexia. *Bulletin of the Orton Society, 19,* 18–58.

Ingram, T.T.S., Mason, A.W., & Blackburn, I. (1970). A retrospective study of 82 children with reading disability. *Developmental Medicine and Child Neurology, 12,* 271–290.

Johnson, O.J., & Myklebust, H.R. (1967). *Learning disabilities. Educational principles and practices.* New York: Grune & Stratton.

Jordan, D.R. (1977). *Dyslexia in the classroom.* Columbus, OH: Charles E. Merrill.

Jöreskog, K.G., & Sörbom, D. (1981). *Lisrel V: Analysis of linear structural relationships by the method of maximum likelihood. User's Guide.* Mooresville, IN: Scientific Software.

Jorm, A.F. (1979). The cognitive and neurological basis of developmental dyslexia: A theoretical framework and review. *Cognition, 7,* 19–33.

Just, M.A., & Carpenter, P.A. (1980). A theory of reading: From eye fixations to comprehension. *Psychological Review, 87,* 329–354.

Karlsen, B. (1954a). *A comparison of some educational and psychological characteristics of successful and unsuccessful readers at the elementary school level.* Ph.D. dissertation, Minneapolis: University of Minnesota.

Karlsen, B. (1954b). *The Bender-Gestalt Test: An objective scoring system for use with children.* Unpublished. Minneapolis: University of Minnesota Psycho-Education Clinic.

Karlsen, B. (1980). Assessment and diagnosis of reading abilities. In P. Lamb & R. Arnold (Eds.), *Teaching reading* (2nd ed.). New York: R.C. Owen.

Kass, C.E., & Myklebust, H.R. (1969). Learning disability: An educational definition. *Journal of Learning Disabilities, 2,* 377–379.

Kaufman, A.S. (1975). Factor analyses of the WISC-R at eleven age levels between 6½ and 16½ years. *Journal of Consulting and Clinical Psychology, 43,* 135–147.

Kavanagh, L.F., & Mattingly, I.G. (Eds.). (1972). *Language by ear and by eye*. Cambridge, MA: MIT Press.

Keeney, A.H. (1968). Ophthalmological aspects of dyslexia. *Transactions of the American Academy of Ophthalmology*, *72*, 825–829.

Keeney, A.H., & Keeney, V.T. (1968). *Dyslexia. Diagnosis and treatment of reading disorders*. St. Louis: C.V. Mosby.

Keogh, B.K. (1965). School achievement associated with successful performance on the Bender Gestalt Test. *Journal of School Psychology*, *3*, 37–40.

Keogh, B.K. (1969). The Bender Gestalt with children: Research implications. *Journal of Special Education*, *3*, 15–22.

Keogh, B.K. (1974). Optometric vision training programs for children with learning disabilities: Review of issues and research. *Journal of Learning Disabiities*, *7*, 219–231.

Kerr, J. (1897). School hygiene in its mental, moral and physical aspects. *Journal of the Royal Statistical Society*. *60*, 613–680.

Kinsbourne, M., & Warrington, E.K. (1963a). Developmental factors in reading and writing backwardness. *British Journal of Psychology*, *54*, 145–156.

Kinsbourne, M., & Warrington, E.K. (1963). The development of finger differentiation. *Quarterly Journal of Experimental Psychology*, *15*, 132.

Klasen, E. (1972). *The syndrome of specific dyslexia*. Lancaster, England: Medical and Technical.

Kline, C., & Kline, C. (1975). Follow-up study of 211 dyslexic children. *Bulletin of the Orton Society*, *25*, 127–144.

Kluckhohn, C., & Murray, H.A. (1949). *Personality in nature, society and culture*. New York: Knopf.

Knights, R.M., & Bakker, D.J. (1980). *Treatment of hyperactive and learning disordered children. Current research*. Baltimore: University Park Press.

Koppitz, E.M. (1964). *The Bender Gestalt Test of young children*. New York: Grune & Stratton.

Koppitz, E.M. (1970). The Visual Aural Digit Span Test with elementary school children. *Journal of Clinical Psychology*, *26*, 349–353.

Koppitz, E.M. (1971). *Children with learning disabilities*. New York: Grune & Stratton.

Koppitz, E.M. (1975). Bender Gestalt Test, Visual Aural Digit Span Test and reading achievement. *Journal of Learning Disabilities*, *8*, 154–158.

Koppitz, E.M. (1977). *The Visual Aural Digit Span Test*. New York: Grune & Stratton.

Koppitz, E.M. (1981). The Visual Aural Digit Span Test for seventh graders: A normative study. The Bender Gestalt and VADS test performance of learning disabled middle school pupils. *Journal of Learning Disabilities*, *14*, 93–98.

Kragh, M.C. (1977). Konsekvenser av ulike vitenskapsteoretiske syn for klinisk psykologisk forskning [The consequences of various theoretical scientific views on research in clinical psychology]. In *Klinisk psykologisk forskning. Konferanserapport*. Oslo: Norsk Almenvitenskapelig Forskningsrad.

Kussmaul, A. (1877). Disturbance of speed. In H. von Ziemssen (Ed.), *Cyclopaedia of practice of medicine*, Vol. *14*. New York: William Wood.

Lapp, E.R. (1957). A study of the social adjustment of slow learning children who were assigned part-time to regular classes. *American Journal of Mental Deficiency*, *62*.

Larsen, C.A. (1960). Om undervisning af börn med laese- og skrivevanskeligheder i de förste skoleår. Undersögelser og overvejelser [Teaching children with reading and writing difficulties in first grade. Research and delibertion]. *Dansk Paedagogisk Tidsskrift*, *8*, 193–252.

Larsen, S.C., Parker, R., & Jorjorian, S. (1973). Differences in self-concept of normal and learning disabled children. *Perceptual and Motor Skills, 37*, 510.

Lashley, K.S. (1929). *Brain mechanisms and intelligence*. Chicago: University of Chicago Press.

Lassen, N.A., Ingvar, D.H., & Skinhöj, E. (1978, October). Brain function and blood flow. *Scientific American, 239*, 50–59.

Leisman, G., & Schwartz, J. (1978). Aetiological factors in dyslexia: 1. Saccadic eye movement control. *Perceptual and Motor Skills, 47*, 403–407.

Leland, H. (1977). Theoretical considerations of adaptive behavior. In W.A. Coulter & H.W. Morrow (Eds.), *The concept and measurement of adaptive behavior within the scope of psychological assessment*. Austin, TX: Regional Research Center.

Levine, M., & Fuller, G. (1972). Psychological, neuropsychological, and educational correlates of reading defect. *Journal of Learning Disabilities, 5*, 563–571.

Liberman, I.Y., Shankweiler, D., Orlando, C., Harris, K.S., & Berti, F.B. (1971). Letter confusion and reversals of sequence in the beginning reader: Implications for Orton's theory of developmental dyslexia. *Cortex, 7*, 127–142.

Lidell, H.J., & Scott, R. (1940). *A Greek–English lexicon* (9th ed.). Oxford, England: Oxford University Press.

Linder, M. (1961, October). Das Problem der legasthenischen Kinder in der deutschen Schweitz [The problem of dyslexic children in German-speaking Switzerland]. *Schweitzer Erziehungsrundschau, 7*, 137–160.

Loevinger, J. (1976). *Ego development*. San Francisco: Jossey Bass.

Lory, P. (1966). *Die Leseschwäche. Entstehung und Formen, ursächliche Zusammenhänge, Behandlung* [Reading disability. Origin and form, causal relationships, treatment]. Munich/Basel: Reinhardt Verlag.

Lovett, M.W. (1984). The search for subtypes of specific reading disability: Reflections from a cognitive perspective. *Annals of Dyslexia, 34*, 155–178.

Luborsky, L. (1953). Intra-individual repetitive measurements (P-technique) in understanding psychotherapeutic change. In O.M. Mowrer (Ed.), *Psychotherapy: Theory and resarch*. New York: Ronald Press.

Lundberg, I. (1981a). *Communication and handicap*. Report of EASE-80. Helsinki: The Finnish Association for Special Education.

Lundberg, I. (1981b). *Läsprosessen i ljuset av aktuell forskning* [The reading process in light of empirical research]. Stockholm: Skolöverstyrelsen. Byrån for pedagogisk forsknings- och utvecklingsarbete.

Lundberg, I. (1983). *Läs- och skrivsvårigheter i ljust av aktuell forskning* [Reading and writing disabilities in light of empirical research]. Stockholm: Skolöverstyrelsen. Planeringssekretariatet IoD-prosjektet.

Lundberg, I., & Olofsson, A. (1981). Dysleksielevers sosiala bakgrund [The social background of pupils with dyslexia]. *Nordisk Tidsskrift för specialpedagogik, 59*, 203–213.

Lundman, L. (1979). *Socioeconomisk differentiering i grundskolan* [Socioeconomic differentiation in the elementary school]. Lund: Liber.

Lyle, J.C. (1970). Certain antecedent, perinatal and developmental variables and reading retardation in middle class boys. *Child Development, 41*, 481–491.

Lytton, H. (1972). Some psychological and sociological characteristics of "good" and "poor" achievers in remedial reading groups: Clinical case studies, I. In J.F. Reid (Ed.), *Reading: Problems and practices*. London: Ward Lock.

Malatesha, R.N., & Dougan, D.R. (1982). Clinical subtypes of developmental dyslexia:

Resolution of an irresolute problem. In R.N. Malatesha & P.G. Aaron (Eds.), *Reading disorders. Varieties and treatment* (pp. 69–92). New York: Academic Press.

Maliphant, R., Supramaniam, S., & Saraga, E. (1971). Acquiring skill in reading: A review of experimental research. *Journal of Child Psychology and Psychiatry and Allied Disciplines, 15*, 175–185.

Malmquist, E. (1958). *Factors related to reading disabilities in the first grade of the elementary school.* Stockholm: Almquist & Wiksell.

Malmquist, E. (1969). *Läs- och skrivsvårigheter hos barn. Analys- och behandlingsmetodik* [Reading and writing disabilities among children. Methods for diagnosis and treatment]. Lund, Sweden: Gleestrup.

Mann, P., & Suiter, P. (1978). *Handbook in diagnostic teaching.* Boston: Allyn & Bacon.

Marceil, J.C. (1977). Implicit dimensions of ideography and nomothesis: A reformulation. *American Psychologist, 32*, 1046–1055.

Marshall, J.C., & Newcombe, F. (1973). Patterns of paralexia: A psycholinguistic approach. *Journal of Psycholinguistic Research, 2*, 175–199.

Mathewson, C. (1979). The moderating effect of extrinsic motivation upon the attitude/comprehension relationship in reading. In Clifford Pennock (Ed.), *Reading comprehension at four linguistic levels* (pp. 8–20). Newark, DE: International Reading Association.

Mattis, S. (1978). Dyslexia syndromes: A working hypothesis that works. In A.L. Benton & D. Pearl (Eds.), *Dyslexia: An appraisal of current knowledge.* New York, London: Oxford University Press.

Mattis, S. (1981). Dyslexia syndromes in children: Toward the development of syndrome-specific treatment programs. In F.J. Pirozzolo & M.C. Wittrock (Eds.), *Neuropsychological and cognitive process in reading.* New York: Academic Press.

Mattis, S., French, J.H., & Rapin, I. (1975). Dyslexia in children and adults: Three independent neuropsychological syndromes. *Developmental Medicine and Child Neurology, 17*, 150–163.

McCusker, L., Bias, R.G., & Hillinger, M.L. (1981). Phonological recording and reading. *Psychological Bulletin, 89*, 217–245.

McKinney, J.D., & Feagans, L. (1983). Adaptive classroom behavior of learning disabled students. *Journal of Learning Disabilities, 16*, 360–364.

McKinney, J.D., McClure, S., & Feagans, L. (1982). Classroom behavior of learning disabled children. *Learning Disability Quarterly, 5*, 45–52.

McNeil, M.R., & Hamre, C.E. (1974). A review of measures of lateralized cerebral hemispheric functions. *Journal of Learning Disabilities, 7*, 51–59.

Meehl, P.E. (1954). *Clinical versus statistical prediction. A theoretical analysis and a review of evidence.* Minneapolis: University of Minnesota Press.

Meyerowitz, J. (1962). Self-derogation in young retardates and special class placement. *Child Development, 33*, 443–451.

Michael-Smith, H., Morgenstern, M., & Karp E. (1970). Dyslexia in four siblings. *Journal of Learning Disabilities, 3*, 185–192.

Miles, T.R., & Ellis, N.C. (1981). A lexical encoding deficiency, II: Clinical observations. In G.T. Pavlidis & T.R. Miles (Eds.), *Dyslexia research and its applications to education.* Chichester: Wiley.

Mitchell, D.C., & Green, D.W. (1978). The effects of context and content on immediate processing in reading. *Quarterly Journal of Experimental Psychology, 30*, 609–636.

Monroe, M. (1928). Methods for diagnosis and treatment of cases of reading disability. *Genetic Psychology Monographs*, *4*, (Nos. 4 and 5).

Monroe, M. (1932). *Children who cannot read*. Chicago: University of Chicago Press.

Morgan, W.P. (1896). A case of congenital word-blindness. *British Medical Journal*, *11*, 378.

Müller, R.G.E. (1958). Die Schreib-Lese-Schwäche als neurotoide Legasthenie und als Regressphänomen [The writing-reading disability as neurotic dyslexia and as regression phenomenon.]. *Schule und Psychologie*, *5*, 266–270.

Myklebust, H.R. (1971). *The pupil rating scale. Screening for learning disabilities*. New York: Grune & Stratton.

Myklebust, H.R. (1978). Toward a science of dyslexiology. In H.R. Myklebust (Ed.), *Progress in learning disabilities*, Vol. 4. New York: Grune & Stratton.

Myklebust, H.R., & Boshes, B. (1969). *Minimal brain damage in children*. Washington, DC: U.S. Department of Health, Education, and Welfare. Public Health Service.

Myklebust, H.R., Boshes, B., Olson, D., & Cole, C. (1969). *Minimal brain damage in children. Final Report*. Evanston, IL: Northwestern University Publications.

Naidoo, S. (1972). *Specific dyslexia: The research report of the ICAA word blind center for dyslectic children*. New York: Wiley.

Neisser, U. (1967). *Cognitive psychology*. New York: A.C.C. Meredith.

Newman, S.P., Wadsworth, J.F., Archer, R., & Hockly, R. (1985). Ocular dominance, reading, and spelling ability in school children. *British Journal of Ophthalmology*, *69*, 228–232.

Nober, L. (1973). Auditory discrimination and classroom noise. *The Reading Teacher*, *27*, 288–291.

Nordisk ministerråd (1982). *Bergen-prosjektet. Et nordisk forskningssamarbeid om laereproblemer hos barn, III. Rapporter, artikler og hjelpemidler. En oversikt* [The Bergen Project. A Scandinavian joint research effort of children's learning disabilities, III. Reports, articles, and teaching aids. An overview]. Copenhagen: "Nord."

Norn, M.S., Rindziunski, E., & Skydsgaard, H. (1969). Ophthalmologic and orthoptic examinations of dyslectics. *Acta Ophthalmologica*, *47*, 147–160.

Norri, E. (1954). Ordblindhedens (dyslexiens) arvegang [The heritability of dyslexia]. *Laesepedagogen*, *5*, 71–76.

Noss, H. (1977). Underyting i grunnskolen. En undersökelse blant et elevkull i et distrikt i Bergen [Underachievement in the elementary school. A study of a cohort of pupils in a school district in Bergen]. Unpublished paper. University of Bergen, Norway.

Nunnally, J.C. (1967). *Psychometric theory*. New York: McGraw-Hill.

Nygaard, H.D. (1978). Problemet underyting: Forsök på en naermere avklaring med grunnlag i litteraturstudier [The under-achievement problem: An explanation based upon analysis of the literature]. In *Bergen-prosjektet. Et nordisk forskningssamarbeid om laereproblemer hos barn. Rapport nr. 1: Virkninger av Specialundervisning*. Copenhagen: Sekretariatet for Nordisk kulturelt samarbejde.

Nygaard, H.D. (1982). Underyting og laerevansker i skolen [Underachievement and learning disabilities in the schools]. In H.J. Gjessing, H.D. Nygaard, R. Solheim, & A. Aasved (Eds.), *Bergen-prosjektet I. Laerevansker som samspillsproblem*. Bergen-Oslo-Tromsö: Universitetsforlaget.

Nygaard, H.D. (1984a). Skolefaglig utvikling fra overgangen 1.-2 klasse til overgangen 3.-4 klasse [Growth in school achievement from grade 1-2 to grade 3-4]. In R. Solheim et al., *Bergen-prosjektet II. Sökelys på småskolealderen*. Bergen-Oslo-Stavanger-Tromsö: Universitetsforlaget.

Nygaard, H.D. (1984b). Elevgrunnlag og prövemateriell [Sample selection and test materials]. In R. Solheim et al., *Bergen-prosjektet II. Sökelys på småskolealderen.* Bergen-Oslo-Tromsö: Universitetsforlaget.

Obrzut, J. (1972). Reexamination of Koppitz's developmental Bender scoring system. *Perceptual and Motor Skills, 34*, 279–282.

Olson, W.C. (1949). *Child development.* Boston: Heath.

Orton, S.T. (1925). Word-blindness in school children. *Archives of Neurology and Psychiatry, 14*, 581–615.

Orton, S.T. (1928). Specific reading disability— Strephosymbolia. *Journal of American Medical Association, 90*, 1095–1099.

Österling, O. (1967). *The efficacy of special education. A comparative study of classes for slow learners.* Upsala, Sweden: Studia sciential peadagogical Upsaliensia.

Park, G.E. (1948). Reading difficulty (dyslexia) from the ophthalmic point of view. *American Journal of Ophthalmology, 31*, 28–34.

Pavlov, I.P. (1927). *Conditioned reflexes.* London: Oxford University Press.

Pelosi, P.L. (1977). The roots of reading. In H.A. Robinson (Ed.), *Reading and writing instruction in the United States: Historical trends.* Newark: DE: International Reading Association.

Peterson, I., & Eeg-Olofssen, O. (1971). The development of the electroencephalogram in normal children from the age of 1 through 15 years: Non paroxysmal activity. *Neuropadiatrie, 2*, 247.

Petrauskas, R., & Rourke, B. (1979). Identification of subgroups of retarded readers: A neuropsychological multivariate approach. *Journal of Clinial Neuropsychology, 1*, 17–37.

Pirozzolo, F.J. (1979). *The neuropsychology of developmental reading disorders.* New York: Praeger.

Preston, M.S., Guthrie, J.T., & Childs, B. (1974). Visual evoked responses (VERs) in normal and disabled readers. *Psychophysiology, 11*, 452–457.

Preston, M.S., Guthrie, J.T., Kirsch, J.T., Gertman, D., & Childs, B. (1977). VERs in normal and disabled adult readers. *Psychophysiology, 14*, 8–14.

Preston, R.C., & Yarrington, D.J. (1967). Status of fifty retarded readers 8 years after reading clinic diagnosis. *Journal of Reading, 11*, 122–124.

Rabinovitch, R.D. (1956). A research approach to reading retardation. *Neurology and Psychiatry in Childhood, 34*, 363–396.

Rabinovitch, R.D. (1968). Reading problems in children: Definitions and classifications. In A.H. Keeney & V.T. Keeney (Eds.), *Dyslexia: Diagnosis and treatment of reading disorders* (pp. 1–10). St. Louis: C.V. Mosby.

Rasmussen, P. (1982). *Neuropediatric aspects of seven-year-old children with perceptual, motor and attentional deficits.* Doctoral dissertation. Gothenburg, Sweden: University of Gothenburg.

Rawson, M. (1968). *Developmental language disability: Adult accomplishments of dyslexic boys.* Baltimore: Johns Hopkins University Press.

Reed, D.W. (1965). A theory of language, speech and writing. *Elementary English, 42*, 347–352.

Reitan, R.M., & Davison, L.A. (1974). *Clinical neuropsychology: Current status and applications.* Washington, DC: Winston and Sons.

Richards, J.C. (Ed.) (1974). *Error analysis. Perspectives on second language acquisition.* London: Longman.

Riding, R.J., & Pugh, J.G. (1977). Iconic memory and reading performance in nine-year-old children. *British Journal of Educational Psychology, 47*, 132–137.

Robinson, H.M. (1946). *Why pupils fail in reading.* Chicago: University of Chicago Press.

Robinson, H.M., & Smith, H.D. (1962). Reading clinic: Ten years after. *Elementary School Journal*, *63*, 22–27.

Rosenshine, B., & Berliner, D. (1978). Academic engaged time. *British Journal of Teacher Education*, *4*, 3–16.

Rosenthal, F.H. (1973). Self-esteem in dyslectic children. *Academic Therapy*, *9*, 27–39.

Rourke, B.P. (1975). Brain-behavior relationships in children with learning disabilities: A research program. *American Psychologist*, *30*, 911–920.

Rubino, C.A., & Minden, H.A. (1973). An analysis of eye-movements in children with reading disability. *Cortex*, *9*, 217–220.

Rucker, C.N., Howe, D.E., & Snider, B. (1969). The participation of retarded children in junior high academic and non-academic regular classes. *Exceptional Children*, *26*.

Rugel, R. (1974a). WISC subtest scores of disabled readers: A review with respect to Bannatyne's recategorization. *Journal of Learning Disabilities*, *7*, 48–58.

Rugel, R. (1974b). The factor structure of the WISC in two populations of disabled readers. *Journal of Learning Disabilities*, *7*, 581–585.

Rummelhart, D.E. (1977). Toward an interactive model of reading. In S. Dornic (Ed.), *Attentions and performance, VI*. Hillsdale, NJ: Lawrence Erlbaum.

Rutter, M. (1978). Prevalence and types of dyslexia. In A.L. Benton & D. Pearl (Eds.), *Dyslexia: An appraisal of current knowledge*. New York, London: Oxford University Press.

Rutter, M., Graham, P., & Yule, W. (1970). A neuropsychiatric study in childhood. *Clinics in Developmental Medicine*, *35/36*. London: Spastics International Medical Publications.

Rutter, M., Tizzard, J., & Whitmore, K. (1970). *Education, health and behavior*. London: Longman.

Rutter, M., & Yule, W. (1975). The concept of specific reading retardation. *Journal of Child Psychology and Psychiatry*, *16*, 161–197.

Rychlak, J.F. (1968). *A philosophy of science for personality theory*. Boston: Houghton Mifflin.

Samuels, S.J. (1977). Introduction to theoretical models of reading. In W. Otto et al. (Eds.), *Reading problems: A multidisciplinary perspective*. Reading, MA: Addison-Wesley.

Sandven, J. (1968). Students in general and school-rejecting students compared. *Scandinavian Journal of Educational Research*, *12*, 91–140.

Sasanuma, S. (1974). Impairment of written language in Japanese aphasics. *Journal of Chinese Linguistics*, *2*, 141–157.

Satz, P., & Morris, R. (1981). Learning disability subtypes. A review. In F.J. Pirozzolo & M.C. Wittrock (Eds.), *Neuropsychological and cognitive processes in reading*. New York, London: Academic Press.

Scranton, T., & Ryckman, D. (1979). Sociometric status of learning disabled children in an integrative program. *Journal of Learning Disabilities*, *12*, 402–407.

Schenk-Danziger, L. (1959). Was ist Legasthenie? [What is dyslexia?]. *Zeitschrift fur Heilpädagogik*, *3*, 34–36.

Schenk-Danziger, L. (1968). *Handbuch der Legasthenie im Kindesalter* [Handbook on dyslexia in childhood]. Weinheim, Berlin: Verlag Julius Beltz.

Schilder, P. (1944). Congenital alexia and its relation to optic perception. *Journal of Genetic Psychology*, *65*, 67–88.

Schonhaut, S., & Satz, P. (1983). Prognosis for children with learning disabilities. A review of follow-up studies. In M. Rutter (Ed.), *Behavioral syndromes of brain dysfunction in childhood*. New York: Guilford Press.

Senf, G.M. (1969). Development of immediate memory for bisensory stimuli in normal children with learning disorders. *Developmental Psychology Monograph*, *1*, No. 6.

Shallice, T. (1981). Neurological impairment of cognitive processes. *British Medical Bulletin*, *37*, 187-192.

Shapiro, M.B. (1966). The single case in clinical psychological research. *Journal of general Psychology*, *74*, 3-23.

Shearer, R.V. (1966). Eye findings in children with reading difficulties. *Journal of Pediatric Ophthalmology*, *3*(4), 47-53.

Shepard, L.A., Smith, M.L., & Vojir, C.P. (1983). Characteristics of pupils identified as learning disabled. *American Educational Research Journal*, *20*, 309-331.

Singer, H., & Ruddell, R.B. (Eds.). (1970). *Theoretical models and processes of reading*. Newark, DE: International Reading Association.

Singer, H., & Ruddell, R.B. (Eds.). (1976). *Theoretical models and processes of reading* (2nd ed.). Newark, DE: International Reading Association.

Singer, H., & Ruddell, RB. (Eds.). (1985). *Theoretical models and processes in reading* (3rd ed.). Newark, DE: International Reading Association.

Skydsgaard, H.B. (1942). *Den konstitusjonelle dyslexi. "Ordblindhed". En klinisk studie* [Constitutional dyslexia. "Wordblindness." A clinical study]. Copenhagen: Nyt Nordisk Forlag.

Smith, D.E.P., & Carrigan, P.M. (1959). *The nature of reading disability*. New York: Harcourt Brace.

Smith, F. (1971). *Understanding reading: A psycholinguistic analysis of reading and learning to read*. New York: Holt, Rinehart & Winston.

Smith, F. (1973). *Psycholinguistics and reading*. New York: Holt, Rinehart & Winston.

Smith, H.P., & Dechant, E.V. (1961). *Psychology in teaching reading*. Englewood Cliffs, NJ: Prentice-Hall.

Smith, M. (1970). *Patterns of intellectual abilities in educationally handicapped children*. Unpublished doctoral dissertation. Claremont, CA: Claremont College.

Sneath, P.H.A., & Sokal, R.R. (1973). *Numerical taxonomy: The principles and practice of numerical classification*. San Francisco: Freeman.

Soar, R., & Soar, R. (1977). An attempt to identify measures of teacher effectiveness from four studies. *Journal of Education*, *27*, 3.

Solheim, R. (1984a). Hva bestemmer den skolefaglige laeringen? [What determines school achievement?]. In R. Solheim et al., *Bergen-prosjektet II. Sökelys på småskolealderen*. Bergen-Oslo-Stavanger-Tromsö: Universitetsforlaget.

Solheim, R., Nygaard, H.D., Aasved, H., et al. (1984b). *Bergenprosjektet II. Sökelys på småskolealderen* [The Bergen Project II. Focus on the primary grades]. Bergen: Universitetsforlaget.

Sperling, G. (1960). The information available in brief visual presentations. *Psychological Monographs*, *43*, 93-120.

Spreen, O. (1978). *Learning-disabled children growing up*. Final report to Health and Welfare Canada. Ottawa: Health and Welfare Canada, Health Programs Branch.

Spreen, O. (1982). Adult outcomes of reading disorders. In R.N. Malatesha & P.G. Aaron (Eds.), *Reading disorders. Varieties and treatments* (pp. 473-498). New York, London: Academic Press.

Stangvik, G. (1970). *Effecten av spesialundervisning. En kritisk oversikt og et empirisk grunnlag* [The effect of special education. A critical review and an empirical base]. Gothenburg, Sweden: Pedagogiska institutionen.

Stephenson, W. (1953). *The study of behavior: Q-technique and its methodology*. Chicago: University of Chicago Press.

Stromberg, E.L. (1938). The relationship of measures of visual acuity and ametropia to reading speed. *Journal of Applied Psychology, 22,* 70–78.

Subirana, A. (1958). The prognosis in aphasia in relation to cerebral dominance and handedness. *Brain, 81,* 415–425.

Svendsen, D. (1979). Norskkunnskaper og sosiale gruppeforskjeller på begynnertrinnene i grunnskolen [Achievement in Norwegian and social group differences in the primary grades]. *Norsk Pedagogisk Tidsskrift, 63,* 272–282.

Tamm, A. (1925). *Kongenitale Wortblindheit und verwandte Störungen* Bericht über den 2. Kongress für Heilpädagogik, Munich, 1925.

Tarnopol, L., & Tarnopol, M. (1976). *Reading disabilities: An international perspective.* Baltimore: University Park Press.

Tarver, S.D., & Dawson, M.M. (1978). Modality preference and the teaching of reading: A review. *Journal of Learning Disabilities, 11,* 17–29.

Taylor, H.G., Satz, P., & Friel, J. (1979). Developmental dyslexia in relation to other childhood reading disorders: Significance and utility. *Reading Research Quarterly, 15,* 84–101.

Thorndike, R.L. (1963). *The concepts of over- and underachievement.* New York: Bureau of Publications, Columbia University.

Thweatt, R.C., Obrzut, J.E., & Taylor, H.D. (1972). The development and validation of a soft-sign scoring system for the Bender Gestalt. *Psychology in the schools, 9,* 170–174.

Tordrup, S.A. (1967). Laeseudviklingen hos elever med store laesevanskeligheder [Reading development in pupils with severe reading disabilities]. *Skolepsykologi, 4* (spesialnummer).

Torgesen, J.K. (1977). The role of non-specific factors in the task performance of learning disabled children: A theoretical assessment. *Journal of Learning Disabilities, 10,* 27–34.

Torgesen, J.K., & Dice, C. (1980). Characteristics of research on learning disabilities. *Journal of Learning Disabilities, 13,* 5–9.

Touwen, B.C.L. (1979). Examination of the child with minor neurological dysfunction (2nd ed.). *Clinics in Developmental Medicine,* Vol. 71, London: Spastic International Medical Publications.

Tranöy, K.E. (1977). Om verdinöytralitet og objektivitet [Neutrality of values and objectivity]. In M.C. Kragh (Ed.), *Klinisk psychologisk forskning.* Conference report. Oslo: Norsk Almenvitenskapelige Forskningsråd.

Trites, R., & Fiedorowicz, C. (1976). Follow-up study of children with specific (or primary) reading disability. In R. Knights & D.J. Bakker (Eds.), *The neuropsychology of learning disorders: Theoretical approaches.* (Proceedings of NATO Conference). Baltimore: University Park Press.

Tzeng, O.J.L., & Wang, W.S.Y. (1985). The first two Rs. In H. Singer & R.B. Ruddell (Eds.), *Theoretical Models and processes of reading* (3rd ed.). Newark, DE: International Reading Association.

Udnaes, I., Bruun, S., & Espeland, A. (1977, April). Dyslexia og öyedominans [Dyslexia and eye dominance]. Foredrag Norsk Oftalmologisk Forening [Lecture at Norwegian Ophthalmological Association].

Uhl, W.L. (1916). The use of the results of reading tests as bases for planning remedial work. *Elementary School Journal, 17,* 266–275.

Uhler, E.S. (1977). A validity study of the Visual Aural Digit Span Test and selected subtests of the Detroit Tests of Learning Aptitude. Texas Woman's Univeristy. *Dissertation Abstracts International, 37,* 4291A.

Underwood, B.J. (1975, February). Individual differences as a crucible in story construction. *American Psychologist*, 128–134.

Undheim, O.J. (1978). *Wechsler Intelligence Scale for Children – Revised* (Norwegian edition). Oslo: Norsk Psykologforening.

Valtin, R. (1978). Dyslexia: Deficit in reading or deficit in research? *Reading Research Quarterly, 14*, 203–221.

Vellutino, F.R. (1979). *Dyslexia. Theory and Research*. Cambridge: MA: MIT Press.

Vernon, M.D. (1971). *Reading and its difficulties*. Cambridge, England: Cambridge University Press.

Vinje, F.E. (1976). *Språkplanlegging. Mål og metoder* [Planning of language instruction. Objectives and methods]. Oslo: Tapir.

Vogel, S. (1974). Syntactic abilities in normal and dyslexic children. *Journal of Learning Disabilities, 7*, 103–109.

Walker, L., & Cole, E.M. (1965). Familial patterns of expression of specific reading disability in a population sample. Part I: Prevalence, distribution and persistence. *Bulletin of the Orton Society, 15*, 12–24.

Warrington, E.K. (1967). The incidence of verbal disability associated with retardation in reading. *Neuropsychologia, 5*, 175–179.

Weber, R.M. (1968). The study of oral reading errors: A review of the literature. *Reading Research Quarterly, 4*, 96–119.

Weintraub, S. (1970-). Summary of investigations relating to reading. *Reading Research Quarterly*.

Wiener, M., & Cromer, W. (1967). Reading and reading difficulty: A conceptual analysis. *Harvard Educational review, 37*, 620–643.

Williams, J.P. (1973). Learning to read: A review of theories and models. *Reading Research Quarterly, 8*, 121–146.

Wylie, R. (1974). *The self concept. Review of methodological considerations and measuring instruments*. Lincoln, NE: University of Nebraska Press.

Yeni-Komshian, G.H., Isenberg, D., & Goldberg, H. (1975). Cerebral dominance and reading disability: Left visual field deficit in poor readers. *Neuropsychologia, 13*, 83–94.

Zaidel, E., & Peters, A.M. (1981). Phonological encoding and ideographic reading by the disconnected right hemisphere: Two case studies. *Brain and Language, 14*, 205–234.

Zangwill, O.L. (1962). Dyslexia in relation to cerebral dominance. In J. Money (Ed.), *Reading disability: Progress and research needs in dyslexia* (pp. 103–114). Baltimore: Johns Hopkins University Press.

Underwood, V.L. (1975). February. Individual differences as a crucible in theory construction. *American Psychologist*, 134-140.

Undheim, J.O. (1976). Ability structure in 10-12 year old children and the theory of fluid and crystallized intelligence. *Journal of Educational Psychology*, 68.

Vellis, R. (1982). Psychology: Differences in cognition of children in classes. *Journal of Research*, 14, 20-200.

Valentine, J.R. (1976). *Psychology, Theory and Research*. Cambridge, MA: MIT Press.

Vernon, M.D. (1971). *Reading and its difficulties*. Cambridge, England: Cambridge University Press.

Videen, P. (1979). *Verbal rehearsing and recall by children of language generation*. Objectives and methods, Univ. dip.

Vygotsky, L. (1978). *Relations in natural and developmental instruction*. Cambridge, MA: Harvard University Press.

Weiner, B. (1974). (Ed.) Fruitful patterns of expectation of specific reading ability in a population sample. Part 1. *Psychological distribution and assessment*. Research report 1, 14, 12-28.

Whittington, M.C. (1987). The background of verbal disorder: A relationship with attention in reading. *Dyslexia*, 14.

Weber, R.M. (1982). The analysis of oral reading errors: A review of the literature. *Reading Research Quarterly*, 4, 96-119.

Weinstein, R. (1970). *The study of the cognitive system in reading*. *Reading Research Quarterly*.

Wiggins, R. (Ed.) (1983). Reading and remedial difficulty: A review of studies. *The Harvard Educational Review*, 7, 670-683.

Williams, J.P. (1973). Learning to read: A review of theories and models. *Harvard Educational Review*, 8, 331-347.

Weber, T. (1974). *An advantage: Reading, remedial, applied comprehension and memory processes*. Eugene, OR: University of Oregon Press.

Von Nostrand, G.H., Saubert, E., & Goldberg, H. (1980). Comprehension and reading disability: Instruction in learning to read aloud. *Merrill, Oregon*, 44, 35-98.

Zafael, M., & Foster, R.M. (1983). Phonological awareness and phonographic reading in the associated child developmental: Two case studies. *Developmental Review*, 14, 203-240.

Zinner, H.O. (1982). Developmental relation to general development. In J. Illance (Ed.), *Reading disability: Process and practice for beginners* (pp. 103-126). Eugene, OR: University Press.

Index